T0253317

Amazon

December 2, 2017: "Concise and comprehensive. I revisit it regularly to remind myself of various aspects to keep in mind for my adolescent with a diagnosis."

March 10, 2018: "I am a licensed mental health clinician . . . Without a doubt the best book I've read on schizophrenia if you're interested in helping a family member or if you are a professional working in a clinical setting. I highly recommend it."

October 7, 2017: "I am a clinical supervisor and therapist. I read this book 23 years ago, when I began my career, and it explained to me what exactly my clients/patients were going through, and helped me to understand something (schizophrenia) that is not always articulated in graduate school. I suggest this book to all new therapists and interns, as a guide."

July 13, 2017: "This book is so informational and on point with everything you need to know about schiz and it's a great book for family and caring friends to read. I highly recommend this book for those with schiz and also family and friends to learn about your illness to help take care of you and know what you're going through."

June 9, 2017: "What a great book. Full of compassion, experience and full of knowledge. Gives you a better understanding of the disease."

February 20, 2017: "A must read for individuals, families and any member of every community. My 2 brothers have suffered from schizophrenia . . . This book is well written and thoughtful and I found it reflected so many of my family's experiences."

December 19, 2014: "This is a clearly written, compassionate guide to the entire scary world of serious mental illness."

December 14, 2016: "This book is so informative, heartbreaking and also encouraging."

July 22, 2016: "Very, very good information. Would highly recommend this book for anyone who has any connection or is associated with a person who has Schizophrenia. It is user friendly and the information is so straightforward and easy to absorb."

March 22, 2016: "I'm now in my late 40s, but as a child I was ashamed to be the daughter of a schizophrenic mother . . . someone recommended an earlier edition of this book, and it literally changed my life. I came to have a better understanding of the world my mother lived in. I developed a stronger compassion for her constant struggle to differentiate her experiences from what the rest of the world experienced."

January 29, 2016: "Torrey's voice is powerful and informed. Since he's both a healthcare provider and family member of a person with schizophrenia, he can speak about the mental health treatment system and the havoc the disease wreaks on patients/families. After reading, I am more understanding of what my mom, who has had schizophrenia for 25 years, is going through and how to help her."

November 11, 2015: "I like this reference, my sister is ill and this helps me to know what is really going on with her, which in return lets us interact together more . . . thank you . . ."

October 24, 2015: "This book is a must have for a family trying to understand schizophrenia. Dr. Torrey seems to anticipate your questions and answer them before you ask. He speaks not only as a specialist who has devoted his life to helping individuals with schizophrenia, the families who love them and the clinicians who serve them, but also as a brother who has lived with a family member struggling with the illness."

October 7, 2015: "So far this is an excellent resource to understanding the disorder. It helps me to understand what is happening in my son's mind. There is so much material I have not read through it all yet. I like the examples of cases presented from a patient's perspective too. I wish I had ordered this months ago."

December 6, 2014: "This is a great read. Especially for people like me who are schizophrenic. I've been ill for years but never wanted to explore this part of my Schizoaffective Disorder. This book takes a complex issue and makes it easier to understand. I'm much more at ease with myself now."

July 14, 2014: "This is a great book for people learning about schizophrenia/schizo-affective disorder whether they are learning because of a family member or because they just want to know more. It has many examples of different people with the disorder and tries to explain things in a way that would be easy to understand, usually by comparing to something in life that is common."

Goodreads
September 28, 2017: "If you or a family member is diagnosed with Schizophrenia, this is probably among the first books you should grab. It attempts to tackle the illness from many different angles, etiology, treatment, social support, activism, misconceptions, and even a rather extensive review of accurate and inaccurate movies and books about the disease."

September 26, 2016: "An excellent book on schizophrenia. The history of the disease, a definition of the disease, how laws and insurance have affected the care of people suffering from the disease, and what we can do to help."

November 11, 2016: "This is an amazing manual to help anyone understand what it is like to suffer from schizophrenia, current research, treatment, practical issues in living with the disease for both patients and family and how the disease is depicted in popular culture. I love that the book ends with advocacy issues, as there are many to work on."

April 19, 2015: "This book is an absolutely amazing reference for anyone who loves someone with this very complicated brain disease."

October 24, 2013: "It was amazing. Really an outstanding walk-through of what is and isn't known about this most feared mental illness."

September 26, 2011: "This must be one of the best books about schizophrenia. I learned a lot. I highly recommend it to everyone."

June 11, 2011: "Although written as a practical, information manual (and succeeding very well!), it turns out to also be always compassionate, at times sorrowful, and many times scathing towards the insanity of the mental health care system in the US. He intersperses quotations from literature, from poetry, and best, from accounts from schizophrenics. I couldn't put it down."

July 14, 2009: "Outstanding. Treats you like you are an intelligent reader. Learned more here about schizophrenia— causes, issues, treatment, meds—than any other source."

February 8, 2008: "Especially good for family members."

Surviving
Schizophrenia

ALSO BY E. FULLER TORREY, M.D.

Surviving Schizophrenia

A FAMILY MANUAL

Seventh Edition

E. Fuller Torrey, M.D.

HARPER PERENNIAL

NEW YORK • LONDON • TORONTO • SYDNEY • NEW DELHI • AUCKLAND

HARPER ● PERENNIAL

SURVIVING SCHIZOPHRENIA (SEVENTH EDITION). Copyright
© 1983, 1988, 1995, 2001, 2006, 2013, 2019 by E. Fuller
Torrey. All rights reserved. Printed in the United States of
America. No part of this book may be used or reproduced
in any manner whatsoever without written permission
except in the case of brief quotations embodied in critical
articles and reviews. For information, address HarperCollins
Publishers, 195 Broadway, New York, NY 10007.

HarperCollins books may be purchased for educational,
business, or sales promotional use. For information, please email
the Special Markets Department at SPsales@harpercollins.com.

First Harper Perennial edition published 2019.

Library of Congress Cataloging-in-Publication
Data has been applied for.

ISBN 978-0-06-288080-2

23 24 25 26 27 LBC 12 11 10 9 8

As for me, you must know that I shouldn't precisely have chosen madness if there had been any choice.

Vincent Van Gogh, 1889, in a letter to his brother,
written while he was involuntarily confined in the
psychiatric hospital at St. Remy

This edition of *Surviving Schizophrenia* is dedicated to Faith Dickerson and Bob Yolken, valued friends and research colleagues.

All royalties from this edition have been assigned to the Treatment Advocacy Center.

CONTENTS

PHOTOGRAPHS

MRIs from identical twins, one with schizophrenia and the other well

ILLUSTRATIONS

PREFACE TO THE
SEVENTH EDITION

I feel fortunate to have lived long enough to write a seventh edition of this book. It is very satisfying to see it continue to be widely used in the United States and in other English-speaking countries, as well as in translations in Spanish, Italian, Russian, Chinese, and Japanese. Such satisfaction, however, is tempered by disappointment that we do not yet understand the precise causes of schizophrenia nor do we yet have definitive treatments. When I wrote the first edition of this book thirty-five years ago I had thought that by now we would be much further along research-wise than we are. For this failure I blame my psychiatric colleagues for not demanding more attention to this disease and the federal government, especially the National Institute of Mental Health, for failing to do sufficient research. Despite my disappointment, I am hopeful that, at this time, we are on the verge of major research breakthroughs.

There are several new features in this revised edition. In Chapter 7 I have outlined a specific treatment plan for a person who has developed a psychosis for the first time. The plan attempts to make sense of how the twenty antipsychotics available in the United States should be used. I have also updated what is known about causes, especially emphasizing exciting new research pointing to inflammatory, infectious, and immunological antecedents (Chapter 5). There is a new chapter on "What Good Services Should Look Like" (Chapter 9) and new sections on "Successful Schizophrenia" (Chapter 4) and "Exercise" (Chapter 8). For advocates I have updated controversial issues such as anosognosia (Chapter 1), the Hearing Voices Network (Chapters 2 and 3), the recovery model (Chapter 4), brain disease deniers (Chapter 5), and the HIPAA law on confidentiality (Chapter 10).

Thus it is my hope that this book will continue to be useful to those who have schizophrenia, their families, and those who are involved in the treatment care system. As I wrote in the Preface of the first edition, I hope that this book will help bring schizophrenia out of the Slough of Despair and into the mainstream of American medicine.

ACKNOWLEDGMENTS

I have had the pleasure of working with HarperCollins for thirty-five years. From 1983, when Carol Cohen and Lou AvRutick initially launched this book, to the present when Emily Taylor and Gail Winston shepherded the new edition, the staff has been consistently kind, competent, and helpful. They have made my job much easier.

I am also indebted to those who contributed ideas and corrections to this edition, including John Davis, Faith Dickerson, Bob Drake, Pete Earley, Jeffrey Geller, Mike Knable, Dick Lamb, Cam Quanbeck, Brian Stettin, Maree Webster, Mark Weiser, and Bob Yolken. Shannon Flynn, Daniel Laitmen, and the late Fred Frese were generous in sharing their life stories as examples of "successful schizophrenia." I owe a huge debt to D. J. Jaffe for sorting out the confusing and ever-changing websites that are relevant for schizophrenia in Appendix B. My research assistant, Wendy Simmons, did an excellent job of keeping track of all the pieces and making sure that they fit together. Most important, I continue to be indebted to my wife, Barbara, for the ineffable ingredients that make writing a book possible.

In addition to these, I gratefully acknowledge the following:

P. J. Kavanagh for permission to quote from the *Collected Poems of Ivor Gurney.*

Joseph H. Berke for permission to reprint excerpts from *Mary Barnes: Two Accounts of a Journey Through Madness*.

Malcolm B. Bowers and Science Press for permission to reprint excerpts from *Retreat from Sanity: The Structure of Emerging Psychosis*.

Andrew McGhie and the British Psychological Society for permission to reprint excerpts from an article in the *British Journal of Medical Psychology*.

British Journal of Psychiatry for permission to reprint excerpts from an article by James Chapman.

Journal of Abnormal and Social Psychology for permission to reprint excerpts from an article by Anonymous.

Anchor Press and Doubleday for permission to reprint excerpts from *These Are My Sisters* by Lara Jefferson.

Presses Universitaires de France for permission to reprint excerpts from *Autobiography of a Schizophrenic Girl* by Marguerite Sechehaye.

W. W. Norton and Company for permission to reprint excerpts from *In a Darkness* by James A. Wechsler.

National Schizophrenia Fellowship for permission to reprint excerpts from *Coping with Schizophrenia* by H. R. Rollin.

G. P. Putnam and Sons for permission to reprint excerpts from *This Stranger, My Son* by Louise Wilson.

University Books for permission to reprint excerpts from *The Witnesses* by Thomas Hennell.

J. G. Hall and *Lancet* for permission to quote from an article.

Nancy J. Hermon and Colin M. Smith for permission to quote from a presentation at the 1986 Alberta Schizophrenia Conference.

Psychological Bulletin and *Schizophrenia Bulletin* for permission to quote from articles.

The purpose of this book is to make you aware of the progress of schizophrenia and the possible ways in which it may develop. The assessment of symptoms requires an expert. For proper diagnosis and therapy of all symptoms, real or apparent, connected with schizophrenia, please consult your doctor. In my discussion of cases, I have changed all names and identifying details while preserving the integrity of the research findings.

Surviving
Schizophrenia

1

The Inner World of Madness:
View from the Inside

What then does schizophrenia mean to me? It means fatigue and confusion, it means trying to separate every experience into the real and the unreal and not sometimes being aware of where the edges overlap. It means trying to think straight when there is a maze of experiences getting in the way, and when thoughts are continually being sucked out of your head so that you become embarrassed to speak at meetings. It means feeling sometimes that you are inside your head and visualising yourself walking over your brain, or watching another girl wearing your clothes and carrying out actions as you think them. It means knowing that you are continually "watched," that you can never succeed in life because the laws are all against you and knowing that your ultimate destruction is never far away.

Patient with schizophrenia, quoted in Henry R. Rollin,
Coping with Schizophrenia

When tragedy strikes, one of the things that make life bearable for people is the sympathy of friends and relatives. This can be seen, for example, in a natural disaster like a flood and with a chronic disease like cancer. Those closest to the person afflicted offer help, extend their sympathy, and generally provide important solace and support in the person's time of need. "Sympathy," said Emerson, "is a supporting atmosphere, and in it we unfold easily and well." A prerequisite for sympathy is an ability to put oneself in the place of the person afflicted. One must be able to imagine oneself in a flood or getting cancer. Without this ability to put oneself in the place of the person afflicted, there can be abstract pity but not true sympathy.

Sympathy for those afflicted with schizophrenia is sparse because it is difficult to put oneself in the place of the sufferer. The whole disease process is mysterious, foreign, and frightening to most people. As noted by Roy Porter in *A Social History of Madness*, "*strangeness* has typically been the key feature in the fractured dialogues that go on, or the silences that intrude, between the 'mad' and the 'sane.' Madness is a foreign country."

Schizophrenia, then, is not like a flood, where one can imagine all one's possessions being washed away. Nor like a cancer, where one can imagine a slowly growing tumor, relentlessly spreading from organ to organ and squeezing life from your body. No, schizophrenia is madness. Those who are afflicted act bizarrely, say strange things, withdraw from us, and may even try to hurt us. They are no longer the same person—they are *mad!* We don't understand why they say what they say and do what they do. We don't understand the disease process. Rather than a steadily growing tumor, which we can understand, it is as if the person has lost control of his/her brain. How can we sympathize with a person who is possessed by unknown and unseen forces? How can we sympathize with a madman or a madwoman?

The paucity of sympathy for those with schizophrenia makes it that much more of a disaster. Being afflicted with the disease is bad enough by itself. Those of us who have not had this disease should ask ourselves, for example, how we would feel if our brain began playing tricks on us, if unseen voices shouted at us, if we lost the capacity to feel emotions, and if we lost the ability to reason logically. As one individual with schizophrenia noted: "My greatest fear is this brain of mine. . . . The worst thing imaginable is to be terrified of one's own mind, the very matter that controls all that we are and all that we do and feel." This would certainly be burden enough for any human being to have to bear. But what if, in addition to this, those closest to us began to avoid us or ignore us, to pretend that they didn't hear our comments, to pretend that they didn't notice what we did? How would we feel if those we most cared about were embarrassed by our behavior each day?

Because there is little understanding of schizophrenia, so there is little sympathy. For this reason it is the obligation of everyone with a relative or close friend with schizophrenia to learn as much as possible about what the disease is and what the afflicted person is experiencing. This is not merely an intellectual exercise or a way to satisfy one's curiosity but rather the means to make it possible to sympathize with the person. For friends and relatives who want to be helpful, probably the most important thing to do is to learn about the inner workings of the brain of a person with schizophrenia. One mother wrote me after listening to her afflicted son's descriptions of his hallucinations: "I saw into the visual hallucinations that plagued him and frankly, at times, it raised the hair on my neck. It also helped me to get outside of *my* tragedy and to realize how horrible it is for the person who is afflicted. I thank God for that painful wisdom. I am able to cope easier with all of this."

With sympathy, schizophrenia is a personal tragedy. Without sympathy, it becomes a family calamity, for there is nothing to knit people together, no balm for the wounds. Understanding schizophrenia also helps demystify the disease and brings it from the realm of the occult to the daylight of reason. As we come to understand it, the face of madness slowly changes before us from one of terror to one of sadness. For the sufferer, this is a significant change.

The best way to learn what a person with schizophrenia experiences is to listen to someone with the disease. For this reason I have relied heavily upon patients' own accounts in describing the signs and symptoms. There are some excellent descriptions scattered throughout English literature; the best of these are listed at the end of this chapter. By contrast one of the most widely read books, Hannah Green's *I Never Promised You a Rose Garden*, is not at all helpful, as is explained in Appendix A. It describes a patient who, according to one analysis, should not even have been diagnosed with schizophrenia but rather with hysteria (now often referred to as somatization disorder).

When one listens to persons with schizophrenia describe what they are experiencing and observes their behavior, certain abnormalities can be noted:

1. Alterations of the senses
2. Inability to sort and interpret incoming sensations, and an inability therefore to respond appropriately
3. Delusions and hallucinations
4. Altered sense of self
5. Changes in emotions
6. Changes in movements
7. Changes in behavior
8. Decreased awareness of illness

No one symptom or sign is found in all individuals; rather, the final diagnosis rests upon the total symptom picture. Some people have much more of one kind of symptom, other people another. Conversely, there is no single symptom or sign of schizophrenia that is found exclusively in that disease. All symptoms and signs can be found at least occasionally in other diseases of the brain, such as brain tumors and temporal lobe epilepsy.

Alterations of the Senses

In Edgar Allan Poe's "The Tell-Tale Heart" (1843), the main character, clearly lapsing into a schizophrenia-like state, exclaims to the reader, "Have I not told you that what you mistake for madness is but overacuteness of the senses?" An expert on the dark recesses of the human mind, Poe put his finger directly on a central theme of madness. Alterations of the senses are especially prominent in the early stages of breakdown in individuals with schizophrenia and can be found, according to one study, in almost two-thirds of all patients. As the authors of the study conclude: "Perceptual dysfunction is the most invariant feature of the early stage of schizophrenia." It can be elicited from patients most commonly when they have recovered from a psychotic episode; rarely can patients who are acutely or chronically psychotic describe these changes.

Alterations of the senses as a hallmark of schizophrenia were also noted by Poe's professional contemporaries. In 1862 the director of the Illinois State Hospital for the Insane wrote that insanity "either entirely reverses or essentially changes the mind in its manner of receiving impressions." The alterations may be either enhancement (more common) or blunting; all sensory modalities may be affected. For example, Poe's protagonist was experiencing predominantly an increased acuteness of hearing:

> True!—nervous—very, very dreadfully nervous I had been and am! But why will you say that I am mad? The disease had sharpened my senses—not destroyed—not dulled them. Above all was the sense of hearing acute. I heard all things in the heaven and in the earth. I heard many things in hell. How, then, am I mad? Harken! and observe how healthily—how calmly—I can tell you the whole story.

Another described it this way:

> During the last while back I have noticed that noises all seem to be louder to me than they were before. It's as if someone had turned up the volume. . . . I notice it most with background noises—you know what I mean, noises that are always around but you don't notice them.

Visual perceptual changes are even more common than auditory changes. One patient described it as follows:

> Colours seem to be brighter now, almost as if they are luminous paintings. I'm not sure if things are solid until I touch them. I seem to be noticing colours more than before, although I am not artistically minded. . . . Not only the colour of things fascinates me but all sorts of little things, like markings in the surface, pick up my attention too.

And another noted both the sharpness of colors as well as the transformation of objects:

Everything looked vibrant, especially red; people took on a dev-
ilish look, with black outlines and white shining eyes; all sorts of
objects—chairs, buildings, obstacles—took on a life of their own; they
seemed to make threatening gestures, to have an animistic outlook.

In some instances the visual alterations improved the appearance:

Lots of things seemed psychedelic; they shone. I was working in a
restaurant and it looked more first class than it really was.

In other cases the alterations made the object ugly or frightening:

People looked deformed, as if they had had plastic surgery, or were
wearing makeup with different bone structure.

Colors and textures may blend into each other:

I saw everything very bright and rich and pure like the thinnest line
possible. Or a shiny smoothness like water but solid. After a while
things got rough and shadowed again.

Sometimes both hearing *and* visual sensations are increased, as happened to this young woman:

These crises, far from abating, seemed rather to increase. One day,
while I was in the principal's office, suddenly the room became
enormous. . . . Profound dread overwhelmed me, and as though lost,
I looked around desperately for help. I heard people talking, but I
did not grasp the meaning of the words. The voices were metallic,
without warmth or color. From time to time, a word detached itself
from the rest. It repeated itself over and over in my head, absurd, as
though cut off by a knife.

Closely related to the overacuteness of the senses is the flooding
of the senses with stimuli. It is not only that the senses become more
sharply attuned but that they see and hear everything. Normally our
brain screens out most incoming sights and sounds, allowing us to con-

centrate on whatever we choose. This screening mechanism appears to become impaired in many persons with schizophrenia, releasing a veritable flood of sensory stimuli into the brain simultaneously.

This is one person's description of flooding of the senses with auditory stimuli:

> Everything seems to grip my attention although I am not particularly interested in anything. I am speaking to you just now, but I can hear noises going on next door and in the corridor. I find it difficult to shut these out, and it makes it more difficult for me to concentrate on what I am saying to you.

And with visual stimuli:

> Occasionally during subsequent periods of disturbance there was some distortion of vision and some degree of hallucination. On several occasions my eyes became markedly oversensitive to light. Ordinary colors appeared to be much too bright, and sunlight seemed dazzling in intensity. When this happened, ordinary reading was impossible, and print seemed excessively black.

Frequently these two things happen together:

> My focus was a bit bizarre. I could do portraits of people who were walking down the street. I remembered license numbers of cars we were following into Vancouver. We paid $3.57 for gas. The air machine made eighteen dings while we were there.

> An outsider may see only someone "out of touch with reality." In fact we are experiencing so many realities that it is often confusing and sometimes totally overwhelming.

As these examples make clear, it is difficult to concentrate or pay attention when so much sensory data are rushing through the brain. In one study more than half the people who had had schizophrenia recalled impairments in attention and in keeping track of time. One patient expressed it as follows:

> Sometimes when people speak to me my head is overloaded. It's too much to hold at once. It goes out as quick as it goes in. It makes you forget what you just heard because you can't get hearing it long enough. It's just words in the air unless you can figure it out from their faces.

Because of this sensory overload, it is often difficult for individuals with schizophrenia to socialize. As one young man noted:

> Social situations were almost impossible to manage. I always came across as aloof, anxious, nervous, or just plain weird, picking up on inane snippets of conversation and asking people to repeat themselves and tell me what they were referring to.

Sensory modalities other than hearing and vision may also be affected in schizophrenia. Mary Barnes in her autobiographical account of "a journey through madness" recalled how "it was terrible to be touched. . . . Once a nurse tried to cut my nails. The touch was such that I tried to bite her." A medical student with schizophrenia remembered that "touching any patient made me feel that I was being electrocuted." Another patient described the horror of feeling a rat in his throat and tasting the "decay in my mouth as its body disintegrated inside me." Increased sensitivity of the genitalia is occasionally found, explained by one patient as "a genital sexual irritation from which there was no peace and no relief." I once took care of a young man with such a sensation who became convinced that his penis was turning black. He countered this delusional fear by insisting that doctors—or anyone within sight—examine him every five minutes to reassure him. His hospitalization was precipitated by his having gone into the local post office where a girlfriend worked and asking her to examine him in front of the customers.

Another aspect of the overacuteness of the senses is a flooding of the mind with thoughts. It is as if the brain is being bombarded both with external stimuli (e.g., sounds and sights) and with internal stimuli as well (thoughts, memories). One psychiatrist who has studied this area extensively claims that we have not been as aware of the internal stimuli in persons with schizophrenia as we should be:

My trouble is that I've got too many thoughts. You might think about something, let's say that ashtray, and just think, oh! yes, that's for putting my cigarette in, but I would think of it and then I would think of a dozen different things connected with it at the same time.

My concentration is very poor. I jump from one thing to another. If I am talking to someone they only need to cross their legs or scratch their heads and I am distracted and forget what I was saying. I think I could concentrate better with my eyes shut.

And this person describes the flooding of memories from the past:

Childhood feelings began to come back as symbols, and bits from past conversations went through my head. . . . I began to think I was hypnotized so that I would remember what had happened in the first four and a half years of my life.

Perhaps it is this increased ability of some patients to recall childhood events that in the past mistakenly led psychoanalysts to assume that the recalled events were somehow causally related to the schizophrenia. There is no scientific evidence to support such theories, however, and much evidence to support contrary theories.

A variation of flooding with thoughts occurs when the person feels that someone is inserting the flood of thoughts into his/her head. This is commonly referred to as thought insertion and when present is considered by many psychiatrists to be an almost certain symptom of schizophrenia:

All sorts of "thoughts" seem to come to me, as if someone is "speaking" them inside my head. When in any company it appears to be worse.

In college, I "knew" that everyone was thinking and talking about me and that a local pharmacist was tormenting me by inserting his thoughts into my head and inducing me to buy things I had no use for.

With this kind of activity going on in a person's head, it is not surprising that it would be difficult to concentrate:

> I was invited to play checkers and started to do so, but I could not go on. I was too much absorbed in my own thoughts, particularly those regarding the approaching end of the world and those responsible for the use of force and for the charge of homicidal intent.

The alterations of the senses can also be very frightening, as described by Esso Leete, who has written many useful articles from a patient's point of view:

> It was evening and I was walking along the beach near my college in Florida. Suddenly my perceptions shifted. The intensifying wind became an omen of something terrible. I could feel it becoming stronger and stronger; I was sure it was going to capture me and sweep me away with it. Nearby trees bent threateningly toward me and tumbleweeds chased me. I became very frightened and began to run. However, though I knew I was running, I was making no progress. I seemed suspended in space and time.

When all aspects of overacuteness of the senses are taken together, the consequent cacophony in the brain must be frightening, and it is so described by most patients. In the very earliest stage of the disease, however, before this overacuteness becomes too severe, it may be a pleasant experience. Many descriptions of the initial days of developing schizophrenia are descriptions of heightened awareness, commonly called "peak experiences"; such experiences are also common in manic-depressive illness (bipolar disorder) and in getting high on drugs. Here is one patient's description:

> Suddenly my whole being was filled with light and loveliness and with an upsurge of deeply moving feeling from within myself to meet and reciprocate the influence that flowed into me. I was in a state of the most vivid awareness and illumination.

Many patients interpret such experiences within a religious framework and believe they are being touched by God:

> I was in a higher and higher state of exhilaration and awareness. Things people said had hidden meaning. They said things that applied to life. Everything that was real seemed to make sense. I had a great awareness of life, truth, and God. I went to church and suddenly all parts of the service made sense.

In view of such experiences it is hardly surprising to find excessive religious preoccupation listed as a common early sign of schizophrenia. One study of individuals in the early stages of schizophrenia reported that "nearly all patients complained of ineffability of their experiences; and a great majority reported preoccupations with metaphysical, supernatural, or philosophical issues."

Sensations can be blunted, as well as enhanced, in schizophrenia. Such blunting is more commonly found late in the course of the disease, whereas enhancement is often one of the earliest symptoms. The blunting is described "as if a heavy curtain were drawn over his mind; it resembled a thick deadening cloud that prevented the free use of his senses." One's own voice may sound muted or faraway, and vision may be wavy or blurred: "However hard I looked it was as if I was looking through a daydream and the mass of detail, such as the pattern on a carpet, became lost."

One sensation that may be blunted in schizophrenia is that of pain. Although it does not happen frequently, when such blunting does occur it may be dramatic and have practical consequences for those who are caring for the person. It is now in vogue to attribute such blunting to medication, but in fact it was clearly described by Dr. John Haslam as early as 1798 in his book *Observations on Insanity*. In older textbooks, for example, there are many accounts of surgeons being able to do appendectomies and similar procedures on some patients with schizophrenia with little or no anesthesia. One of my patients did not realize she had a massive breast abscess until the fluid from it seeped through her dress; although this is normally an exceedingly painful condition, she insisted she had felt no pain whatsoever. Nurses who have cared for patients with schizophrenia over many years can recite stories of fractured bones, perforated ulcers, or ruptured appendixes the patients said nothing about. Practically, it is important to be aware of this possibility so that medical help can be sought for persons if they look sick, even if they are not complaining of pain. It is also the reason that some people with schizophrenia burn their fingers when they smoke cigarettes too close to the end.

It may well be that there is a common denominator for all aspects of the alterations of the senses discussed thus far. All sensory input into the brain passes through the thalamus in the lower portion of the brain. This area is suspected of being involved in schizophrenia, as will be described in chapter 5, and it is likely that disease of this part of the brain accounts for many symptoms. Norma MacDonald, a woman who published an account of her illness in 1960, foresaw this possibility in a particularly clear manner several years before psychiatrists and neurologists understood it, and she wrote about her conception of the breakdown in the filter system:

> The walk of a stranger on the street could be a sign to me which I must interpret. Every face in the windows of a passing streetcar would be engraved on my mind, all of them concentrating on me and trying to pass me some sort of message. Now, many years later, I can appreciate what had happened. Each of us is capable of coping with a large number of stimuli, invading our being through any one of the senses. We could hear every sound within earshot and see every object, hue, and colour within the field of vision, and so on. It's obvious that we would be incapable of carrying on any of our daily activities if even one-hundredth of all these available stimuli invaded us at once. So the mind must have a filter which functions without our conscious thought, sorting stimuli and allowing only those which are relevant to the situation in hand to disturb consciousness. And this filter must be working at maximum efficiency at all times, particularly when we require a degree of concentration. What had happened to me in Toronto was a breakdown in the filter, and a hodge-podge of unrelated stimuli were distracting me from things which should have had my undivided attention.

Inability to Interpret and Respond

In normal people the brain functions in such a way that incoming stimuli are sorted and interpreted; then a correct response is selected and sent out. Most of the responses are learned, such as saying "thank you" when a gift is given to us. These responses also include logic, such as being able to predict what will happen to us if we do not arrive for work at the time we are supposed to. Our brains sort and interpret incoming stimuli and send out responses hundreds of thousands of times each day.

A fundamental defect in schizophrenia is a frequent inability to sort, interpret, and respond. Textbooks of psychiatry describe this as a thought disorder, but it is more than just thoughts that are involved. Visual and auditory stimuli, emotions, and some actions are misarranged in exactly the same way as thoughts; the brain defect is probably similar for all.

We do not understand the human brain well enough to know precisely how the system works; but imagine a telephone operator sitting at an old plug-in type of switchboard in the middle of your brain. He or she receives all the sensory input, thoughts, ideas, memories, and emotions coming in, sorts them, and determines those that go together. For example, normally our brain takes the words of a sentence and converts them automatically into a pattern of thought. We don't have to concentrate on the individual words but rather can focus on the meaning of the whole message.

Now what would happen if the switchboard operator decided not to do the job of sorting and interpreting? In terms of understanding auditory stimuli, two patients describe this kind of defect:

When people are talking I have to think what the words mean. You see, there is an interval instead of a spontaneous response. I have to think about it and it takes time. I have to pay all my attention to people when they are speaking or I get all mixed up and don't understand them.

I can concentrate quite well on what people are saying if they talk simply. It's when they go on into long sentences that I lose the meanings. It just becomes a lot of words that I would need to string together to make sense.

One pair of researchers described this defect as a receptive aphasia similar to that found in some patients who have had a stroke. The words are there, but the person cannot synthesize them into sentences, as explained by this person with schizophrenia:

> I used to get the sudden thing that I couldn't understand what people said, like it was a foreign language.

Difficulties in comprehending visual stimuli are similar to those described for auditory stimuli:

> I have to put things together in my head. If I look at my watch I see the watchstrap, watch, face, hands and so on, then I have got to put them together to get it into one piece.

One patient had similar problems when she looked at her psychiatrist, seeing "the teeth, then the nose, then the cheeks, then one eye and the other. Perhaps it was this independence of each part that inspired such fear and prevented my recognizing her even though I knew who she was."

It is probably because of such impairments in visual interpretation that some persons with schizophrenia misidentify someone and say he or she looks like someone else. My sister with schizophrenia did this frequently, claiming to have seen many friends from childhood who I know in fact could not have been present. Another patient with schizophrenia added a grandiose flair to the visual misperception:

> This morning, when I was at Hillside [Hospital] I was making a movie. I was surrounded by movie stars. The X-ray technician was Peter Lawford. The security guard was Don Knotts.

In addition to difficulties in interpreting individual auditory and visual stimuli in coherent patterns, many persons with schizophrenia have difficulty putting the two kinds of stimuli together:

I can't concentrate on television because I can't watch the screen and listen to what is being said at the same time. I can't seem to take in two things like this at the same time especially when one of them means watching and the other means listening. On the other hand I seem to be always taking in too much at the one time and then I can't handle it and can't make sense of it.

I tried sitting in my apartment and reading; the words looked perfectly familiar, like old friends whose faces I remembered perfectly well but whose names I couldn't recall; I read one paragraph ten times, could make no sense of it whatever, and shut the book. I tried listening to the radio, but the sounds went through my head like a buzz saw. I walked carefully through traffic to a movie theater and sat through a movie which seemed to consist of a lot of people wandering around slowly and talking a great deal about something or other. I decided, finally, to spend my days sitting in the park watching the birds on the lake.

These persons' difficulties in watching television or movies are very typical. In fact, it is striking how few patients with schizophrenia on hospital wards watch television, contrary to what is popularly believed. Some may sit in front of it and watch the visual motion, as if it were a test pattern, but few of them can tell you what is going on. This includes patients of all levels of intelligence and education, among them college-educated persons who, given little else to do, might be expected to take advantage of the TV for much of the day. On the contrary, you are more likely to find them sitting quietly in another corner of the room, ignoring the TV; if you ask them why, they may tell you that they cannot follow what is going on, or they may try to cover up their defect by saying they are tired. One of my patients was an avid New York Yankees baseball fan prior to his illness, but he refused to watch the game even when the Yankees were on and he was in the room at the time, because he could not understand what was happening. As a practical aside, the favorite TV programs and movies of many persons with schizophrenia are cartoons and travelogues; both are simple and can be followed visually without the necessity of integrating auditory input at the same time.

But the job of the switchboard operator in our brain does not end with sorting and interpreting the incoming stimuli. The job also includes hooking up the stimuli with proper responses to be sent back outside. For example, if somebody asks me, "Would you like to have lunch with me today?" my brain focuses immediately on the overall content of the question and starts calculating: Do I have time? Do I want to? What excuses do I have? What will other people think who see me with this person? What will be the effect on this person if I say no? Out of these calculations emerges a response that, in a normal brain, is appropriate to the situation. Similarly, news of a friend's death gets hooked up with grief, visual and auditory stimuli from a funny movie are hooked up with mirth, and a new idea regarding the creation of the universe is hooked up with logic and with previous knowledge in this area. It is an orderly, ongoing process, and the switchboard operator goes on, day after day, making relatively few mistakes.

The inability of patients with schizophrenia to not only sort and interpret stimuli but also select out appropriate responses is one of the hallmarks of the disease. It led Swiss psychiatrist Eugen Bleuler in 1911 to introduce the term "schizophrenia," meaning in German a splitting of the various parts of the thought process. Bleuler was impressed by the inappropriate responses frequently given by persons with this disease; for example, when told that a close friend has died, a person with schizophrenia may giggle. It is as if the switchboard operator not only gets bored and stops sorting and interpreting but becomes actively malicious and begins hooking the incoming stimuli up to random, usually inappropriate, responses.

The inability to interpret and respond appropriately is also at the core of patients' difficulties in relating to other people. Not being able to put the auditory and visual stimuli together makes it difficult to understand others; if in addition you cannot respond appropriately, then interpersonal relations become impossible. One patient described such difficulties:

> During the visit I tried to establish contact with her, to feel that she was actually there, alive and sensitive. But it was futile. Though I certainly recognized her, she became part of the unreal world. I knew her name and everything about her, yet she appeared strange, unreal,

like a statue. I saw her eyes, her nose, her lips moving, heard her voice and understood what she said perfectly, yet I was in the presence of a stranger. To restore contact between us I made desperate efforts to break through the invisible dividing wall but the harder I tried, the less successful I was, and the uneasiness grew apace.

It is for this reason that many persons with schizophrenia prefer to spend time by themselves, withdrawn, communicating with others as little as possible. The process is too difficult and too painful to undertake except when absolutely necessary.

Just as auditory and visual stimuli may not be sorted or interpreted by the person's brain and may elicit inappropriate responses, so too may actions be fragmented and lead to inappropriate responses. This will be discussed in greater detail in a subsequent section, but it is worth noting that the same kind of brain deficit is probably involved. For example, compare the difficulties this patient has in the simple action of getting a drink of water with the difficulties in responding to auditory and visual stimuli described above:

> If I do something like going for a drink of water, I've got to go over each detail—find cup, walk over, turn tap, fill cup, turn tap off, drink it. I keep building up a picture. I have to change the picture each time. I've got to make the old picture move. I can't concentrate. I can't hold things. Something else comes in, various things. It's easier if I stay still.

It suggests that there may be relatively few underlying brain deficits leading to the broad range of symptoms the disease of schizophrenia comprises.

When schizophrenia thought patterns are looked at from outside, as when they are being described by a psychiatrist, such terms as "disconnectedness," "loosening of associations," "concreteness," "impairment of logic," "thought blocking," and "ambivalence" are used. To begin with disconnectedness: one of my patients used to come into the office each morning and ask my secretary to write a sentence on paper for him. One request was: "Write all kinds of black snakes looking like raw onion, high strung, deep down, long winded, all kinds of sizes." This patient had put together several apparently disconnected ideas that a normally functioning brain would not have joined. Another patient wrote:

> My thoughts get all jumbled up, I start thinking or talking about something but I never get there. Instead I wander off in the wrong direction and get caught up with all sorts of different things that may be connected with the things I want to say but in a way I can't explain. People listening to me get more lost than I do.

Sometimes there may be a vague connection between the jumbled thoughts in schizophrenia thinking; such instances are referred to as loose associations. For example, in the sentence about black snakes above, it may be that the patient juxtaposed onions to black snakes because of the onionlike pattern on the skin of some snakes. On another occasion I was drawing blood from a patient's arm and she said, "Look at my blue veins. I asked the Russian women to make them red," loosely connecting the color of blood with the "Reds" of the former Soviet Union.

Occasionally the loose association will rest not upon some tenuous logical connection between the words but merely upon their similar sound. For example, one young man presented me with a written poem:

> *I believe we will soon*
> *achieve world peace. But*
> *I'm still on the lamb.*

He had confused the lamb associated with peace with the expression "on the lam," the correct spelling of which he apparently did not know. There is no logical association between "lamb" and "lam" except for their similar sound; such associations are referred to as clang associations. Another example of such thinking was sent to me by a young man with schizophrenia. He wanted to share with me a letter he had written to an official to whom he was trying to explain his symptoms:

Schizophrenics are not necessarily stupid, as some would have you believe. Schizophrenics can be very intelligent. I, for example, look at a sentence and see it in three dimensions. I see every letter combination in the sentence and see words not intended to be seen. These hidden words can ultimately turn into a hidden sentence with a completely unrelated meaning to the original sentence. An example of this may baffle the most studious observer. Simple words such as *eye* can be substituted for *I* and *to* for *too* or *two*. Homonyms have significant meaning to the schizophrenic, as you can see, or should I say sea. Words like *no* and *know* can be used interchangeably. So when I answer a question "no" I may very well be simply asking the question "know?" As in "do you know?" So you can see how confusing it may be for a doctor to enter my world as a schizophrenic and evaluate me. It is as if the rules of logic are altered.

Another characteristic of schizophrenia thinking is concreteness. This can be tested by asking the person to give the meaning of proverbs, which require an ability to abstract, to move from the specific to the general. When most people are asked what "People who live in glass houses shouldn't throw stones" means, they will answer something like: "If you're not perfect yourself, don't criticize others." They move without difficulty from the specific glass house and stones to the general concept.

But the person with schizophrenia frequently loses this ability to abstract. I asked a hundred patients with schizophrenia to explain the proverb above; less than one-third were able to think abstractly about it. The majority answered simply something like: "It might break the windows." In many instances the concrete answer also demonstrated some disconnected thinking:

> Well, it could mean exactly like it says 'cause the windows may well be broken. They do grow flowers in glass houses.

> Because if they did they'd break the environment.

A few patients personalized it:

> People should always keep their decency about their living arrangements. I remember living in a glass house but all I did was wave.

Others responded with totally irrelevant answers that illustrated many facets of the thinking disorder in schizophrenia:

> Don't hit until you go—coming or going.

A few patients were able to think abstractly about the proverb, but in formulating their reply incorporated other aspects of thinking typical of schizophrenia:

> People who live in glass houses shouldn't forget people who live in stone houses and shouldn't throw glass.

> If you suffer from complexities, don't talk about people. Don't be agile.

The most succinct answer came from a quiet, chronically ill young man who pondered it solemnly, looked up and said, "Caution."

Concrete thinking can also occur during the everyday life of some persons. For example, one day I was taking a picture of my sister, who had schizophrenia. When I said, "Look at the birdie," she immediately looked up to the sky. Another patient, passing a newspaper stand, noticed a headline announcing that a star had fallen from a window. "How could a big thing like a star get into a window?" he wondered, until he realized it referred to a movie star.

An impairment of the ability to think logically is another facet of thinking characteristic of schizophrenia, as illustrated in several of the previous examples. One young man wrote: "It seemed the part of my mind that controlled logic went out the door." Another example was a patient under my care who, in psychological testing, was asked, "What would you do if you were lost in a forest?" He replied, "Go to the back of the forest, not the front." Similarly, many patients lose the ability to reason causally about events. One, for example, set his home on fire with his wheelchair-confined mother in it; when questioned carefully he did not seem to understand the fact that he was endangering her life.

Given this impairment of causal and logical thinking in many persons with this disease, it is not surprising that they frequently have difficulty with daily activities, such as taking a bus, following directions, or planning meals. It also explains the fantastic ideas that some patients offer as facts. One of my patients, for example, wrote me a note about "a spider that weighs over a ton" and "a bird which weighs 178 pounds and makes 200 tracks in the winter and has only one foot." The writer was college-educated.

In addition to disconnectedness, loosening of associations, concreteness, and impairment of logic, there are other features of the thought processes in individuals with schizophrenia. Neologisms—made-up words—are occasionally heard. They may sound like gibberish to the listener, but to those saying them they are a response to an inability to find the words they want:

> Big magnified thoughts come into my head when I am speaking and put away words I wanted to say. . . . I've got a lot to say but I can't focus the words to come out so they come out jumbled up.

Another uncommon but dramatic form of thinking in schizophrenia is called a word salad; the person just strings together a series of totally unrelated words and pronounces them as a sentence. One of my patients once turned to me solemnly and asked, "Bloodworm Baltimore frenchfry?" It's difficult to answer a question like that!

Generally it is not necessary to analyze the thought pattern in detail to know that something is wrong with it. The overall effect on the listener is both predictable and indicative. In its most common forms, it makes the listener feel that something is fuzzy about the thinking, as if the words have been slightly mixed up. John Bartlow Martin wrote a book about mental illness called *A Pane of Glass*, and Ingmar Bergman portrayed the recurrence of the symptoms of schizophrenia in his *Through a Glass Darkly* (see chapter 13). Both were referring to this opaque quality in speech and thinking. The listener hears all the words, which may be almost correct, but at the end of the sentence or paragraph realizes that it doesn't "make sense." It is the feeling evoked when, puzzled by something, we squint our eyes, wrinkle our forehead, and smile slightly. Usually we exclaim "What?" as we do this. It is a reaction evoked often when we listen to people with schizophrenia who have a thinking disorder:

> I feel that everything is sort of related to everybody and that some people are far more susceptible to this theory of relativity than others because of either having previous ancestors connected in some way or other with places or things, or because of believing, or by leaving a trail behind when you walk through a room you know. Some people might leave a different trail and all sorts of things go like that.

There can, of course, be all degrees of these thinking disorders in patients. Especially in the early stages of illness there may be only a vagueness or evasiveness that defies precise labeling, but in the full-blown illness the impairment usually is quite clear. It is an unusual patient who does not have some form of thinking disorder. Some psychiatrists even question whether schizophrenia is the correct diagnosis if the person's thinking pattern is completely normal: they would say that schizophrenia, by definition, must include some disordered thinking. Others claim that it is possible, though unusual, to have genuine schizophrenia with other symptoms but without a thinking disorder.

A totally different type of thinking disorder is also commonly found in persons with schizophrenia: blocking of thoughts. To return to the metaphor of the telephone operator at the switchboard, it is as if she suddenly dozes off for a few moments and the system goes dead. The person is thinking or starting to respond and then stops, often in midsentence, and looks blank for a brief period. John Perceval described this as long ago as 1840:

> For instance, I have been often desired to open my mouth, and to address persons in different manners, and I have begun without premeditation a very rational and consecutive speech . . . but in the midst of my sentence, the power had either left me, or words have been suggested contradictory of those that went before: and I have been deserted, gaping, speechless, or stuttering in great confusion.

Other people have given these accounts:

> I may be thinking quite clearly and telling someone something and suddenly I get stuck. You have seen me do this and you may think I am just lost for words or that I have gone into a trance, but that is not what happens. What happens is that I suddenly stick on a word or an idea in my head and I just can't move past it. It seems to fill my mind and there's no room for anything else. This might go on for a while and suddenly it's over.

Everyone who has spent time with persons with schizophrenia has observed this phenomenon. James Chapman claims it occurs in 95 percent of all patients. Some of the patients explain it by saying the thoughts are being taken out of their head. This symptom—called thought withdrawal—is considered by many psychiatrists to be strongly suggestive of a diagnosis of schizophrenia when it is present.

Ambivalence is another common symptom of thinking in schizophrenia. Although now a fashionable term used very broadly, it was originally used in a narrower sense to describe patients with schizophrenia who were unable to resolve contradictory thoughts or feelings, holding opposites in their minds simultaneously. A person with schizophrenia might think: "Yes, they are going to kill me and I love them." One woman described the contradictory thoughts as follows:

> I am so ambivalent that my mind can divide on a subject, and those two parts subdivide over and over until my mind feels like it is in pieces and I am totally disorganized.

Sometimes the ambivalence gets translated into actions as well. For example, one of my patients frequently left the front door of the building, turned right, then stopped, took three steps back to the left and stopped, turned back and started right, sometimes continuing in this way for a full five minutes. It is not found as dramatically in most patients but is of sufficient frequency and severity for Bleuler to have named it as one of the cardinal symptoms of schizophrenia. It is as if the ability to make a decision has been impaired. Normally our brain assesses the incoming thoughts and stimuli, makes a decision, and then initiates a response. The brains of some persons with schizophrenia are apparently impaired in this respect, initiating a response but then immediately countermanding it with its opposite, then repeating the process. It is a truly painful spectacle to observe.

Delusions and Hallucinations

Delusions and hallucinations are probably the best-known symptoms of schizophrenia. They are dramatic and are therefore the behaviors usually focused on when schizophrenia is being represented in popular literature or movies. The person observed talking to himself or to in-animate objects has been, until recently, a sine qua non for schizophrenia; now, however, the person may merely be talking on a cell phone! Nevertheless, the image of talking to oneself is the image evoked in our minds when the term "crazy" or "mad" is used.

And certainly delusions and hallucinations are very important and common symptoms of this disease. However, it should be remembered that they are not essential to it; indeed no *single* symptom is essential for the diagnosis of schizophrenia. There are many people with schizophrenia who have a combination of other symptoms, such as a thought disorder, disturbances of affect, and disturbances of behavior, who have never had delusions or hallucinations. It should also be remembered that delusions and hallucinations are found in brain diseases other than schizophrenia, so their presence does not automatically mean that schizophrenia is present.

Finally, it is important to realize that most delusions and hallucinations, as well as distortions of the body boundaries, are a direct outgrowth of overacuteness of the senses and the brain's inability to interpret and respond appropriately to stimuli. In other words, most delusions and hallucinations are logical outgrowths of what the brain is experiencing. They are "crazy" only to the outsider; to the person experiencing them they form part of a logical and coherent pattern. This was clearly illustrated by John Nash, who won the 1994 Nobel Prize in economics and who also had schizophrenia, when he was being queried by Professor George Mackey regarding his delusional beliefs:

"How could you," began Mackey, "how could you, a mathematician, a man devoted to reason and logical proof . . . how could you believe that extraterrestrials are sending you messages? How could you believe that you are being recruited by aliens from outer space to save the world? How could you . . . ?"

Nash looked up at last and fixed Mackey with an unblinking stare as cool and dispassionate as that of any bird or snake. "Because," Nash said slowly in his soft, reasonable southern drawl, as if talking to himself, "the ideas I had about supernatural beings came to me the same way that my mathematical ideas did. So I took them seriously."

Delusions are simply false ideas believed by the patient but not by other people in his/her culture and that cannot be corrected by reason. They are usually based on some kind of sensory experience that the person misinterprets. This may be as simple as brief static on the radio or a flicker of the television screen that the person interprets as a signal. Family members often wonder where the delusional ideas in the affected person came from.

One simple form of a delusion is the conviction that random events going on around the person all relate in a direct way to him or her. If you are walking down the street and a man on the opposite sidewalk coughs, you don't think anything of it and may not even consciously hear the cough. The person with schizophrenia, however, not only hears the cough but may immediately decide it must be a signal of some kind, perhaps directed to someone else down the street to warn him that the person is coming. The schizophrenia sufferer *knows* this is true with a certainty that few people experience. If you are walking with such a person and try to reason him/her past these delusions, your efforts will probably be futile. Even if you cross the street, and in the presence of the same person question the man about his cough, the individual will probably just decide that you are part of the plot. Reasoning with people about their delusions is like trying to bail out the ocean with a bucket. If, shortly after the cough incident, a helicopter flies overhead, the delusion may enlarge. Obviously the helicopter is watching the person, which further confirms suspicions about the cough. And if in addition to these happenings, the person arrives at

the bus stop just too late to catch the bus, the delusional system is confirmed yet again; obviously the person who coughed or the helicopter
pilot called the bus driver and told him to leave. It all fits together into
a logical, coherent whole.

Normal persons would experience these events and simply curse
their bad luck at missing the bus. The person with schizophrenia, however, is experiencing different things so the events take on a different
meaning. The cough and the helicopter noise may be very loud to him/
her and even the sound of the bus may be perceived to be strange.
While the normal person responds correctly to these as separate and
unrelated events, similar to the stimuli and events of everyday life, the
person with schizophrenia puts them together into a pattern. Thus,
both overacuteness of the senses and impaired ability to logically interpret incoming stimuli and thoughts may lie behind many of the
delusions experienced by afflicted minds. To them the person who
cannot put these special events together must be crazy, not the other
way around.

There are many excellent examples of delusional thinking in
literature. Chekhov, in his well known "Ward No. 6," described it as
follows:

> A policeman walking slowly passed by the windows: that was not for
> nothing. Here were two men standing still and silent near the house.
> Why? Why were they silent? And agonizing days and nights followed
> for Ivan Dmitritch. Everyone who passed by the windows or came
> into the yard seemed to him a spy or a detective.

In many cases the delusions become more complex and integrated. Rather than simply being watched, the person becomes convinced that he/she is being controlled by other persons, manipulated,
or even hypnotized. Such persons are constantly on the alert for confir-
matory evidence to support their beliefs; needless to say, they always
find it from among the myriad visual and auditory stimuli perceived by
all of us each day. A good example of this was a kind, elderly Irish lady
who was a patient on my ward. She believed that she had been wired
by some mysterious foreign agents in her sleep and that through the
wires her thoughts and actions could be controlled. In particular she

pointed to the ceiling as the place from which the control took place. One morning I was dismayed to come onto the ward and discover workmen installing a new fire alarm system; wires were hanging down in all colors and in all directions. The lady looked at me, pointed to the ceiling, and just smiled; her delusions had been confirmed forever!

Delusions of being wired or radio-controlled are relatively common. Often it is the FBI or the CIA that is the suspected perpetrator of the scheme. In recent years, an increasing number of delusions have involved the Internet. One patient was convinced that a radio had been sewn into his skull when he had had a minor scalp wound sutured and had tried to bring legal suit against the FBI innumerable times. Another man, at one time a highly successful superintendent of schools, became convinced that a radio had been implanted in his nose. He went to dozens of major medical centers, even to Europe, seeking a surgeon who would remove it. He even had an X-ray of his nose showing a tiny white speck that he was convinced was the radio.

Friends of the unfortunate people often try to reason them out of their delusions. Rarely is this successful. Questions about why the FBI would want to control them are deftly brushed aside as irrelevant; the important point is that they do, and the person is experiencing sensations (such as strange noises) that confirm the fact. Reasoning a person with schizophrenia out of a delusion is hampered by the distorted stimuli he/she is perceiving and also by the fact that the thinking processes may not be logical or connected. A further impediment is the fact that delusions frequently become self-fulfilling. Thus, someone who believes others are spying on him/her finds it logical to act furtively, perhaps running from corner to corner and peering anxiously into the faces of passersby. Such behavior inevitably invites attention and leads to the delusional person's actually being watched by other people. As the saying goes, "I used to be paranoid but now people really *are* watching me."

Delusions in which the person is being watched, persecuted, or attacked are commonly called paranoid delusions. Paranoia is a relative concept; everybody experiences bits and pieces of it from time to time. Among the general population, paranoid thinking is quite common, especially among groups that do not trust the government. On the Internet there are websites that support paranoid thinking, such as www.stopcovertwar.com. In some places a little paranoia even has survival value; the fellow who works across the hall may really be stealing your memos, because he wants your job. Paranoid thinking by itself is not schizophrenia; it is only when it becomes a frank delusion (unaffected by reason) that it *may* be. Even then, however, it must be remembered that paranoid delusions can occur in brain diseases other than schizophrenia.

Paranoid delusions may on occasion be dangerous. "During the paranoid period I thought I was being persecuted for my beliefs, that my enemies were actively trying to interfere with my activities, were trying to harm me, and at times even to kill me." The paranoid person may try to strike first when the threat is perceived as too close. Facilities for the criminally insane in every state include among their inmates a large number of persons with schizophrenia who have committed a crime in what they believed to be self-defense. It is this subgroup that has produced the general belief that people with schizophrenia as a whole are dangerous. As will be discussed in chapter 10, when we take into consideration all persons with schizophrenia, this subgroup is very small. Most persons with schizophrenia are not dangerous at all, and I would far rather walk the halls of any mental hospital than walk the streets of any inner city.

Delusions may be of many types other than paranoid; grandiose delusions are quite common: "I felt that I had power to determine the weather, which responded to my inner moods, and even to control the movement of the sun in relation to other astronomical bodies." This often leads to a belief by the person that he/she is Jesus Christ, the Virgin Mary, the President, or some other exalted or important person. One admission in our hospital believed himself to be Mao Ze-dong. We began him on medication and, by the next day, knew he was getting better because he had become only the brother of Mao Ze-dong.

Grandiose delusions can on occasion be dangerous. People who believe that they can fly, or stop bullets with their chest, may place themselves in a position to demonstrate the truth of their belief with predictably tragic consequences.

There is one particular type of grandiose delusion that, although not seen commonly, is so distinctive that it has acquired its own name. It is the delusion that another person, usually famous, is deeply in love with the patient. Such cases, originally called *psychoses passionnelles* by Dr. Gaëtan G. de Clerambault, a French psychiatrist, now often bear the designation of de Clerambault syndrome, or erotomania. One of my patients, who believed that Senator Edward Kennedy was in love with her, spent all her time and money following him around but always staying at a distance; she produced a multitude of incredible reasons why he could not acknowledge her presence. Another patient believed she was engaged to a man whom she had met once casually several years before, and spent all day walking the city streets looking for him. Most patients with such delusions have schizophrenia, although a few may have bipolar disorder. These patients have a pathos to their lives that is unusually affecting.

A relatively common delusion is that a person can control other people's minds. One young woman I saw had spent five years at home because each time she went into the street she believed that her mind compelled other people to turn and look at her. She described the effect of her mind as "like a magnet—they have no choice but to turn and look." Another patient believed he could change people's moods by "telepathic force": "I eventually felt I could go into a crowded restaurant and while just sitting there quietly, I could change everyone's mood to happiness and laughter."

Another variant is the delusional belief that one's thoughts are radiating out of one's head and being broadcast over radio or television; this is called thought broadcasting and is considered to be an almost certain indication of schizophrenia. One woman described it as follows: "I believed I had a ticker tape going in one ear and coming out the other, with all my thoughts written on it." And a young man recalled:

> I was really upset the other night because the people on the news were saying what my thoughts were. I know this is true because they sent me messages on what they were doing. I hate it when they can tell my thoughts to everyone who is watching them. I also hate it when people can hear my thoughts and know everything about me.

Occasionally such individuals call or go to the radio or television station and ask them to stop broadcasting their thoughts. A 1999 study of radio and television stations reported that such contacts are relatively common.

In evaluating delusions, it is very important to keep in mind that their content is culture-bound. It is not the belief per se that is delusional but how far the belief differs from the beliefs shared by others in the same culture or subculture. A man who believes he is being influenced by others who have "worked roots" (put a hex) on him may be completely normal if he grew up in lowland South Carolina, where "working roots" is a widespread cultural belief. If he grew up in affluent Scarsdale, New York, on the other hand, his belief in being influenced by "worked roots" is more likely to suggest schizophrenia. Minority groups in particular may have a culturally induced high level of paranoid belief, and this belief may be based on real discrimination and real persecution. In other subcultural groups it may be difficult to assess the pathological nature of delusional thinking, for instance regarding grandiose delusions among the deeply religious and paranoid delusions among employees of the intelligence community. Imagine, for example, the dilemma of a Mother Superior in evaluating a novice who claims to have a special relationship with the Virgin Mary or a supervisor at the CIA who is told by one of his undercover employees that he is being watched all the time. Beliefs of persons suspected of having schizophrenia must *always* be placed within a cultural context and regarded as only one facet of the disease.

One other aspect of delusions is important to note. Delusions may be fixed and static in some individuals with schizophrenia, but in others the delusions may be labile and held with varying degrees of conviction. I recall one patient, for example, who believed that another patient was trying to kill him. On one day he would avoid the feared person completely, on the next day he would socialize with him pleasantly, and on the following day he would avoid him again. This lack of consistency was also noted in 1890 by Dr. Pliny Earle, whose patient believed she had "millions and billions of children . . . and that persons are constantly engaged in murdering them. . . . Yet this woman is always quiet and gentle, makes no outward show of grief or unhappiness, and never attempts to force or find her way into the presence of her imaginary children." This lack of consistency in response to delusional thinking is difficult to understand for families of individuals with schizophrenia.

Hallucinations are very common in schizophrenia and are the end of that spectrum that begins with overacuteness of the senses. To take vision as an example: the spectrum has overacuteness of vision at one end of it, that is, lights are too bright, colors take on a more brilliant hue. In the middle of the spectrum are gross distortions of visual stimuli (also called illusions), such as a dog that takes on the appearance of a tiger. And at the far end of the spectrum are things that are seen by the person with schizophrenia when there is nothing there; this is a true hallucination. The experiences described by patients are usually a mixture of different points on the spectrum.

Gross distortions of visual or auditory stimuli are not uncommon experiences in schizophrenia:

> This phenomenon can perhaps best be depicted by a description of the first time I experienced it. I was one of four men at a bridge table. On one of the deals, my partner bid three clubs. I looked at my hand: I had only one small club. Though my hand was weak, I had to bid to take him out. My bid won. When my partner laid down his cards, he showed only two small clubs in his hand. I immediately questioned why he had bid three clubs. He denied having made such a bid. The other two men at the table supported him. . . . Furthermore, the man had actually declared a different bid at the time I had heard him bidding three clubs. This bid I had not heard. Somewhere along the line of my nervous system the words which he had actually spoken were blocked and the hallucinatory words substituted.

In this instance there was a stimulus of some kind, but the person saw or heard it in a grossly distorted way. It is as if the person's brain is playing tricks.

Even worse tricks are played in forming true hallucinations, in which there is no initial stimulus at all. The brain makes up what it hears, sees, feels, smells, or tastes. Such experiences may be very real for the person. People who hallucinate voices talking to them may hear the voices just as clearly as, or even more clearly than, the voices of real people talking to them, and people with schizophrenia frequently talk back to the voices. There is a tendency for people close to patients to scoff at the "imaginary" voices, to minimize them and not believe the persons really hear them. But they do, and in the sense that the brain hears them, they are real. The voices are but an extreme example of the malfunctioning of the sufferer's sensory apparatus.

Auditory hallucinations are by far the most common form of hallucination in schizophrenia. They are so characteristic of the disease that a person with true auditory hallucinations should be assumed to have schizophrenia until proven otherwise. They may take a variety of forms. They may be a simple swishing or thumping sound, such as the beating of the heart in Poe's famous short story:

> No doubt I now grew very pale;—but I talked fluently, and with a heightened voice. Yet the sound increased and what could I do? It was a low, dull, quick sound—much such a sound as a watch makes when enveloped in cotton. I gasped for breath—and yet the officers heard it not. I talked more quickly—more vehemently; but the noise steadily increased. Why would they not be gone? I paced the floor to and fro with heavy strides, as if excited to fury by the observation of the men—but the noise steadily increased.

They may be a single voice: "Thus for years I have heard daily in hundredfold repetition incoherent words spoken into my nerves without any context, such as 'Why not?' 'Why, if,' 'Why, because I,' 'Be it,' 'With respect to him.'"

Or they may be multiple voices or even a choir:

> There was music everywhere and rhythm and beauty. But the plans were always thwarted. I heard what seemed to be a choir of angels. I thought it the most beautiful music I had ever heard. . . . This choir of angels kept hovering around the hospital and shortly afterward I heard something about a little lamb being born upstairs in the room just above mine.

The hallucinations may be heard only occasionally or they may be continuous. When occasional, the most common time for them, in my clinical experience, is at night when going to sleep:

> For about almost seven years—except during sleep—I have never had a single moment in which I did not hear voices. They accompany me to every place and at all times; they continue to sound even when I am in conversation with other people, they persist undeterred even when I concentrate on other things, for instance read a book or a newspaper, play the piano, etc.; only when I am talking aloud to other people or to myself are they of course drowned by the stronger sound of the spoken word and therefore inaudible to me.

I have taken care of people with similar manifestations. One unfortunate woman had heard voices continuously for twenty years. They became especially loud whenever she tried to watch television, so she couldn't watch it at all.

In the vast majority of cases, the voices are male voices and are unpleasant. They are often accusatory, reviling the victims for past misdeeds, either real or imagined. Often they curse them, and I have had many people refuse to tell me what the voices say to them because they were embarrassed by it. One patient, who ultimately committed suicide, described her voices as "a constant state of mental rape." Understandably, many patients react to their voices:

> I don't just sit there and let the voices beat up on me. I fight back the best I can. Sometimes I scream at them so hard and loud that a nurse at my psychiatric group home has to give me a shot. Sometimes I calm down on my own. I don't scream at the voices as much as I used to. If I can't ignore them, I try to talk back to them in a voice that's only slightly louder than theirs.

In a minority of cases the voices may be pleasant, as in the example with lovely music cited above. Occasionally they are even helpful, as with a woman who announced to me one day that she was getting well: "I know I am, because my voices told me so."

The precise mechanism of auditory hallucinations is now reasonably well understood. Recent studies using magnetic resonance imaging (MRI) scans on individuals with schizophrenia who have persistent auditory hallucinations, compared to normal controls, found that auditory hallucinations are associated with activation of an area of the brain at the junction of the superior temporal gyrus and the inferior parietal lobule, especially on the right side. The area is often referred to as the temperoparietal junction (TPJ), and contains one of the brain's two auditory areas. Its association with auditory hallucinations is consistent with other evidence linking that area to the brain network that is thought to be primarily involved in causing the symptoms of schizophrenia, as will be discussed in chapter 5. It is also of interest that individuals who are born deaf and who later develop schizophrenia can experience auditory hallucinations.

Visual hallucinations also occur but much less frequently. One patient described the variety of these hallucinations:

> At an early stage the appearance of colored flashes of light was common. These took the form either of distant streaks or of near-by round glowing patches about a foot in diameter. Another type, which took place five or six times, was the appearance of words or symbols on blank surfaces. Closely connected with this was the occasional substitution of hallucinatory matter for the actual printed matter in books which I have been reading. On these occasions, the passage which I have been seeing has dissolved while I have been looking at it and another and sometimes wholly different passage has appeared in its place.

Visual hallucinations usually appear in conjunction with auditory hallucinations. When only visual hallucinations appear, it is unlikely that schizophrenia is the cause. Many other brain diseases, notably drug intoxications and alcohol withdrawal, cause purely visual hallucinations and are the more likely diagnosis in such cases.

Like delusions, hallucinations must always be evaluated within their cultural context. In medieval times and today among some religious groups, visual hallucinations are not uncommon and do not necessarily suggest mental illness. Dr. Silvano Arieti attempted to distinguish the hallucinations of the profoundly religious from those of schizophrenia by proposing the following criteria: (a) religious hallucinations are usually visual, while those in schizophrenia are predominantly auditory; (b) religious hallucinations usually involve benevolent guides or advisers who issue orders to the person; and (c) religious hallucinations are usually pleasant.

Hallucinations of smell or taste are unusual but do occur. One patient gave this description of hallucinations of smell:

> On a few occasions, I have experienced olfactory hallucinations. These have consisted of the seeming smelling of an odor as though originating from a source just outside the nose. Sometimes this odor has had a symbolical relationship with the thoughts-out-loud, as for instance, the appearance of an odor of sulphur in connection with a threat of damnation to hell by the thoughts-out-loud.

Hallucinations of taste usually consist of familiar food tasting differently. I have had patients with paranoid schizophrenia, for example, who decided that they were being poisoned when their food began tasting "funny." Certainly if one's food suddenly starts changing in taste, it is logical to suspect that somebody is adding something to it.

Hallucinations of touch are also found among individuals with schizophrenia, although not commonly. I provided care for one woman who felt small insects crawling under the skin on her face; it is an understatement to say that this was very upsetting to her. Another patient experienced hallucinatory pain:

> To the person who experiences hallucinatory pains, the pains feel identical with actual pains. . . . The person who feels it undergoes real suffering.

Altered Sense of Self

Closely allied with delusions and hallucinations is another complex of symptoms that is characteristic of many patients with schizophrenia. Normal individuals have a clear sense of self; they know where their bodies stop and where inanimate objects begin. They know that their hand, when they look at it, belongs to them. Even to make a statement like this strikes most normal persons as absurd because they cannot imagine its being otherwise.

But many persons with schizophrenia can imagine it, for alterations in their sense of self are not uncommon in this condition. As one man described it: "I have no contact to myself. I feel like a zombie. . . . I am almost nonexistent." Such alterations are frequently associated with alterations in bodily sensations, such as was described by one man with schizophrenia who wrote to me:

> My body has the same forms of distortions as my vision and these are manifested throughout my anatomy. My body feels like there are indentations, ridges, and agonizing disfigurements all over. Strands of hair falling down on my forehead feel much larger, heavier, and more noticeable. . . . Hands, arms, and legs sometimes feel an inch to the side of where they really are at. Fingers at times feel and look longer or shorter than usual. My face can feel twice as long as it is.

Alterations of the self may range from such somatic perceptual distortions to, on the other end of the spectrum, confusion in distinguishing oneself from another person:

> A young man was frequently confused in a conversation, being unable to distinguish between himself and his interlocutor. He tended to lose the sense of whose thoughts originated in whom, and felt "as if" his interlocutor somehow "invaded him," an experience that shattered his identity and was intensely anxiety provoking. When walking on the street, he scrupulously avoided glancing at his mirror image in the windowpanes of the shops, because he felt uncertain on which side he really was.

In extreme cases, a few patients with schizophrenia are unable to recognize photographs of themselves. When one such man was shown a picture of himself and asked who it was, he answered: "It is a man."

A patient's body parts may develop lives of their own, as if they have become disassociated and detached. One patient described this feeling:

> I get shaky in the knees and my chest is like a mountain in front of me, and my body actions are different. The arms and legs are apart

and away from me and they go on their own. That's when I feel I am the other person and copy their movements, or else stop and stand like a statue.

One woman also described confusion regarding where her body stopped and the rest of the world began: "This was equally true in body functions. When I urinated and it was raining torrents outside, I was not at all certain whether it was not my own urine bedewing the world, and I was gripped by fear."

Confusion about one's sexual characteristics is also not uncommonly found among people with schizophrenia, as in this man who believed his body was acquiring a feminine appearance:

My breast gives the impression of a pretty well-developed female bosom; this phenomenon can be *seen* by anybody who wants to observe me *with his own eyes*. . . . A brief glance would not suffice. The observer would have to go to the trouble of spending ten or fifteen minutes near me. In that way anybody would notice the periodic swelling and diminution of my bosom.

The altered sense of self may be further aggravated if hallucinations of touch or delusions about the body are also present. One possible example of this is Kafka's famous story "The Metamorphosis," in which Gregor awakens in the morning and slowly realizes that he has been transformed into a huge beetle. Such passages in Kafka have led some scholars to speculate that Kafka himself may have had symptoms of schizophrenia. The origin of such sensory changes is now known to be tied to brain areas involved in the schizophrenia disease process, as will be discussed in chapter 5.

Changes in Emotions

Changes in emotions—or affect, as it is often called by professionals—are one of the most common and characteristic changes in schizophrenia. In the early stages of the illness, depression, guilt, fear, and rapidly fluctuating emotions may all be found. In the later stages, flattening of emotions are more characteristic, often resulting in individuals who appear to be unable to feel emotions at all. This in turn makes it more difficult for us to relate to them, so we tend to shun them even more.

Depression is a very common symptom early in the course of the disease but is often overlooked. In one study it was reported that "81 percent of the patients . . . presented a well defined episode of depressive mood." In half of the patients, the symptoms of depression preceded the onset of delusions or hallucinations. Most such depression is biologically based, caused by neurochemical changes in the brain as part of the disease process, although some of it may also be a reaction of the person to the realization that he/she is becoming sick. One of the tragic and not uncommon sequelae of such depression is suicide, which is discussed in chapter 10.

Early in the course of illness the person with schizophrenia may also feel widely varying and rapidly fluctuating emotions. Exaggerated feelings of all kinds are not unusual, especially in connection with the peak experiences described previously.

> During the first two weeks of my psychosis, religious experience provided that dominant factor of the psychotic phenomena. The most important form of religious experience in that period was religious ecstasy. The attempts of the thoughts-out-loud to persuade myself to adopt a messianic fixation formed the hallucinary background. In affective aspects, a pervasive feeling of well-being dominated the complex. I felt as though all my worries were gone and all my problems solved. I had the assurance that all my needs would be satisfied. Connected with this euphoric state, I experienced a gentle sensation of warmth over my whole body, particularly on my back, and a sensation of my body having lost its weight and gently floating.

Guilt is another commonly felt emotion in these early stages:

> Later, considering them appropriate, I no longer felt guilty about these fantasies, nor did the guilt have an actual object. It was too pervasive, too enormous, to be founded on anything definite, and it demanded punishment. The punishment was indeed horrible, sadistic—it consisted, fittingly enough, of being guilty. For to feel

oneself guilty is the worst that can happen, it is the punishment of punishments.

And fear is frequently described by patients, often a pervasive and nameless fear that exists without any specific object. It is well described by a young man with schizophrenia:

> I sat in my basement with a fear that I could not control. I was totally afraid—just from watching my cat look out the window.

Exaggerated feelings usually are not found in patients beyond the early stages of the disease. If they are, they should raise questions as to whether schizophrenia is the correct diagnosis. It is the *retention* of such feelings and emotions that is one of the sharpest dividing lines between schizophrenia and bipolar disorder (see chapter 2). If the person retains exaggerated feelings to a prominent degree beyond the early stages of the disease, it is much more likely that the correct diagnosis will turn out to be bipolar disorder.

In addition to the exaggerated emotions that are experienced by individuals with schizophrenia, there is also evidence that some people affected with this disease have difficulties in assessing emotions in other people. A review of studies in this area asserted that "there has been a growing literature suggesting that schizophrenics differ substantially from controls in processing emotional communication." One research technique used to demonstrate this is to ask individuals with schizophrenia to describe the emotions of people in photographs, which is frequently a difficult task for them. For example, in one study of patients with schizophrenia, the "patients performed worse than comparison subjects on recognition of all emotions and neutral faces combined, including mild and extreme expressions." This impaired ability to judge emotions in others is a major reason why many people with schizophrenia have trouble in social communications and forming friendships.

The most characteristic changes in emotions in schizophrenia are inappropriate emotions or flattened emotions. It is an unusual patient who does not have one or the other—and sometimes both—by the time the disease is full-blown.

Inappropriate emotions are to be expected in light of the previous analogy of the telephone operator at the switchboard. Just as he/she hooks up the wrong thoughts with incoming stimuli, so he/she also hooks up wrong emotions. The incoming call may carry sad news, but he/she hooks it up with mirth and the patient laughs. In other instances a patient responds with an inappropriate emotion because of the other things going on in his/her head that cause laughter.

> Half the time I am talking about one thing and thinking about half a dozen other things at the same time. It must look queer to people when I laugh about something that has got nothing to do with what I am talking about, but they don't know what's going on inside and how much of it is running round in my head. You see I might be talking about something quite serious to you and other things come into my head at the same time that are funny and this makes me laugh. If I could only concentrate on the one thing at the one time I wouldn't look half so silly.

These inappropriate emotions produce one of the most dramatic aspects of the disease—the victim suddenly breaking out in cackling laughter for no apparent reason. It is a common sight to those who have worked or lived with people with this disease.

The flattening of emotions may be subtle in the earlier stages of the disease. Chapman claims that "one of the earliest changes in schizophrenic experience involves impairment in the process of empathy with other people." The person with schizophrenia loses the ability to put him/herself in the other person's place or to feel what the other person is feeling. As the disease progresses this flattening or blunting of the emotions may become more prominent: "During my first illness I did not feel the emotions of anger, rage, or indignation to nearly as great an extent as I would have normally. Attitudes of dislike, estrangement, and fear predominated."

Emotions may become detached altogether from specific objects, leaving the victim with a void, as poignantly described by this patient:

> Instead of wishing to do things, they are done by something that seems mechanical and frightening, because it is able to do things and

yet unable to want to or not to want to. All the constructive healing parts that could be used healthily and slowly to mend an aching torment have left, and the feeling that should dwell within a person is outside, longing to come back and yet having taken with it the power to return.

And Michael Wechsler summarized it neatly in a statement to his father: "I wish I could wake up feeling really bad—it would be better than feeling nothing."

In the advanced stage of flattening of the emotions, there appear to be none left at all. This does not happen frequently, but when it does it is an unforgettable experience for those who interact with the victims. I have had two such patients in whom I was unable to elicit *any* emotion whatsoever under any circumstances. They were polite, at times stubborn, but never happy or sad. It is uncannily like interacting with a robot. One of these patients set fire to his house, then sat down placidly to watch TV. When it was called to his attention that the house was on fire, he got up calmly and went outside. Clearly the brain damage in these cases has seriously affected the centers mediating emotional response. Fortunately, most persons with schizophrenia do not have such complete damage to this area of the brain.

One must be cautious, however, in assuming that a person with schizophrenia who apparently is experiencing no emotions *really* is experiencing no emotions. A study of individuals with schizophrenia who were videotaped while watching emotion-laden films found that the individuals "reported experiencing as much positive and negative emotion" despite the fact that they expressed much less of the emotion. Jean Bouricius, the mother of a young man with schizophrenia, published excerpts from her son's writings that demonstrated that he was experiencing intense, although unexpressed, emotions at the same time that mental health professionals were rating him as being emotionally very flat. His writings included: "Loneliness needs a song, a song of love and pain, sweet release and hope for the future," and "I close my eyes softly and become that part of midnight winds where emotion is choked and no cries can emerge." It is becoming increasingly apparent that some individuals with schizophrenia, who on the surface appear to be experiencing no emotions, are inwardly feeling intense emotions.

Often associated with a flattening of emotions are apathy, slowness of movement, underactivity, lack of drive, and a paucity (usually called poverty) of thought and speech. This composite picture is frequently seen in patients who have been sick for many years and is frequently referred to as the "negative" symptoms of schizophrenia, as will be discussed in chapter 2. These patients appear to be desireless, apathetic, seeking nothing, wanting nothing. It is as if their will had eroded, and indeed something like that probably does happen as part of the disease process. One especially insightful man described this condition with a sense of humor: "I still have what I call 'the poverties,' like poverty of thought, emotion, friends, and hard cash."

It is fashionable nowadays to believe that much of the flattening of emotions and apathy common in patients with schizophrenia are side effects of the drugs used to treat the disease. In fact, there is only a little truth to this. Many of the drugs used to treat schizophrenia do have a calming or sedative effect (see chapter 7). Most of the flattening of emotions and weakening of motivation, however, are products of the disease itself and not the effect of the drugs. This can easily be proved by reviewing descriptions of patients in the literature prior to the introduction of these drugs. Emotional flattening and apathy are just as prominent in those early descriptions as they are today.

Changes in Movements

In recent years changes in movements have been closely linked in people's minds with the side effects of drugs used to treat schizophrenia. And indeed the antipsychotic drugs and lithium may cause changes in movements, varying from a fine tremor of the fingers to gross jerky movements of the arms or trunk.

But it is important to keep in mind that the schizophrenia disease process can also cause changes in movements, and that these were clearly described in accounts of the disease for many years before modern drugs became available. One study of changes of movements in schizophrenia found that they occur "in virtually all cases of conser-

vatively defined schizophrenia" and concluded that they were consequences of the disease process and not of the medication being taken
by the patients. In another study half the patients in remission remembered changes in their movements. In some cases their movements
appeared to speed up, while in others they slowed down. A feeling
of awkwardness or clumsiness is relatively common, and persons with
this disease may spill things, or stumble while walking, much more
commonly than before they became sick.

Another change in movement is decreased spontaneity, and the
person may be aware of this. One recalled: "I became the opposite
of spontaneous, as a result of which I became very diffident, very la-
bored." Some patients with schizophrenia have decreased spontaneous swinging of their arms when they walk, a finding that has led
some researchers to theorize that the cerebellum or basal ganglia por-
tions of the brain may be affected in this disease.

Repetitious movements such as tics, tremors, tongue movements,
and sucking movements are also seen. In the majority of patients in
whom they occur, these are side effects of the medication being given
the patient, but in a minority they will not be due to the medication
but rather to the disease process. Even subtle body movements like
eye blinking may be affected in schizophrenia. Some patients with the
disease blink much less often than normal people. Drugs can account
for some of this decrease but not for all of it. Balzac noted it in a patient
in the early years of the nineteenth century: "[He] stood, just as I now
saw him, day and night, with fixed eyes, never raising or lowering the
lids, as others do."

The most dramatic change of movements in schizophrenia, of
course, is catatonic behavior. A patient may remain motionless for
hours, and if the person's arm is passively moved, the arm will often
remain in its new position for an hour or longer. Catatonic forms of
schizophrenia were seen more commonly in the earlier years of this
century but have become much less common; the availability of antipsychotic medication may be one reason for this, as catatonic symptoms usually respond promptly to medication.

Changes in Behavior

Changes in behavior are usually secondary rather than primary symptoms of schizophrenia; that is, the behaviors shown by persons with this illness are most often a response to other things occurring in their brains. For example, if the person with schizophrenia is beset by over-acuteness of the senses and an inability to synthesize incoming stimuli, it makes perfect sense for him/her to withdraw into a corner. Many of the other behaviors seen in this disease can be similarly and logically explained.

Withdrawing, remaining quietly in one place for long periods, and immobility are all common behaviors in this illness. The extreme versions of such behaviors are catatonia, where the person remains rigidly fixed in one position for long periods of time, and mutism, where the person does not speak at all. Catatonia and mutism are part of a continuum that includes the less blatant forms of withdrawal and immobility so commonly seen in the disease.

A person with schizophrenia may withdraw and remain silent for any one of a number of reasons. Sometimes this occurs when the person becomes lost in deep thought:

> When I am walking along the street it comes on me. I start to think deeply and I start to go into a sort of trance. I think so deeply that I almost get out of this world.

Or it may be adopted in order to slow down the incoming sensory stimuli so the brain can sort them out:

> I don't like moving fast. I feel there would be a breakup if I went too quick. I can only stand that a short time and then I have to stop. If I carried on I wouldn't be aware of things as they really are. I would just be aware of the sound and noise and the movements. Everything would be a jumbled mass. I have found that I can stop this happening by going completely still and motionless. When I do that, things are easier to take in.

The movements may also be slowed so as to allow them to be integrated into a whole in exactly the same way that visual and auditory stimuli may need to be integrated:

> I am not sure of my own movements any more. . . . If I am going to sit down, for example, I have got to think of myself and almost see myself sitting down before I do it. It's the same with other things like washing, eating, and even dressing—things that I have done at one time without even bothering or thinking about at all. . . . All this makes me move much slower now.

Other unusual behaviors are also found in persons with schizophrenia. Ritualistic behaviors are not uncommon. Some patients repeatedly walk in circles, and I know one who walked through all doors backward. There are reasons why they do such things, as explained by this woman who felt compelled to beat eggs a certain way when making a cake:

> As the work progressed, a change came. The ingredients of the cake began to have a special meaning. The process became a ritual. At certain stages the stirring must be counter-clockwise; at another time it was necessary to stand up and beat the batter toward the east; the egg whites must be folded in from the left to the right; for each thing that had to be done there were complicated reasons. I recognized that these were new, unfamiliar, and unexpected, but did not question them. They carried a finality that was effective. Each compelling impulse was accompanied by an equally compelling explanation.

Certain gestures may be repeated often, for reasons that are quite logical to the person doing them but that appear bizarre to the onlooker. One patient shook his head rhythmically from side to side to try and shake the excess thoughts out of his mind. Another massaged his head "to help to clear it" of unwanted thoughts. It is because of such ritualistic and repetitive behaviors that occasional patients with schizophrenia may be misdiagnosed with obsessive-compulsive disorder. Obsessions and compulsions are indeed frequently present in schizophrenia; however, a person with true obsessive-compulsive disorder will not have the thought disorder, delusions, hallucinations, or other symptoms that are also present in schizophrenia.

Specific postures may also be adopted by persons with schizophrenia. One of my patients marched endlessly up and down the sidewalk with his left hand placed awkwardly on his left shoulder. It appeared to be uncomfortable, but he invariably returned to it for reasons I was never able to ascertain.

Occasionally a person with schizophrenia will repeat like a parrot whatever is said to him/her. In psychiatric language this is called echolalia. Chapman believes that repeating the words probably is useful to the patient because it allows time to absorb and synthesize what was said. Much rarer is the occurrence of behavior that is parroted, called echopraxia. When it occurs, it may be the consequence of a dissolution of boundaries of the self so that the person does not know where his/her body leaves off and where the body of the other person begins.

Most worrisome to friends and relatives of individuals with schizophrenia, for obvious reasons, are socially inappropriate behaviors. Fortunately, most patients who act inappropriately on hospital wards may act quite appropriately when taken out of the hospital on trips. It is always impressive to see patients from even the most regressed hospital wards go to public places; they are usually more distinguishable by their dress (characteristically poorly fitting) than by their behavior. A small number of patients are so ill that they continue inappropriate behaviors (such as random urination, open masturbation, spitting on others) even in public, but such patients are comparatively rare. Some—but not all—of them can be improved by proper medication or conditioning techniques.

It should always be remembered that the behavior of persons with schizophrenia is internally logical and rational; they do things for reasons that, given their disordered senses and thinking, make sense *to them*. To the outside observer the behavior may appear irrational, "crazy," "mad," the very hallmark of the disease. To the ill person, however, there is nothing "crazy" or "mad" about it at all. For example, a woman with schizophrenia who believed that a pharmacist was controlling her mind decided "the only way I could escape his influence and radiation was to walk a circuit a mile in diameter around his drugstore." And an Ohio man who believed he was "the Abominable Snowman" stole "a street sweeper so he could drive to Alaska and 'save the world.'"

Although most bizarre behavior of individuals with schizophrenia is caused by their disordered thinking processes, some of it may also be caused by disease-related physiological brain changes. For example, many individuals with schizophrenia have dysregulation of their body temperature. As a consequence of this, some patients dress in many layers of clothing, even in hot weather.

Indeed, almost everything a person with schizophrenia says and does may be, to them, rational. It is "crazy" only to the outsider who sits on the sidelines and observes from afar. To someone who will take the time to listen, a person with schizophrenia is not "crazy" at all if by "crazy" one means irrational. The "craziness" has its roots in the disordered brain function that produces erroneous sensory data and disordered thinking.

Decreased Awareness of Illness: Anosognosia

Some people with schizophrenia are aware of the malfunctioning of their brain; this is what is called awareness of illness, or insight. A few of them even tell those around them in the early stages of illness that something is going wrong with their head. One mother remembered her son holding his head and pleading: "Help me, Mom, something is wrong in my head." One young lady, only twelve years old, asked her parents if she could see a psychiatrist and asked him if she had schizophrenia. John Hinckley wrote a letter to his parents (but never sent it), in which he said: "I don't know what's the matter. Things are not going well. I think there's something wrong with my head." One of the most poignant stories I have ever heard concerned a very bright teenage boy who realized that something was going wrong with his brain in the earliest stages of the disease and then spent months in the local medical libraries researching the illness before his symptoms became too severe. In another instance a parent told me that her son "had diagnosed himself as having schizophrenia" before anyone in the family fully realized that he was sick.

Such awareness of illness in the early stages is often lost as the disease becomes fully manifest. This is not surprising since it is the brain that is malfunctioning, and it is also the brain that we use to think about ourselves. In fact, I am always surprised at the many patients with schizophrenia who have awareness of their illness. Even in the stage of chronic illness an occasional person with schizophrenia will exhibit surprising insight. One woman, afflicted by schizophrenia for many years, wrote me that she would gladly "sacrifice my right arm to make my brain work." Another woman who had had severe schizophrenia for seven years, when I asked her what she was asking for at Christmas, looked at me sadly, paused for a moment, and then replied: "A mind."

Decreased awareness of illness is also found in other diseases of the brain. In Alzheimer's disease, for example, the affected individual is often aware of the illness when it first begins but then loses awareness as it progresses. Former president Ronald Reagan publicly announced his illness when it began, but as the disease progressed he lost all awareness and was even unable to identify members of his family. Decreased awareness of illness is also seen in other forms of dementia and in some individuals following strokes. Some post-stroke victims will even deny that their arm or leg is paralyzed, despite the obvious visible evidence that it is. Decreased awareness of illness is officially referred to in neurological terms as anosognosia.

It is known that decreased awareness of illness is caused by damage to specific parts of the brain. At least 25 studies have compared the brains of people with schizophrenia who have anosognosia to those who do not have anosognosia and almost every study reported differences in the brains between the two. These studies are summarized on the website of the Treatment Advocacy Center (www.treatment advocacycenter.org) under "Background Papers." The areas that appear to be malfunctioning in individuals with anosognosia are the medial frontal lobe, including the anterior cingulate, and insula, and the inferior parietal lobule, especially on the right side. These areas are all part of the brain network involved in the schizophrenia disease process, as will be described in chapter 5. Thus, some individuals with schizophrenia have complete awareness of their illness, others have partial awareness, and some have no awareness, depending on the specific brain areas affected. It is also known that awareness of illness may fluctuate in some individuals over time; during periods of remission, when the disease process is quiescent, the person may have good awareness, but during relapses, when the disease process is active, this awareness may be lost.

Decreased awareness of illness in individuals with schizophrenia has been observed for many years but only recently studied. In 1869 the *American Law Review* noted: "Generally, insane persons do not regard themselves as insane, and, consequently, can see no reason for their confinement other than the malevolent designs of those who have deprived them of their liberty." Since the 1990s there has been an outpouring of research on awareness of illness in schizophrenia; many of these are summarized in *Insight and Psychosis* and *I Am Not Sick, I Don't Need Help*, listed at the end of this chapter. Scales to assess such awareness have been developed and have revealed that approximately half of all individuals with schizophrenia have either moderately or severely impaired awareness of their illness.

The consequences of decreased awareness of illness for individuals with schizophrenia are legion. On the positive side, it has been shown that those with decreased awareness of their illness are less depressed and probably have a lower incidence of suicide, as one would expect. On the negative side, lack of awareness of illness is the largest single cause of the need for involuntary hospitalization and medication, major problems that are discussed in chapter 10.

The Black-Red Disease

Schizophrenia, then, is a disorder of the brain. The distinguished neurologist C. S. Sherrington once referred to a normal brain as "an enchanted loom," taking the threads of experience and weaving them into the fabric of life. For persons whose brains are afflicted with schizophrenia the loom is broken, and in some cases appears to have been replaced by a Waring blender that produces jumbled thoughts and loose associations. Given the resulting cerebral cacophony, is it any wonder that patients with this disease often describe their life as like being in the Twilight Zone?

Imagine what it would be like to have the alterations of the senses; the inability to interpret incoming stimuli; the delusions and hallucinations; and changes in bodily boundaries, emotions, and movements that are described above. Imagine what it would be like to no longer be able to trust your brain when it told you something. As one very articulate woman with schizophrenia explained to me, the problem is one of "a self-measuring ruler"—that is, you must use your malfunctioning brain to assess the malfunction of your brain. Is it any wonder that people with this disease get depressed? Is it any wonder that they frequently feel humiliated by their own behavior? If a worse disease than schizophrenia exists, it has not come to light.

How can family and friends of persons with schizophrenia understand what they are going through? Taking mind-altering drugs will produce alterations of the senses and even delusions that may resemble schizophrenia briefly, but it is not recommended that families use these drugs. A better way to understand the experience of having schizophrenia is to take a walk by yourself through an art museum and pretend that you are inside some of the pictures.

Begin with works by Vincent van Gogh painted in late 1888 and 1889 when he was undergoing a psychosis; "The Starry Night" and "Olive Grove with White Cloud" especially illustrate van Gogh's distorted perception of light, colors, and texture. Van Gogh was especially insightful about his illness. In describing his painting "The Garden of St. Paul's Hospital," done in 1889 while he was hospitalized, he wrote:

> You will realize that this combination of red-ocher, of green gloomed over by gray, the black streaks surrounding the contours, produces something of the sensation of anguish, called "noir-rouge," from which certain of my companions in misfortune frequently suffer.

This, then, is the "noir-rouge," or black-red disease.

Many other artists, although they themselves were not psychotic, included in their artistic creations elements that are reminiscent of the perceptions of people with schizophrenia. Joan Miró, for example, in paintings such as "Portrait IV, 1938," "Head of a Woman, 1938," and "Head of a Catalan Peasant," shows facial features as grossly distorted and disjointed. The viewer of a painting such as "Nude Woman" by Pablo Picasso is faced with the perplexing task of synthesizing the individual pieces into a whole, a task not unlike that faced every day by some individuals with schizophrenia. Marcel Duchamp's "Nude Descending a Staircase" suggests the jerky movements, lack of coordination, and clumsiness complained of frequently by persons with schizophrenia; this painting was specifically cited by one woman with schizophrenia symptoms from viral encephalitis to illustrate to the doctor how she felt.

Distorted emotions are evoked in several paintings of Henri Rousseau. Imagine yourself in "The Dream," for example, with eyes staring at you and unnamed terrors lurking behind every bush. Move on to lithographs or paintings by Edvard Munch, such as "The Scream," which mirrors the depression, despair, and loneliness of schizophrenia; the woman in the picture is covering her ears just as some patients do to try to shut out the auditory hallucinations. Finally, end your tour of the art museum at Hieronymus Bosch's "Garden of Earthly Delights." Study the tortures designed by Bosch for the "Hell" portion of the triptych, and think about the fact that the experience of having schizophrenia can be worse than anything Bosch ever imagined.

In summary, schizophrenia is a disease in which the brain, the essence of being, plays cruel tricks on the person affected. Kathy Bick, in the earliest stages of what was to become severe schizophrenia, poignantly captured that strangeness in her diary: "Something inside me is going thru this funny, alien state, a sense of being at the mercy of some strange force, and this pathetic scarecrow figure inside me at the mercy of other forces." Given the disordered brain function as a starting point, many persons with schizophrenia are heroic in their attempts to keep a mental equilibrium. And the proper response of those who care about the unfortunate persons with this disease is patience and understanding. Perhaps nowhere is this better illustrated than by Balzac's heroine in "Louis Lambert," a young woman who married a man who developed schizophrenia. She then dedicates her life to caring for him:

"No doubt Louis appears to be 'insane,'" she said, "but he is not so, if the word insanity is applied only to those whose brain, from unknown causes, becomes vitiated, and who are, therefore, unable to give a reason for their acts. The equilibrium of my husband's mind is perfect. If he does not recognize you corporeally, do not think that he has not seen you. He is able to disengage his body and to see us under another form, I know not of what nature. When he speaks, he says marvellous things. Only, in fact often, he completes in speech an idea begun in the silence of his mind, or else he begins a proposition in words and finishes it mentally. To other men he must appear insane; to me, who lives in his thought, all his ideas are lucid. I follow the path of his mind; and though I cannot understand many of its turnings and digressions, I nevertheless reach the end with him. Does it not often happen that while thinking of some trifling matter, we are drawn into serious thought by the gradual unfolding of ideas and recollections? Often, after speaking of some frivolous thing, the accidental point of departure for rapid meditation, a thinker forgets, or neglects to mention the abstract links which have led him to his conclusions, and takes up in speech only the last rings in the chain of reflections. Common minds to whom this quickness of mental vision is unknown, and who are ignorant of the inward travail of the soul, laugh at dreamers and call them madmen if they are given to such forgetfulness of connecting thoughts. Louis is always so; he wings his way through the spaces of thought with the agility of a swallow; yet I can follow him in all his circlings. That is the history of his so-called madness."

Such dedication and understanding, unachievable except in fiction, is a worthy ideal. It exists to some degree in many families and among some professionals who must care for such individuals on psychiatric wards or in outpatient clinics. As Louis Lambert's wife illustrates, compassion follows understanding. It is therefore incumbent on us to understand as best we can; the burden of disease will become lighter for all.

Recommended Further Reading

Amador, X. F., and A. S. David, eds. *Insight and Psychosis*, 2nd ed. New York: Oxford University Press, 2004.

Amador, X. F., and A.-L. Johanson. *I Am Not Sick, I Don't Need Help.* Peconic, N.Y.: Vida Press, 2000.

Chapman, J. "The Early Symptoms of Schizophrenia." *British Journal of Psychiatry* 112 (1966): 225–51.

Cutting, J., and F. Dunne. "Subjective Experience of Schizophrenia." *Schizophrenia Bulletin* 15 (1989): 217–31.

DeVries, M. W., ed. *The Experience of Psychopathology.* Cambridge: Cambridge University Press, 1992.

Dworkin, R. H. "Pain Insensitivity in Schizophrenia: A Neglected Phenomenon and Some Implications." *Schizophrenia Bulletin* 20 (1994): 235–48.

Freedman, B. J. "The Subjective Experience of Perceptual and Cognitive Disturbances in Schizophrenia: A Review of Autobiographical Accounts." *Archives of General Psychiatry* 30 (1974): 333–40.

Kaplan, B., ed. *The Inner World of Mental Illness.* New York: Harper & Row, 1964.

McGhie, A., and J. Chapman. "Disorders of Attention and Perception in Early Schizophrenia." *British Journal of Medical Psychology* 34 (1961): 103–16.

Morgan K. *Mind Without a Home: A Memoir of Schizophrenia.* Center City, MN: Hazeldon, 2013.

North, C. *Welcome Silence: My Triumph over Schizophrenia.* New York: Simon & Schuster, 1987.

Parnas, J., and P. Handest. "Phenomenology of Anomalous Self-Experience in Early Schizophrenia." *Comprehensive Psychiatry* 44 (2003): 121–134.

Plaze, M., M.-L. Paillère-Martinot, J. Penttilä, et al. "'Where Do Auditory Hallucinations Come From?'—A Brain Morphometry Study of Schizophrenia Patients with Inner or Outer Space Hallucinations." *Schizophrenia Bulletin* 37 (2011): 212–21.

Potvin, S., and S. Marchand. "Hypoalgesia in Schizophrenia Is Independent of Antipsychotic Drugs: A Systematic Quantitative Review of Experimental Studies." *Pain* 138 (2008): 70–78.

Prigatano, G. P., ed. *The Study of Anosognosia.* New York: Oxford University Press, 2010.

Sechehaye, M. *Autobiography of a Schizophrenic Girl.* New York: Grune & Stratton, 1951. Paperback by New American Library. Part 2 of the book, a psychoanalytic interpretation of the woman's symptoms, should be skipped.

Snyder, K., R.E. Gur, L.W. Andrews. *Me, Myself and Them: A Firsthand Account of One Young Person's Experience with Schizophrenia.* New York: Oxford University Press, 2007.

Sommer, R., J. S. Clifford, and J. C. Norcross. "A Bibliography of Mental Patients' Autobiographies: An Update and Classification System." *American Journal of Psychiatry* 155 (1998): 1261–64.

2

Defining Schizophrenia:
View from the Outside

To one who is mad, the world is still real, but it has a new meaning; people are real too, close and powerful and perhaps dangerous, but among them all the individual is alone. That is the central feature when we penetrate insanity. Not that the world is less with us, but that another world pervades it too, and we, seeing and experiencing life upon a different plane, are cut off from communication with the sane around us: the sane and blinkered folk who do not see and must not know or would never believe the vast, vital, urgent and perhaps cataclysmic truths of which we, alone among them, are aware.

Morag Coate, 1965

The definition of most diseases of mankind has been accomplished. We can define typhoid fever by the presence of the bacteria that cause it, kidney failure by a rise in certain chemicals in the blood, and cancers by the appearance of the cells under the microscope. In most diseases there is something that can be seen or measured, and this can be used to define the disease and separate it from nondisease states.

Not so with schizophrenia! Although there are numerous abnormalities in brain structure and function, there is no single thing that can be measured and from which we can then say: Yes, that is schizophrenia. Because of this, the definition of the disease is a source of continuing debate. This situation is exacerbated because of the probability that schizophrenia includes more than one disease entity.

Since we do not yet have any definitive measures for schizophrenia, we must define it by its symptoms. This may be misleading, however, for different diseases may cause the same symptoms. For example, a pain in the abdomen is a symptom, but the diseases that may cause this symptom number well over one hundred. Thus, to use symptoms to define diseases is risky. Such is the state of the art with schizophrenia; yet precise diagnosis is of utmost importance. It both determines the appropriate treatment for the patient and provides the patient and family with an informed prognosis. It also makes research on the disease easier because it allows researchers to be certain they are talking about the same thing.

Official Criteria for Diagnosis

Although there is no single symptom that is found only in schizophrenia, there are several that are found very uncommonly in diseases other than schizophrenia. When these are present they should elevate the index of suspicion considerably. Eugen Bleuler, a Swiss psychiatrist, believed that loosening of associations in the thinking process was central to the disease. Similarly, Kurt Schneider, a German psychiatrist, proposed a list of symptoms that he called "first rank" symptoms, meaning that when one or more of them are present they point strongly toward schizophrenia as the diagnosis.

These symptoms are used informally in European countries for the diagnosis of schizophrenia, but less so in the United States. Studies have shown that at least three-quarters of patients with schizophrenia have one or more of these symptoms. However, they cannot be considered as definitive for schizophrenia because they are also found in at least one-quarter of patients with bipolar disorder.

Until 1980, the term "schizophrenia" was used much more loosely and broadly in the United States than in most European countries. In

---

SCHNEIDER'S FIRST RANK SYMPTOMS FOR SCHIZOPHRENIA

1. Auditory hallucinations in which the voices speak one's thoughts aloud
2. Auditory hallucinations with two voices arguing
3. Auditory hallucinations with the voices commenting on one's actions
4. Hallucinations of touch when the bodily sensation is imposed by some external agency
5. Withdrawal of thoughts from one's mind
6. Insertion of thoughts into one's mind by others
7. Believing one's thoughts are being broadcast to others, as by radio or television
8. Insertion by others of feelings into one's mind
9. Insertion by others of irresistible impulses into one's mind
10. Feeling that all one's actions are under the control of others, like an automaton
11. Delusions of perception, as when one is certain that a normal remark has a secret meaning for oneself

---

fact, the only other country in the world where schizophrenia was diagnosed as loosely was the former Soviet Union, where it was abused as a label to discredit and stigmatize opponents of the government.

American psychiatry took a major step forward in 1980 when it adopted a revised system of diagnosis and nomenclature in the third edition of the *Diagnostic and Statistical Manual of Mental Disorders*, usually referred to as *DSM-III*. This was followed by revisions in 1987 (known as *DSM-III-R*) and then by further revisions in 1994 *(DSM-IV)* and 2013 *(DSM-V)*. The DSM diagnostic criteria are very similar to, but not exactly the same as, the diagnostic criteria used in European countries, called the *International Classification of Diseases* (ICD).

The DSM criteria for schizophrenia have achieved wide acceptance in the United States and may be utilized by families who are seeking a definition of the disease. If these criteria are not met, an official diagnosis of schizophrenia should not be made.

Lists of symptoms such as the above give the impression that schizophrenia is relatively easy to diagnose. In its fully developed form it usually is, but in the earlier stages it may be difficult to diagnose with certainty. The symptoms may appear intermittently or may be relatively mild, and the affected individual may be able to cover up some manifestations of the disease. It is therefore quite common for mental

CRITERIA FOR THE DIAGNOSIS
OF SCHIZOPHRENIA UNDER *DSM-V*

A. Two or more of the following symptoms must be present for a significant portion of time during a one-month period.
   1. delusions
   2. hallucinations
   3. disorganized speech
   4. catatonia or other grossly abnormal psychomotor behavior
   5. "negative" symptoms, e.g., restricted affect, asociality
B. Significant decreased function at work, in interpersonal relations, or in self-care.
C. At least one month of active symptoms (criteria A) unless successfully treated and at least six months of all symptoms (prodromal, active, and residual).
D. Does not meet criteria for schizoaffective disorder, and symptoms of psychosis are not caused by substance abuse.

illness professionals to write "rule out schizophrenia" on their initial encounter with a patient, which simply means that their diagnosis is tentative until the clinical picture is clearer.

Requiring that symptoms be present for at least six months before schizophrenia can be diagnosed is a sharp departure from traditional American practice. It is a useful advance, however, for schizophrenia is a serious diagnosis and should not be applied indiscriminately to someone with any schizophrenia-like symptom, however brief, as happened frequently in the past. For persons with schizophrenia-like symptoms of less than six months' duration, the *DSM-V* recommends the use of schizophreniform disorder as a diagnosis. If the duration is less than one month, a diagnosis of brief psychotic disorder is used.

Although the DSM criteria have been valuable in clarifying the diagnosis of schizophrenia, problems persist. Diagnosis continues to be based on the psychiatrist's subjective evaluation of patients' behavior and what patients say they are experiencing. What is clearly needed, and may be available before many years, are objective measures for diagnosis, such as laboratory tests of blood and cerebrospinal fluid. Until that time, criteria for the diagnosis of schizophrenia will continue to be debated and will require skilled clinical judgment.

A highly publicized experiment carried out by Dr. David L. Rosenhan, a psychologist at Stanford University, in 1973 illustrates some of the ongoing diagnostic problems. Rosenhan had volunteers go to psychiatric hospitals seeking admission and claiming to be hearing voices that had lasted for three weeks. Auditory hallucinations of any kind are unquestionably important and common symptoms of schizophrenia, with the majority of patients experiencing them at some point in the course of their illness. They are so important as symptoms that most psychiatrists take their presence as an indication of schizophrenia until proven otherwise. Thus, it should not have been surprising that all the volunteers were admitted as genuine patients. Rosenhan used this study to mock psychiatrists and their ability to diagnose patients, but this is erroneous. It would have been much *more* disturbing if these volunteers, who said they were being greatly troubled by the voices, had *not* been admitted for further investigation. Auditory hallucinations are to schizophrenia what abdominal pain is to appendicitis or vomiting blood is to a peptic ulcer. They are all danger signs suggesting that more definitive studies need to be done. The late Dr. Seymour Kety illustrated the fallacy of the Rosenhan study nicely:

> If I were to drink a quart of blood and, concealing what I had done, come to the emergency room of any hospital vomiting blood, the behavior of the staff would be quite predictable. If they labeled and treated me as having a bleeding ulcer, I doubt that I could argue convincingly that medical science does not know how to diagnose that condition.

Subtypes of Schizophrenia

During the last half of the nineteenth century different subtypes of what we now call schizophrenia were described as separate diseases. Thus, paranoid psychosis was initially characterized in 1868, hebephrenia in 1871, and catatonia in 1874. These three were grouped together in 1896 by Emil Kraepelin and called dementia praecox (dementia of early life). Bleuler changed the name to schizophrenia in 1911 and added the simple schizophrenia subtype as well.

For many years these subtypes of schizophrenia continued to be widely used. Their differentiation was based exclusively on the symptoms of the illness. Thus, paranoid schizophrenia was characterized by delusions and/or hallucinations with a predominantly persecutory or, less commonly, a grandiose content. Hebephrenic schizophrenia, called the "disorganized type" in the *DSM-IV* nomenclature, had as its predominant symptoms disorganized speech, disorganized behavior, and flat or inappropriate affect. Catatonic schizophrenia was diagnosed when the outstanding features of the disease were behavioral disturbances, such as posturing, rigidity, stupor, and often mutism, but this subtype is now rarely seen. And simple schizophrenia, not included as a separate entity under *DSM-IV,* was characterized by an insidious loss of interest and initiative, withdrawal, blunting of emotions, and the absence of delusions or hallucinations.

The validity and utility of these subtypes were very questionable despite their widespread usage. Few patients fall cleanly into one subtype or another, with most having some mix of symptoms. For these reasons, these subtypes of schizophrenia have been dropped by both the American DSM and the European ICD classifications and are no longer used.

Probably the most valid subtyping of schizophrenia is into deficit and nondeficit categories. This division, originally proposed by Dr. William Carpenter et al. in 1988, has slowly gained adherents. Deficit schizophrenia is one in which the "negative" symptoms predominate. The person has a restricted ("flat") affect and diminished social drive, says little, and has few interests. The "positive" symptoms, such as delusions and hallucinations, may be present but are not as prominent as the "negative" symptoms. Approximately 15 percent of individuals with schizophrenia fall into the deficit subtype. Studies have reported that individuals with deficit schizophrenia can be differentiated from other individuals with schizophrenia through neuropsychological tests, family history (they have a greater family history of schizophrenia), season of birth (more summer births), genetic findings, and serum markers of inflammation. Deficit schizophrenia also tends to be treatment-resistant. Whether this subtype of schizophrenia has a different cause remains to be ascertained.

Other researchers have argued that trying to subtype schizophrenia by its clinical symptoms is a waste of time. Subtyping should rather be done based on the presence of specific biological findings, referred to as endophenotypes, such as electrophysiological, neuroimaging, or cognitive abnormalities. Thus all patients with certain cognitive findings would be regarded as a subtype.

The Schizophrenia Spectrum: Do We All Have a Little?

What are the outer boundaries of the schizophrenia disease spectrum? This is an ongoing and hotly debated question, and there are, in fact, few murkier diagnostic lands to enter than the shadowy terrain lying at the borderlands of schizophrenia. Travelers to this region must have a high tolerance for ambiguity.

Increasingly, it has become evident that full-blown schizophrenia is just one end of a spectrum. Other areas of the spectrum include the following:

Delusional Disorder: These individuals have delusions but do not meet the full criteria for schizophrenia. Such delusions may be paranoid delusions (e.g., the belief that you are being followed), delusions of jealousy (e.g., the belief that your spouse is being unfaithful), delusions of erotomania (e.g., the belief that a famous person is in love with you), or somatic delusions (e.g., the belief that you have a fatal disease). The hallmark of a delusional disorder is that the delusion is untrue but not unreasonable, that apart from the delusion the person's functioning is not impaired, and that hallucinations are either absent or not prominent.

The precise relationship of delusional disorders to schizophrenia is still to be determined. Most clinicians and researchers suspect that delusional disorders are a less developed form of schizophrenia, but this is not proven. Delusional disorder is included in *DSM-V*.

Schizotypal Personality Disorder: These individuals were in the past said to have such things as borderline schizophrenia, ambulatory schizophrenia, pseudoneurotic schizophrenia, latent schizophrenia, subclinical schizophrenia, and schizophrenic character. They have oddities and eccentricities of perception, thinking, speech, and behavior. To meet criteria for this diagnosis under *DSM-V* the individual should have some of the following:

- ideas of reference, meaning that the person frequently thinks that other people are talking about him/her
- odd beliefs or magical thinking that influence behavior and are inconsistent with subcultural norms (e.g., superstitiousness, belief in clairvoyance, telepathy, or "sixth sense"; in children and adolescents, bizarre fantasies, or preoccupations)
- unusual perceptual experiences, including bodily illusions
- odd thinking and speech (e.g., vague, circumstantial, metaphorical, overelaborate, or stereotyped)
- suspiciousness or paranoid ideation
- inappropriate or constricted affect
- behavior or appearance that is odd, eccentric, or peculiar
- lacks close friends or confidants other than first-degree relatives
- excessive social anxiety that does not diminish with familiarity and tends to be associated with paranoid fears rather than negative judgments about self

Schizoid Personality Disorder: These individuals are loners and have virtually no friends. They avoid social situations and seek employment in which they do not have to interact with others (e.g., forest ranger, computer programmer). Schizoid men rarely marry. Such individuals appear incapable of experiencing feelings for others, either those of affection or those of hostility, and are relatively indifferent to praise or criticism. Some also appear to be detached from their environment as if in a perpetual fog. This is not included in *DSM-V.*

Paranoid Personality Disorder: These individuals are known for their hypersensitivity, mistrust, and suspiciousness of other people's motivations. They are always on guard, easily slighted, and quick to take offense. They believe that others are trying to trick or harm them, and will go to great lengths to prove it. They question the loyalty of others and often see plots where nobody else can see them. They are often rigid, argumentative, and litigious. Many are interested in electronics and mechanical devices that can be used for spying. They appear to have few tender feelings, disdain weak people, and lack any sense of humor. The dividing line between a paranoid personality disorder and a paranoid delusional disorder is a very narrow one, with the latter having a fully developed delusion. This is not included in *DSM-V*.

Controversy continues regarding the validity of these personality disorders and their relationship to schizophrenia. It is widely acknowledged that the personality disorders overlap and that many individuals have combinations of these traits. Studies of families of individuals with schizophrenia have found more relatives with schizotypal and paranoid personality disorders, suggesting that they are probably genetically related to schizophrenia. They can, in a theoretical sense, be considered mild forms of the disease. This possibility, generally referred to as the "spectrum concept" of schizophrenia, implies that there may be individuals at all points on the spectrum between schizoid personality disorder and severe schizophrenia. The concept has received support from recent findings that many individuals with schizotypal personality disorder have structural brain changes (e.g., enlarged ventricles, temporal lobe, and caudate abnormalities) similar to those seen in schizophrenia. In addition, many individuals with schizotypal personality disorder feel better and function better on low doses of antipsychotic drugs.

If there is indeed a schizophrenia spectrum, what are its outer boundaries? This question has become more important in recent years because of claims by some researchers, mostly in Europe, that many people have auditory hallucinations or other psychic experiences similar to the symptoms experienced by individuals with schizophrenia. Community surveys have been carried out using questionnaires that ask such things as: "Have you ever had a feeling that something strange and unexplainable was going on that other people would find hard to believe?" and "Have you ever seen visions or heard voices that others could not see or hear?" Some surveys have reported that as many as 18 percent of people in European countries have had such experiences, although a recently published review of thirty-five such studies reported a median prevalence of psychotic-like experiences of only 5 percent.

The fact that individuals other than those with schizophrenia report having had psychotic-like experiences is well known. Approximately half of individuals with bipolar disorder and one-quarter of individuals with severe depression may have major psychotic symptoms. Individuals with severe anxiety, post-traumatic stress disorder, and less severe forms of depression may also report experiencing minor psychotic symptoms. There are also problems with the community surveys, since the questionnaire most commonly used, the Composite International Diagnostic Interview (CIDI), is known to be unreliable in detecting psychotic symptoms. Then there is the issue of cultural expectations: in some cultures, you would be regarded as abnormal if you did *not* hear the voice of your mother giving you advice. In a cross-national survey, the percentage of people who reported having had visual or auditory hallucinations was 32 percent in Nepal, 14 percent in Brazil, and 12 percent in India, but less than 1 percent in China, Spain, and Pakistan. Also problematic is the fact that most surveys make no distinction between the occasional voice of your dead mother and a voice shouting unpleasant things at you hour after hour, day after day, such as many people with schizophrenia experience.

Predictably, this research has been picked up by individuals with schizophrenia who would like to deny that schizophrenia exists and who claim to be normal. As described in Chapter 8, there are now organized Hearing Voices Networks in Europe that celebrate it. Hearing voices, some say, "should not be thought of as a pathological phenomenon in need of eradication but as a meaningful, interpretable *experience*, intimately linked to the hearer's life story." All of this would seem harmless enough, except that such thinking is spilling over into official diagnostic thinking. Those doing the current revisions of *DSM-V* even considered adding a category called the Attenuated Psychosis Syndrome to include some of these people, but then decided not to do so. Most psychiatrists opposed adding such a syndrome, but the pharmaceutical industry was an enthusiastic backer, envisioning a much-expanded market for antipsychotic drugs.

In summary, schizophrenia is clearly part of a spectrum of disorders in which some people have the full-blown syndrome, while others, such as those diagnosed with schizotypal personality disorder, have lesser degrees of illness. It is also clear that many people in the general population occasionally experience hallucinations or other psychotic-like manifestations. However, there is no evidence that the latter is one end of the schizophrenia spectrum. Schizophrenia appears to be a categorical brain disease, not merely an extreme end of a phenomenological spectrum. There is no evidence that all of us have a little schizophrenia.

Schizoaffective Disorder and Bipolar Disorder

Among psychiatric researchers, the relationship of schizophrenia to schizoaffective disorder and bipolar disorder is just as controversial as the diagnostic entities discussed above.

The division of the psychoses into dementia praecox (now called schizophrenia) and manic-depressive illness was proposed by Emil Kraepelin in 1896 and has continued to be widely accepted in psychiatry. In 1980 the American Psychiatric Association under *DSM-III* proposed changing the name of manic-depressive psychosis to bipolar disorder, but the new term offers no significant advantages, and many of us have resisted giving up the older term.

Bipolar disorder is said to be more prevalent than schizophrenia but it is also over-diagnosed. It has a modest predilection for women over men and is thought to be disproportionately common in higher socioeconomic groups for unknown reasons. It usually begins before age thirty, but, unlike schizophrenia, later onsets are not unusual. Research on the causes of the disease is proceeding along the same lines as that for schizophrenia. A genetic predisposition is clearly established, with some researchers arguing that it is an inherited disease. Biochemical dysfunction in the brain of individuals with bipolar disorder is also established, with interest centered on serotonin and its metabolites rather than on dopamine. Most biological abnormalities found in schizophrenia (e.g., ventricular enlargement on MRI scans, neurological abnormalities) are also found in bipolar disorder, although they usually are not as marked.

The major clinical characteristic of bipolar disorder is episodes of mania, depression, or some combination thereof. Manic episodes consist of an elevated (or occasionally irritable) mood, during which time the person is excessively cheerful, talkative, sociable, expansive, grandiose, energetic, and hypersexual, and often needs little sleep. The person's speech may be rapid (pressured), with ideas thrown out faster than the listener can sort through them (flights of ideas). Grandiosity may proceed to a delusional state (e.g., belief that one is the president), dress may turn flamboyant, and behavior may become dangerous and inappropriate (e.g., buying sprees, foolish investments). Depressive episodes consist of a sad ("dysphoric") mood with hopelessness, poor appetite, sleep disturbances (either insomnia or excessive sleeping), loss of interest in usual activities, loss of sexual desire, loss of energy, slowed thinking, feelings of guilt or worthlessness, and often suicidal ideas. To qualify for these diagnoses under *DSM-V* diagnostic standards, a manic episode must last at least one week (or require hospitalization) and a depressive episode must last at least two weeks.

Although the public stereotype of bipolar disorder is a person who swings from one extreme to the other and back again, this is found only rarely. Some affected persons have a series of manic episodes, some have a series of depressive episodes, while others have the two in every conceivable combination. Many months or even years may separate episodes; between episodes the person is characteristically normal. There are, of course, all gradations of mood swings in either direction within the general population; some people have great energy and cheerfulness as part of their personality, others are chronically self-deprecating and depressed. A person who falls just short of being fully manic is referred to as hypomanic and is diagnosed as having bipolar II disorder. If a person has numerous mood swings that fail to meet the full criteria for bipolar disorder, the psychiatric diagnosis used is cyclothymic disorder. Approximately 15 percent of persons with bipolar disorder commit suicide.

In its classic form, then, bipolar disorder is easy to differentiate from schizophrenia; the predominant clinical symptoms involve disorders of *mood* rather than disorders of *thought*. Patients with bipolar disorder may have delusions or hallucinations, but when they occur they accompany and are congruent with the elevated or depressed mood. Most important, bipolar disorder occurs in discrete episodes with a return to normal functioning between episodes being the rule; schizophrenia rarely occurs in such discrete episodes and residual disability is the rule. Because of their recovery, it is common to find people with bipolar disorder holding important jobs in government, industry, and the entertainment field, and some traits of the hypomanic (e.g., high energy, inflated self-esteem, decreased need for sleep) lead to greater productivity and success in such fields.

Textbooks of psychiatry and psychology usually imply that patients with psychosis fall neatly into either the schizophrenia or the bipolar disorder and that the two can be readily distinguished. Unfortunately, that is not always the case, as a large percentage of patients have symptoms of both diseases. Furthermore, it is not rare to find patients whose symptoms change over time, appearing initially as a textbook case of schizophrenia or bipolar disorder, and a year or two later clearly exhibiting symptoms of the other disease. It has been facetiously suggested that either we need to insist that patients read the psychiatric textbooks and choose the disease they wish to have or we must become more flexible in our psychiatric thinking. I personally have seen patients with virtually every possible combination of symptoms of schizophrenia and bipolar disorder.

The resolution of the problem within the psychiatric establishment has been the creation of an intermediate disease category called *schizoaffective disorder*. Prior to *DSM-III* it was officially included as a subtype of schizophrenia. *DSM-III* classified it independently and noted that "at the present time there is no consensus on how this category should be defined." *DSM-IV* defined schizoaffective disorder as the occurrence of symptoms of major depression or mania concurrent with the symptoms of schizophrenia, but there must be at least a two-week period in which the symptoms of schizophrenia have been present without the depression or mania.

If this sounds like arguments among psychiatrists about how many angels can dance on the head of a pin, to a large extent it is. For patients and families, however, it is often confusing because they think that schizophrenia and schizoaffective disorder are different diagnoses. In fact, they are two aspects of a diagnostic spectrum. At a practical level the diagnosis of schizoaffective disorder implies statistically a somewhat better prognosis than classical schizophrenia, although this may not be true for any given patient. Other than that, the treatments of schizoaffective disorder and schizophrenia are virtually identical, with the same medication being used in both cases.

What, then, is the relationship of schizoaffective disorder and bipolar disorder to schizophrenia? In brief, the answer is not known. In recent years, suggestions have been made increasingly that perhaps Kraepelin was wrong, and that schizophrenia and bipolar disorder are two ends of a spectrum of a single disease rather than two separate diseases. Perhaps the specific symptoms (e.g., more schizophrenia-like or more bipolar-like) are determined by the person's underlying *genetic predisposition*, or *which specific areas of the brain* are predominantly affected in that person, or *when in the course of development* the initial brain damage took place.

One possibility that has received increasingly serious attention in recent years is that the important common denominator is psychotic symptoms. All individuals with schizophrenia have, by definition, psychotic symptoms (e.g., delusions, hallucinations). But only half of all individuals with bipolar disorder have psychotic symptoms. There is increasing evidence that individuals with bipolar disorder who have psychotic symptoms are closely related to individuals with schizophrenia and that their illness may even be part of the same disease category. This appears to be less true for individuals with bipolar disorder who do not have psychotic symptoms.

The following list summarizes ways in which schizophrenia and bipolar disorder are alike and ways in which they are different. As can be seen, the two disorders share many *antecedents,* including seasonality of birth and admissions, excess perinatal complications and developmental abnormalities, some MRI findings, some clinical symptoms, and response to antipsychotic medications. On the other hand, the two disorders differ significantly in their *expression,* especially on neuropsychological abnormalities, some MRI findings, prominence of affective symptoms, clinical course, and response to mood stabilizers such as lithium.

ARE SCHIZOPHRENIA AND BIPOLAR DISORDER ONE DISEASE OR TWO?

A. How are the two alike?

- both disorders have an excess of people affected who were born in the winter and spring
- both disorders have an excess of admissions and readmissions in the summer
- both disorders have an excess of perinatal complications and dermatoglyphic abnormalities, suggesting an *in utero* origin of some cases
- genes on similar chromosomes (e.g., 10, 13, 18, 22) are suspected of being involved in both disorders
- both disorders show increased developmental abnormalities in some individuals, including delayed motor and language milestones, educational problems

and neurological signs such as poorer coordination, although these are more marked in schizophrenia

- on MRI studies, both show enlarged cerebral ventricles and gray matter abnormalities, although these are generally more marked in schizophrenia
- both conditions may have prominent psychotic features such as delusions and hallucinations
- both conditions respond to antipsychotic medication

B. How are the two different?

- bipolar disorder is more prevalent in upper socioeconomic groups
- schizophrenia affects men earlier and more severely, whereas bipolar disorder has a slight predilection for women
- genetic factors are more prominent in bipolar disorder
- individuals with bipolar disorder are found more commonly in families with other members so diagnosed, and individuals with schizophrenia are found more commonly in families with other members so diagnosed, but exceptions to this rule are also found
- geographic, perhaps genetic clustering of cases is more prominent in bipolar disorder
- schizophrenia produces more marked and more generalized neuropsychological dysfunction, especially on tests of memory and frontal lobe function
- many people with bipolar disorder have achieved fame for their creativity in the arts
- on MRI, schizophrenia shows greater decrease in brain volume and specific decrease in medial temporal lobe structures (e.g., hippocampus), whereas bipolar disorder has more white matter hyperintensities
- although neurotransmitters are believed to be involved in both disorders, bipolar disorder is thought to involve serotonin more prominently and schizophrenia is thought to involve dopamine more prominently
- clinically, bipolar disorder is much more likely to have a relapsing and remitting course with periods of normality
- affective (mood) symptoms (e.g., depression, mania) are much more common in bipolar disorder
- bipolar disorder can be successfully treated by mood stabilizers (e.g., lithium), often with no other medication, but this is not true for schizophrenia
- ECT is more effective for bipolar disorder

Recommended Further Reading

Birur, B., N. V. Kraguljac, et al. "Brain Structure, Function, and Neurochemistry in Schizophrenia and Bipolar Disorder—a Systematic Review of the Magnetic Resonance Neuroimaging Literature." *NPJ Schizophrenia* 3 (2017). https://dx-doi-org.lrc1.usuhs.edu/10.1038%2Fs41537-017- 0013-9

Carpenter, W. T. Jr., D. W. Heinrichs, and A.M.I. Wagman. "Deficit and Nondeficit Forms of Schizophrenia: The Concept." *American Journal of Psychiatry* 145 (1988): 578–83.

Diagnostic and Statistical Manual of Mental Disorders: DSM-IV. 4th ed. Washington, D.C.: American Psychiatric Association, 1994.

Dickey, C. C., R. W. McCarley, M. M. Voglmaier, et al. "Schizotypal Personality Disorder and MRI Abnormalities of Temporal Lobe Gray Matter." *Biological Psychiatry* 45 (1999): 1393–1402.

Duke, P., and G. Hochman. *A Brilliant Madness: Living with Manic-Depressive Illness.* New York: Bantam Books, 1992.

Jamison, K. R. *An Unquiet Mind: A Memoir of Moods and Madness.* New York: Vintage Books, 1995.

Ketter, T. A., P. W. Wang, O. V. Becker, et al. "Psychotic Bipolar Disorders: Dimensionally Similar to or Categorically Different from Schizophrenia?" *Journal of Psychiatric Research* 38 (2004): 47–61.

Kirkpatrick, B., R. W. Buchanan, D. E. Ross, et al. "A Separate Disease within the Syndrome of Schizophrenia." *Archives of General Psychiatry* 58 (2001): 165–71.

Lieberman, J. A., T. S. Stroup, D. O. Perkins, eds. *Essentials of Schizophrenia.* Washington: American Psychiatric Publishing, 2012.

Slater, E., and M. Roth. *Clinical Psychiatry.* Baltimore: Williams and Wilkins, 1969. This is the best textbook description of schizophrenia by a wide margin.

Soares, J. C., and S. Gershon, eds. *Bipolar Disorders: Basic Mechanisms and Therapeutic Implications.* Vol. 15 of the series *Medical Psychiatry.* New York: Marcel Dekker, 2000.

Taylor, M. A. "Are Schizophrenia and Affective Disorder Related? A Selected Literature Review." *American Journal of Psychiatry* 149 (1992): 22–32.

Torrey, E. F., and M. B. Knable. "Are Schizophrenia and Bipolar Disorder One Disease or Two? Introduction to the Symposium." *Schizophrenia Research* 39 (1999): 93–94. The entire September 1999 issue of *Schizophrenia Research* (vol. 39, no. 2) is devoted to articles on this subject.

Torrey, E. F., and M. B. Knable. *Surviving Manic Depression: A Manual on Bipolar Disorder for Patients, Families and Providers.* New York: Basic Books, 2002.

Conditions Sometimes Confused with Schizophrenia

What consoles me is that I am beginning to consider madness as an illness like any other, and that I accept it as such.

Vincent van Gogh, 1889, in a letter to his brother, Theo

One way to understand a disease is to describe what it is, which was the task of the last chapter. The alternative is to describe what it is not. In the case of schizophrenia this is especially important to do, for in the past the term has been used broadly and imprecisely both in popular culture and in medicine. If we hope to move forward in our understanding of this disease, then we must first be clear what we are talking about.

A "Split Personality"

Schizophrenia is *not* a multiple or "split personality," although many people mistakenly believe that it is. A "split personality," as in *Sybil* or *The Three Faces of Eve,* is officially called a dissociative disorder. It is much less common than schizophrenia, occurs almost exclusively in women, and is thought in most cases to be a reaction to sexual or physical abuse in childhood.

In recent years, "dissociative disorder" has become a trendy diagnosis among a few psychiatrists and has been applied to individuals with a wide variety of symptoms. It has been greatly overdiagnosed, especially among people who are highly suggestible. A competent mental health professional should never confuse a dissociative disorder with schizophrenia.

Psychosis Caused by Street Drugs:
Can Marijuana Use Cause Schizophrenia?

It is a well-recognized fact that many drugs that are abused for their psychic effects may produce symptoms similar to schizophrenia. Even after ingesting a comparatively mild drug like marijuana, the user may experience strange bodily sensations, loss of body boundaries, and paranoid delusions. There is even a subgroup of people who give up using marijuana because it produces an unpleasant paranoid state after each usage. Stronger drugs, such as LSD and PCP, regularly produce hallucinations (although these are more likely to be visual than auditory), delusions, and disorders of thinking. Occasionally these symptoms become so severe that the person must be hospitalized, and if the history of drug abuse is not known, the person may be diagnosed with schizophrenia by mistake. Amphetamines (speed) in particular are well known for producing transient symptoms that may look identical to those of schizophrenia. Increasing numbers of such cases have been seen in recent years, as the methamphetamine ("crank") epidemic has spread in rural areas in America.

The question naturally arises whether drug abuse can *cause* schizophrenia. It is a question asked frequently by families and relatives of patients with this disease. There is now abundant evidence that chronic and repeated usage of many of the mind-altering drugs can damage the brain, impairing intellectual functions and memory, and exacerbate the symptoms of a person who already has schizophrenia.

Whether street drugs can cause schizophrenia, however, is unclear. In recent years, several European researchers have argued that marijuana can do so, looking to several studies that show an association between marijuana use and schizophrenia. A 2016 review of all the evidence by Gage et al. (see Recommended Further Reading) concluded that, although this association is consistently reported, "establishing causality from observational designs can be problematic." Skeptics point to the widespread marijuana use in the 1960s and argue that if marijuana use causes schizophrenia then the disease should be epidemic in California. Non-skeptics reply that the marijuana available today is up to five times stronger then what was available in the 1960s. The question of marijuana use and schizophrenia is especially relevant at this time as states move toward its legalization. What is clear is that marijuana use, especially heavy use, can precipitate schizophrenia earlier in individuals who are predisposed to getting it; thus those who use marijuana have an earlier age of onset. It is also clear that the use of marijuana by individuals with schizophrenia leads to a worse outcome.

Why, then, is it so common to see schizophrenia begin after a person has used mind-altering drugs? The answer is probably twofold. First, both drug abuse and the onset of schizophrenia occur in the same age range of the late teens and early twenties. The percentage of people in this age range who have at least smoked a few "joints" is very high. Assuming there is no connection whatsoever between drug abuse and schizophrenia, it would still be expected that a considerable number of people developing schizophrenia would also have tried mind-altering drugs.

Second, and more important, is the common sequence of people developing the early symptoms of schizophrenia and then turning to mind-altering drugs to provide a rationalization for what they are experiencing. Hearing voices for the first time in your life, for example, is a very frightening experience; if you then begin using hashish, PCP, or some similar drug, it provides you with a persuasive reason for hearing the voices. Drug use can put off the uncomfortable confrontation with yourself that tells you something is going wrong—very wrong—with your mind. You are, quite literally, losing it. Drugs, and alcohol as well, may also partially relieve the symptoms. In these cases persons can be said to be medicating themselves; this will be discussed in chapter 10.

The best study of the relationship of street drug use to the onset of schizophrenia was carried out by Drs. Hambrecht and Häfner in Germany. In examining 232 individuals who were experiencing their first episode of schizophrenia, they found that 14 percent had used street drugs, predominantly marijuana. Among those who had used street drugs, 27 percent had used drugs prior to any symptom of schizophrenia, 35 percent had started using street drugs in the same month in which their symptoms began, and 38 percent had not used street drugs until at least one month after the onset of their illness.

The families of persons who are developing schizophrenia are often not aware of the earliest symptoms of the disease. Not knowing what their relative is experiencing, all they see is him/her turning to increasingly heavy drug abuse. Three to six months later, the person is diagnosed with schizophrenia and the family immediately concludes that it was caused by the drug abuse. Such reasoning also relieves any burden of guilt on their part by making it clear that they had nothing to do with causing it. This may be especially attractive to relatives if they are faced with a mental health professional who implies that problems of child rearing or problems of family communication contributed to the genesis of the disease. In these cases, relatives will often seize on drug-abuse-causes-schizophrenia as a defense against the professional.

Ted was a promising college student who had his life well planned. Midway through his sophomore year he began having episodes of euphoria, strange bodily sensations, and ideas that he had been sent to save the world. His grades dropped sharply, he began going to church every day, and then began using LSD. Prior to that time he had used marijuana only occasionally at parties. His roommate, college authorities, and finally his parents became alarmed about his turn to drugs. Within one month he was admitted to the local hospital with symptoms of overt schizophrenia. His parents believe it was caused by his drug use and have never been persuaded otherwise.

Psychosis Caused by Prescription Drugs

Our society is a drug-using society; young adults abuse street drugs, while older adults use extraordinary numbers of prescription drugs. One only has to open a medicine cabinet in any American home to realize the number of prescription drugs available for ingestion.

Many of these drugs can cause psychiatric symptoms as side effects, ranging from confusion to depression to paranoid delusions or hallucinations. In the majority of cases the hallucinations will be exclusively visual, suggesting that the symptoms are due to drugs or other organic medical conditions. Occasionally the hallucinations may be auditory and the patient may appear to have a sudden onset of classical schizophrenia. For any first episode of psychosis, therefore, the physician should always ask the question: "What medications are you taking?"

Prescription drugs that cause symptoms of psychosis as a side effect almost always do so when they are first started. The psychotic symptoms will go away, sometimes immediately and in other cases more slowly, as soon as the drug is stopped. Many of these drugs cause such symptoms more commonly in elderly individuals and/or at higher doses. Medications that sometimes cause delusions or hallucinations and may therefore produce a clinical picture that could be confused with schizophrenia are listed on page 75. There are undoubtedly others, and just because a specific drug is not listed here does not mean that it cannot cause such symptoms. The interaction of two or more drugs can also produce such symptoms. This list is taken from the *Medical Letter* (volume 50, December 15, 2008) and lists drugs generically with a common trade name in parenthesis. Many of these drugs have additional trade names.

Psychosis Caused by Other Diseases

There are several diseases of the body that can produce symptoms similar to schizophrenia. In most cases there is no ambiguity because the disease is clearly diagnosable; in a few cases, however, there may be some confusion, especially in the early stages of the disease.

MEDICATIONS THAT SOMETIMES CAUSE DELUSIONS OR HALLUCINATIONS

abacavir *(Ziagen)*

acyclovir *(Zovirax)*

amantadine *(Symmetrel)*

azithromycin *(Zithromax)*

baclofen *(Kemstro)*

bupropion *(Wellbutrin)*

caffeine

chlorambucil *(Leukeran)*

chloroquine *(Aralen)*

clonidine *(Catapres)*

cyclobenzaprine *(Flexeril)*

cycloserine *(Seromycin)*

dapsone

DEET *(Off)*

dextromethorphan *(Robitussin)*

digoxin *(Lanoxin)*

disopyramide *(Norpace)*

disulfiram *(Antabuse)*

dronabinol *(Marinol)*

efavirenz *(Sustiva)*

ganciclovir *(Cytovene)*

ifosfamide *(Ifex)*

interleukin-2 *(Proleukin)*

isoniazid

levodopa *(Sinemet)*

lidocaine *(Xylocaine)*

mefloquine *(Lariam)*

methyldopa

methylphenidate *(Ritalin)*

metronidazole *(Flagyl)*

monafinil *(Provigil)*

nevirapine *(Viramune)*

oseltamivir *(Tamiflu)*

propafenone *(Rythmol)*

pseudoephedrine *(Sudafed)*

quinidine

ramelteon *(Rozerem)*

selegiline *(Eldepryl)*

sibutramine *(Meridia)*

sildenafil *(Viagra)*

sodium oxybate *(Xyrem)*

tizanidine *(Zanaflex)*

trazodone

trimethoprim, sulfamethoxazole *(Bactrim)*

valganciclovir *(Valcyte)*

vincristine

voriconazole *(Vfend)*

zolpidem *(Ambien)*

There is considerable dispute about how often other diseases mimic schizophrenia and go undetected. In a widely quoted study, Hall and his associates in Texas examined 38 hospitalized patients with schizophrenia and found that 9 percent of them had a medical illness that "caused or exacerbated" the schizophrenia. On the other hand, Koran and his colleagues in California thoroughly studied 269 patients with schizophrenia and found only one patient whose disease (temporal lobe epilepsy) had been missed and was apparently causing the schizophrenia-like symptoms. One English study of 318 hospital admissions with a diagnosis of schizophrenia found 8 percent "with antecedent organic cerebral disorders." Another English study of 268 first admissions with schizophrenia found fewer than 6 percent with relevant organic disease findings. A postmortem study of 200 patients with schizophrenia "found organic cerebral disease thought to be causally related in 11 percent." What is clear is that there is a small subgroup of patients with schizophrenia who have other medical diseases that are causing their symptoms, and that some of these other diseases are treatable.

The most important diseases that may produce symptoms of schizophrenia are as follows:

Brain Tumors: Tumors of the pituitary gland are especially likely to cause symptoms of schizophrenia, but other tumors (e.g., a meningioma of the temporal lobe) may also do so. These are usually detectable on MRI scan and often curable by surgery in their early stages.

Viral Encephalitis: It has been known for many years that viral encephalitis can produce schizophrenia-like symptoms following the encephalitis. What is becoming increasingly clear is that encephalitis occasionally mimics schizophrenia in the early stages of illness, before other signs and symptoms of encephalitis become apparent; how often this occurs is unknown. A review of twenty-two such cases identified a variety of viruses as capable of doing this, including herpes simplex, Epstein-Barr virus, cytomegalovirus, measles, coxsackie, and equine encephalitis. If suspected, most such cases can be diagnosed by lumbar puncture and EEG. It is likely that viral encephalitis also causes many cases of brief psychotic disorders, schizophrenia-like syndromes that last for only a few days. Additional discussion regarding the possible relationship of viruses to schizophrenia can be found in chapter 5.

Temporal Lobe Epilepsy: The relationship between epilepsy and schizophrenia has been a controversial issue for many years. There have been reports that epilepsy and schizophrenia share some predisposing genes, and also that the incidence of schizophrenia is elevated among individuals with epilepsy and vice versa. There is agreement, however, that one type of epilepsy—that of the temporal lobe—frequently produces symptoms like schizophrenia. One study found that 17 percent of patients with temporal lobe epilepsy had some symptoms of schizophrenia.

Cerebral Syphilis: Although not seen so much as in the past, syphilis should never be forgotten as a possible cause of schizophrenia-like symptoms. In 2004 three such cases were admitted to a single state psychiatric hospital. A routine blood test will alert one to its possibility, and a lumbar puncture will confirm the diagnosis.

Multiple Sclerosis: Depression and intellectual deterioration are commonly found in the early stages of multiple sclerosis. Occasionally symptoms of schizophrenia may also occur, with one report of a woman who had symptoms of "paranoid schizophrenia" for ten years before her multiple sclerosis became fully manifest.

Huntington's Disease: Schizophrenia is said to be "a common initial diagnosis" and "the most frequent persisting mis-diagnosis" in Huntington's disease, a genetic disease beginning in midlife. Once choreiform movements begin in the patient, the correct diagnosis becomes clear.

AIDS: This is the newest addition to the list of diseases that may present with symptoms resembling schizophrenia. It has been clearly established that AIDS may occasionally manifest itself with symptoms of either schizophrenia or bipolar disorder because of the effect of the human immunodeficiency virus (HIV) on the brain. A test for HIV should be included in all routine first admission diagnostic workups for serious mental illness.

Other Diseases: A large number of other diseases have been recorded as occasionally presenting with symptoms similar to schizophrenia. They include those listed in the table on page 78.

For those interested in diseases that may mimic schizophrenia, see the publications by Coleman and Gillberg, Davison, and Lishman listed at the end of this chapter.

Wilson's disease	progressive supranuclear palsy
acute intermittent porphyria	aqueductal stenosis
metachromatic leukodystrophy	normal pressure hydrocephalus
lupus erythematosus	cerebral vascular accident (stroke)
congenital calcification of basal ganglia	narcolepsy
adrenal disease	thyroid disease
hepatic encephalopathy	insecticide poisoning (e.g., organophosphorus compounds)
pellagra	leptospirosis
sarcoidosis	tropical infections (e.g., trypanosomiasis, cerebral malaria)
pernicious anemia	
metal poisoning (e.g., lead, mercury)	

Psychosis Caused by Head Trauma

Whether or not head injuries can cause psychosis has been hotly debated for more than two hundred years. In 1800 James Hadfield, who was psychotic and had shot at King George in a failed assassination attempt, was acquitted as insane because he had suffered a severe head injury six years previously. The jury was invited to look at the outer covering of Hadfield's brain, still visible through a hole in his skull.

Major changes in personality, including the onset of psychosis, were clearly documented in studies of penetrating head injuries during the Franco-Prussian and the Russo-Finnish wars. Still unresolved, however, is how often head trauma causes psychosis, how severe the trauma must be, what parts of the brain are affected, and how long the period can be between the trauma and the onset of psychosis.

There is some evidence that severe head injuries may contribute to the onset of schizophrenia in some individuals. As a general rule, however, it is extremely unlikely that head trauma could cause psychosis unless the person had been unconscious for at least several hours following the trauma. In addition, most injuries that are likely to produce psychosis will involve the frontal and especially the temporal lobes. An MRI study of three individuals with a schizophrenia-like psychosis reported that all three had abnormalities in the left temporal lobe.

The main problem arises in trying to assess whether the head trauma is related to the onset of the psychosis. Head trauma and schizophrenia are both more common in young adults and so will occur coincidentally from time to time. Most young adults can recall some instance of head trauma, and associating the trauma with the schizophrenia has an appeal to relatives who may be looking for an explanation for the sickness. Further complicating this assessment is the fact that individuals developing early symptoms of schizophrenia may do irrational things that produce head trauma; the family may not have been aware of the early symptoms and so may associate the onset of the schizophrenia with the trauma. Finally there is the confounding issue of whether the trauma produces the psychosis by direct injury to the brain or by acting as a severe stressor, the straw that broke the camel's back.

Psychosis with Mental Retardation

Mental retardation is an impairment of cognitive functions measured by the intelligence quotient (IQ). Depending on the person's IQ, mental retardation is divided into mild (50 to 70), moderate (35 to 49), severe (20 to 34), and profound (below 20). It may be caused by chromosomal abnormalities (e.g., Down's syndrome), metabolic diseases (e.g., phenylketonuria), or brain damage from any cause either prior to or after birth. Most individuals with schizophrenia show a mild loss of IQ as measured by their impaired functioning on tests of cognitive skills; their innate IQ is not necessarily impaired, but their ability to demonstrate their IQ is impaired (see chapter 12).

Occasional individuals may have both schizophrenia and mental retardation. Each may arise independently, with the combination merely occurring by chance, or both may be related to a common cause of brain damage. When this occurs it is virtually impossible to get adequate care for the person because treatment facilities are organized for people with either mental illness or mental retardation. In most states such individuals are passed back and forth from one agency to another, each agency disclaiming ultimate responsibility, with the individual made to feel like a leper's leper. Families of such individuals often achieve heroic heights providing services at home with little or no assistance from mental health officials.

The best-known example of co-occurring mental retardation and psychosis was Rosemary Kennedy, sister to John, Robert, and Edward Kennedy. She was mildly retarded in childhood, eventually reaching a fifth-grade level of achievement. At age twenty-one, however, she had the onset of a schizophrenia-like psychosis that alarmed her family. Since antipsychotic medications were not yet available in 1941, she was given a surgical lobotomy. The results of the lobotomy were a disaster, causing severe retardation and brain damage, and she was confined to a private nursing convent until her death.

Infantile Autism

Infantile autism, a brain disease of infancy, appears to be unrelated to schizophrenia. This syndrome, beginning within the child's first two and a half years, is characterized by severe social withdrawal (e.g., the child resists being held or touched), retarded language development, abnormal responses to sensory stimuli (e.g., sounds may overwhelm the child), and a fascination with inanimate objects (e.g., a faucet, the child's own shadow) or repetitive routines (e.g., spinning). It occurs in approximately 4 children per 10,000 and thus is one-twentieth as common as schizophrenia. At one time it was said that autism was more common in higher socioeconomic groups, but that has been disproved. It occurs four times more often in males than in females. Recent studies suggest that autism may be increasing in incidence in the United States.

Autism is almost certainly a collection of diseases rather than a single disease. Rett's disorder is a milder form, occurring only in girls. Asperger's disorder is another milder form in which there is normal language development. Autism-like behavior may also be observed in children with the fragile X syndrome, phenylketonuria, viral encephalitis, and other diseases. Epilepsy commonly accompanies autism; approximately one-half of children with autism may have some degree of mental retardation; and a higher than expected percentage of children with autism also have blindness or deafness.

The evidence that autism, like schizophrenia, has biological causes has become overwhelming in recent years; older psychogenic theories such as Kanner's "refrigerator mother" now are completely discredited. There definitely appears to be a genetic component to autism: neuropathological abnormalities occur in the brains of these children, especially in the cerebellum. MRI abnormalities have been found in some studies but not in others. Abnormalities in endocrine function and blood chemistry have also been found. One of the most interesting findings that may relate to the causes of autism is that mothers who give birth to children with autism report having had an unusually high frequency of bleeding during pregnancy, compared with controls. In the past some people have claimed that childhood vaccines cause autism, but this has now been disproven.

A variety of medications have been used to treat autism but so far with only modest success. Specialized training appears to produce some improvement in behavior. As the children get older, a small percentage improve and function well. An example of the latter is Temple Grandin, who earned a doctorate and is an assistant professor in the Department of Animal Science at Colorado State University; she documented her illness in her book *Thinking in Pictures*. The majority, however, take on the characteristics of adult schizophrenia with an emphasis on "negative" symptoms (e.g., withdrawal, flattened emotions, poverty of thoughts) rather than "positive" symptoms (e.g., delusions, hallucinations).

Differentiation of infantile autism from childhood schizophrenia is in most cases not difficult. Autism almost always begins before age two and a half, while schizophrenia is rare before five and uncommon before age ten. The child with autism will have prominent withdrawal, language retardation, and repetitive routines, while the child with schizophrenia will have delusions, hallucinations, and thinking disorders. Half the children with autism will be retarded, but far fewer of the children with schizophrenia will be. Finally, children with schizophrenia may have a family history of schizophrenia, but children with autism almost never have such a family history.

Antisocial Personality Disorders and Sexual Predators

There really should not be confusion between antisocial personality disorders, sexual predators, and schizophrenia, but because of court decisions, there is. Individuals with antisocial personality disorder have a pervasive disregard for other individuals, as demonstrated by lying, cheating, breaking laws, injuring others, and feeling no remorse for their actions. They are also referred to as sociopaths, psychopaths, and common criminals. A subset of individuals with antisocial personality disorders also have sexual problems, leading them to rape or to prey on children (pedophilia). They are usually called sexually violent predators, or SVPs.

In 1994 the state of Kansas passed a law allowing the indefinite incarceration of sexually violent predators in public psychiatric hospitals. This law was upheld by the U.S. Supreme Court in 1997 and is usually referred to as the Hendricks decision. In the past, sexually violent predators were handled in the criminal justice system and sentenced to prison, but now they are being sentenced to psychiatric hospitals. At the same time, as described in chapter 14, many individuals with schizophrenia who have been discharged from psychiatric hospitals but who are not receiving treatment may commit crimes as a consequence of their illness and are sentenced to prison. This turnabout of putting prisoners into psychiatric hospitals and psychiatric patients into prisons has led many people to conclude that the psychiatric care system is more thought-disordered than most of the patients.

There is no relationship among antisocial personality disorder, sexually violent predators, and schizophrenia. And a study reported that the incidence of antisocial personality disorder among the relatives of individuals with schizophrenia was no higher than among the general population. Whether or not individuals with antisocial personality disorder and sexually violent predators have damage to their brains remains to be demonstrated; if they do, it will almost certainly be different from the damage that occurs in schizophrenia.

Culturally Sanctioned Psychotic Behavior

Occasionally confusion will arise between schizophrenia and culturally induced or hysterical psychosis. This is an altered state of consciousness usually entered into voluntarily by an individual; while in this altered state of consciousness the person may exhibit symptoms that superficially look like schizophrenia. For example, the person may complain of altered bodily sensations and hallucinations and may behave in an excited and irrational manner. In the United States these conditions are seen most commonly in connection with fundamentalist religious services. In other cultural groups and in other countries, these conditions are known by such names as moth craziness (Navajo Indians), windigo (Cree and Ojibwa Indians), zar (Middle East), koro (China), susto (Latin America), latah (Southeast Asia), and amok (worldwide):

> Cecelia led a perfectly normal life except for the monthly all-night worship service at her fundamentalist church. During the service she claimed to hear voices talking to her, often spoke in tongues, and occasionally behaved in a wild and irrational way so that others had to restrain her. Other members of the congregation regarded her with both fear and awe, suspecting that she was possessed by spirits.

People like Cecelia should not be labeled as having schizophrenia unless there are other symptoms of the disease. Occasionally persons who have schizophrenia will be attracted to fundamentalist religious groups or religious cults, however, since such groups often value hearing voices or "speaking in tongues."

Recommended Further Reading

Achté, K. A., E. Hillbom, and V. Aalberg. "Psychoses Following War Brain Injuries." *Acta Psychiatrica Scandinavica* 45 (1969): 1–18.

Clarke, M. C., A. Tanskanen, M. O. Huttunen, et al. "Evidence for Shared Susceptibility to Epilepsy and Psychosis: A Population-Based Family Study." *Biological Psychiatry* 71 (2012): 836–39.

Coleman, M., and C. Gillberg. *The Biology of the Autistic Syndromes.* New York: Praeger, 1985.

Coleman, M., and C. Gillberg. *The Schizophrenias: A Biological Approach to the Schizophrenia Spectrum Disorders.* New York: Springer, 1996.

David, A. S., and M. Prince, "Psychosis Following Head Injury: A Critical Review." *Journal of Neurology, Neurosurgery, and Psychiatry* 76 (2005): 53–60.

Davison, K. "Schizophrenia-like Psychoses Associated with Organic Cerebral Disorders: A Review." *Psychiatric Developments* 1 (1983): 1–34. An earlier version of the article, widely referenced, was published by Davison and C. R. Bagley as "Schizophrenia-like Psychoses Associated with Organic Disorders of the Central Nervous System" in *Current Problems in Neuropsychiatry,* edited by R. N. Herrington. Ashford, England: Headley Brothers, 1969.

De Hert, M., M. Wampers, T. Jendricko, et al. "Effects of Cannabis Use on Age at Onset in Schizophrenia and Bipolar Disorder." *Schizophrenia Research* 126 (2011): 270–76.

Gage, S. H., M. Hickman, and S. Zammit, "Association Between Cannabis and Psychosis: Epidemiologic Evidence." *Biological Psychiatry* 79 (2016): 549-556.

Grandin, T. *Thinking in Pictures.* New York: Vintage Books, 1996.

Hambrecht, M., and H. Häfner. "Substance Abuse and the Onset of Schizophrenia." *Biological Psychiatry* 40 (1996): 1155–63.

Lishman, W. A. *Organic Psychiatry: The Psychological Consequences of Cerebral Disorder.* Oxford: Blackwell Science, 1998.

McGrath, J., J. Welham, J. Scott, et al. "Association Between Cannabis Use and Psychosis-Related Outcomes Using Sibling Pair Analysis in a Cohort of Young Adults." *Archives of General Psychiatry* 67 (2010): 440–47.

Molloy, C., R. M. Conroy, D. R. Cotter, et al. "Is Traumatic Brain Injury a Risk Factor for Schizophrenia? A Meta-Analysis of Case-controlled Population-based Studies." *Schizophrenia Bulletin* 37 (2011): 1104–10.

Torrey, E. F. "Functional Psychoses and Viral Encephalitis." *Integrative Psychiatry* 4 (1986): 224–36.

4

Onset, Course, and Prognosis

Such a disease, which disorders the senses, perverts the reason and breaks up the passions in wild confusion—which assails man in his essential nature—brings down so much misery on the head of its victims, and is productive of so much social evil—deserves investigation on its own merits, by statistical as well as other methods. . . . We may discover the causes of insanity, the laws which regulate its course, the circumstances by which it is influenced, and either avert its visitations, or mitigate their severity; perhaps in a later age, save mankind from its inflictions, or if this cannot be, at any rate ensure the sufferers early treatment.

Dr. William Farr, 1841

When diagnosed with schizophrenia for the first time, the person and his/her family have many questions. Were there predictors of the illness in childhood? Did they miss the earliest symptoms? What are the chances for complete recovery? How independent is the person likely to be ten years later, or thirty years later? What are the chances of the person spending much of his or her life in a psychiatric hospital or group home? These are important questions, for the answers to them will determine how the person with schizophrenia and his/her family plan for the future.

Childhood Precursors

The idea that the earliest manifestations of schizophrenia begin in childhood is not a new one. John Hawkes, a prominent English physician, noted in 1857 that "it is only too probable that, from a much earlier period than the actual manifestation of disease, the fuel has been laid." Similarly, Emil Kraepelin observed in 1919 that "in a considerable number of cases definite *psychic peculiarities* have come under observation in our patients from childhood up."

Formal studies of childhood precursors of schizophrenia date to the 1930s. Within recent decades, however, there has been an outpouring of information on this subject. Many of the best studies have included large groups of children born at a particular time who were intensively studied and tested as children. Many of these children have now reached the age of risk for schizophrenia and so it is possible to examine the childhood records and compare the records of those who do and those who do not have the disease. The largest such birth cohort included 55,000 children born in the United States between 1959 and 1966 (the National Collaborative Perinatal Project), but smaller birth cohorts have been similarly studied in England, Sweden, Finland, Denmark, New Zealand and Israel.

What these studies show is that there is a subset of children, approximately one-quarter or one-third of those who later develop schizophrenia, who are different as children. These differences include:

1. Delayed developmental milestones in infancy (e.g., slower to walk and talk)
2. More language and speech problems
3. Poorer coordination (e.g., not as good at sports, lower grades in physical education)
4. Poorer academic achievement
5. Poorer social functioning and fewer friends

It should be emphasized that these childhood precursors are merely *statistical associations* and *not predictors for individual cases*. The majority of individuals who develop schizophrenia are not different in childhood, and in fact one study in Finland even found that a disproportionate number of the children who developed schizophrenia had done especially well in school. Conversely, most children who have delayed milestones; language and speech problems; and poor coordination, grades, and social skills will not develop schizophrenia.

Childhood precursors of schizophrenia have also been studied in the offspring of mothers who have schizophrenia (these are so-called "high risk" studies, because it is known that approximately 13 percent of the children will later develop schizophrenia) and among identical twins. In a twin study carried out by the author, for example, among 27 identical twin pairs in which one had schizophrenia and the other twin was well, 7 of the twins who later developed schizophrenia were clearly different from the well twin by age five. Among one pair, for example, both twins could tie their shoes at age four, but a year later one of them had lost that ability and had also developed an odd gait. Although nothing was found on examination at that time, it was that twin who developed schizophrenia at age twenty-six.

Onset and Early Symptoms

One of the questions most frequently asked by families is how to identify the early symptoms of schizophrenia. This question is different from that of relapse of the disease, which is discussed in chapter 11. The question is asked by families who are raising difficult teenage children and are wondering if the children might be developing schizophrenia. It is also asked by families in which an older child has been diagnosed with schizophrenia and the parents are worried about the younger children.

When you are thinking about the early symptoms of schizophrenia, it is helpful to remember that this disease has a strikingly narrow age of onset. In the United States, three-quarters of those who get schizophrenia do so between ages seventeen and twenty-five. Having an initial onset before age fourteen or after age thirty is unusual. There is some evidence that the age of onset now is earlier than it was fifty or a hundred years ago.

Why the onset of schizophrenia occurs in this particular age group is unknown. It should be pointed out, however, that other chronic brain diseases, such as multiple sclerosis and Alzheimer's disease, have particular age ranges of onset, and we do not understand the reasons in these diseases either. There are also suggestions that the average age of onset of schizophrenia may be younger in the United States than it is in Europe, that the age of onset for paranoid schizophrenia is older than for the other subtypes, and that the average age of onset in the United States is younger now than it was in the nineteenth century. Especially interesting was a study showing that the onset of schizophrenia occurs earlier in countries closer to the equator, with a ten-year difference in average age of onset between countries closest (e.g., Colombia) and farthest (e.g., Russia) from the equator.

There are some individuals for whom it is impossible to date the onset of the disease. As noted above, the family says things such as: "She was always different from the other children" or "Throughout childhood his teachers noticed he was eccentric and told us to get him evaluated." The suggestion in such cases is that the disease process began early in life despite the fact that the full-blown thinking disorder, delusions, and hallucinations did not begin until the late teens or early twenties.

This raises the question of when families with an eccentric child should worry. It is known that the majority of individuals who develop schizophrenia have normal childhoods and are not identifiable in their early years. And it is also known that the vast majority of eccentric children will not develop schizophrenia; many, in fact, grow up to be leaders. The problem of separating the eccentricities of normal childhood from the early symptoms of schizophrenia is especially difficult in adolescence, approximately ages eleven to thirteen, when the norms of behavior are very strange indeed. Overacuteness of the senses is a common symptom of schizophrenia, yet how many adolescents have not had some such experiences? Moodiness, withdrawal, apathy, loss of interest in personal appearance, perplexity, the belief that people are watching one, preoccupation with one's body, and vagueness in thoughts may all be harbingers of impending schizophrenia, but they may also be just normal manifestations of early adulthood and its accompanying problems. For this reason families should *not* worry about every quirk in their children but rather should assume they are normal until proven otherwise. This can be particularly difficult for a parent who has already had one child diagnosed with schizophrenia and who is expecting the worst for the younger children, but it is important. A fifteen-year-old has enough to worry about without being told things like "Don't daydream. That's what your brother did and it got him sick and into the hospital."

At what point *should* parents begin to worry that something may be wrong? When do the normal psychological vicissitudes of early adulthood cross the line and enter the realm of early symptoms of schizophrenia? Researchers in Germany and Canada questioned large numbers of individuals in the first stages of schizophrenia and their families to ascertain the earliest symptoms. The results, together with those from other researchers and my own clinical experience, are summarized in the box below. The most important word in this summary is "changes"—in social behavior, sleep or eating patterns, self-care, school performance, or emotional relationships. Parents may say things such as: "John has become a different person over the last six months" or "None of Jennifer's friends come around anymore, and she doesn't seem to want to see anyone." Such changes may of course be caused by

---

THE MOST COMMON EARLY SYMPTOMS OF SCHIZOPHRENIA
AS OBSERVED BY THE FAMILY

- depression
- changes in social behavior, especially withdrawal
- changes in sleep or eating patterns
- suspiciousness or feelings that people are talking about him/her
- changes in pattern of self-care
- changes in school performance
- marked weakness, lack of energy
- headaches or strange sensations in head
- changes in emotional relationships with family or close friends
- confused, strange, or bizarre thinking

things other than schizophrenia; the use of street drugs must always be considered as a possibility in this age group.

It should be emphasized that this list of early symptoms are those observed by the family. The individual who is in the early stages of schizophrenia may be experiencing things that are not visible to their family members, including anxiety, restlessness, difficulty in concentration, and decreased self-confidence. They may also be hearing voices (auditory hallucinations) for weeks or months before family members become aware of it.

Childhood Schizophrenia

It is generally believed that childhood schizophrenia is simply an early version of the adult disease, although much rarer. Approximately two males are affected for every female. Only about 2 percent of individuals with schizophrenia have the onset of their disease in childhood, although that percentage varies depending on where one fixes the childhood-adult line. Schizophrenia beginning before age five is exceedingly rare (see section on infantile autism, chapter 3), and between ages five and ten it increases slowly. From age ten, schizophrenia increases in incidence until age fifteen, when it begins its sharp upward peak as the adult disease.

The symptoms of childhood schizophrenia are very similar to those of adult schizophrenia with the predictable exception that their content is age-related. For example, one study of young children with schizophrenia reported that the source of auditory hallucinations was frequently believed to be pet animals or toys and that "monster themes were common. . . . As age increased, both hallucinations and delusions tended to be more complex and elaborate." The other distinguishing feature of childhood schizophrenia is that the affected child also often has one or more of the following: seizures, learning disabilities, mild mental retardation, neurological symptoms, hyperactivity, or other behavioral problems. In an attempt to resolve this confusion the American Psychiatric Association deleted "childhood schizophrenia" from its official nomenclature and suggested instead using schizophrenia with onset in childhood or "childhood-onset pervasive developmental disorder," a catchall term for many poorly defined brain disorders of childhood.

Like adult schizophrenia, childhood schizophrenia is thought to have genetic antecedents, and many researchers believe that these antecedents are more important than in adult-onset schizophrenia. It is also known that these children have an excess number of minor physical anomalies and mothers' history of having had excess pregnancy and birth complications. The fact that childhood schizophrenia is a brain disease has been demonstrated by findings of MRI and EEG abnormalities. Recent MRI studies have shown that individuals with childhood-onset schizophrenia have brain changes related to their disease during adolescence, including a progressive loss of brain volume in general and of gray matter in particular.

Childhood schizophrenia is treated with the same antipsychotic medication used for adult schizophrenia. A follow-up of ten children with this disease from fourteen to thirty-four years after its onset found them still diagnosed with schizophrenia but with relatively few delusions or hallucinations. Instead they tended to be quiet and withdrawn, with poverty of thought and lack of drive. A minority of children with schizophrenia will recover and do quite well as adults, but what percentage this constitutes is uncertain. In general it is thought that the earlier the age of onset of schizophrenia, the worse the outcome is likely to be, but there are major exceptions to this rule. A fictional description of the onset of schizophrenia in a twelve-year-old boy was written by Conrad Aiken in "Silent Snow, Secret Snow" (see chapter 13). Another brief fictional account is Vladimir Nabokov's short story "Signs and Symbols," a literary gem. Louise Wilson, in *This Stranger, My Son*, provides a good account of what it is like to live with a child with this illness.

Postpartum Schizophrenia

Some degree of depression in mothers following childbirth is relatively common and on occasion may be severe. Much less common, occurring approximately once in every thousand births, are symptoms of psychosis that develop in the mother. These usually begin between three and seven days postpartum and may include delusions (e.g., the mother believes her baby is defective or has been kidnapped) or hallucinations (the mother hears voices telling her to kill the baby). Because of the unpredictability of such patients, the baby is usually separated from the mother until she improves.

The vast majority of such cases of postpartum psychosis are eventually diagnosed with bipolar disorder or major depression with psychotic features. A minority will be diagnosed as having schizophrenia. In a large study in Denmark, 9 percent of the women with postpartum psychosis were diagnosed with schizophrenia. These women had a poor prognosis; 50 percent were rehospitalized within one year of their initial illness, and 98 percent had relapsed within ten years.

It is likely in such cases that the childbirth precipitated schizophrenia that would have developed sooner or later. Childbirth is accompanied by massive hormonal changes, and it is known that some women with schizophrenia are especially sensitive to hormonal fluctuations and become more symptomatic just prior to their menstrual period.

Late-Onset Schizophrenia

Just as there is a form of schizophrenia that begins early in childhood, so there is also a form that begins later in life. Late-onset schizophrenia is variously defined as beginning after the age of forty or forty-five. Its precise incidence is unclear, but it is not rare. Many studies of it have been done by Europeans, with less interest having been shown by American researchers. That fact is especially pertinent since the mean age of onset of schizophrenia in general is almost invariably reported as being older in European studies compared to American studies. It seems possible, therefore, that late-onset schizophrenia is of more interest to European researchers because it occurs more commonly there for reasons that are unknown.

Clinically, late-onset schizophrenia is similar to the earlier onset variety except for having a predominance of females affected; having more schizoid and paranoid personality traits in the person before he/she becomes sick; having more paranoid delusions and more visual, tactile, and olfactory (smell) hallucinations; and having fewer "negative" symptoms or thinking disorders. Neuropsychological tests and MRI scans show deficits similar to other forms of schizophrenia. One study that followed up individuals with late-onset schizophrenia found that in one-third of the cases the schizophrenia progressed to an Alzheimer-type dementia.

Predictors of Outcome

Over the years it has been noted that some persons afflicted with schizophrenia recover completely, others recover partially, and some do not recover at all. This observation has led many professionals to review the clinical data taken at the time of the original hospital admission to determine which factors might have predicted a good outcome and which might have predicted a poor outcome. The result of these efforts has been a series of predictive factors, each of which taken by itself has limited usefulness but which taken together may be very useful. From this a subtyping of schizophrenia into good outcome (good prognosis) and poor outcome (poor prognosis) has emerged and is becoming widely used. It is probably the most valid way to classify the disease that has been found to date.

Patients who are more likely to have a good outcome are those who were considered to be relatively normal prior to getting sick. Thus, if as children they were able to make friends with others, did not have major problems with delinquency, and achieved success levels in school reasonable for their intelligence level, their outcome is more likely to be good. Conversely, if they are described by relatives as "always a strange child," had major problems in school or with their peers, were considered delinquent, or were very withdrawn, they are more likely to fall into the poor outcome group.

It has now been clearly established that women with schizophrenia have a more favorable outcome than men. Patients with the best outcome also have no history of relatives with schizophrenia. The more close relatives who have schizophrenia, the poorer the outcome becomes. If there is a history of depression or bipolar disorder in the family, the person is more likely to have a good outcome. Thus, a good outcome is suggested by a family history with no mental disease or only depression and/or bipolar disorder. A poor outcome is suggested by a family history of schizophrenia.

In general, the younger the age at which schizophrenia develops, the poorer the outcome. A person who is first diagnosed with schizophrenia at age fifteen is likely to have a poorer outcome than a person with the onset at age twenty-five. Persons who are first diagnosed with schizophrenia in older age groups, especially over age thirty, are more likely to fall into the good outcome group.

The type of onset is an important predictor of recovery, with the best outcomes occurring in those patients whose onset is the most sudden. A relative who describes the gradual onset of the person's symptoms over a period of many months is painting a bleak picture, for it is much more likely that the person will fall into the poor outcome group. Conversely, as a practicing psychiatrist I am very happy when a relative tells me that, "John was completely normal up until about a month ago," for I know that such a history bodes well for the future. Awareness of one's illness (insight) is a very good sign, whereas lack of awareness (anosognosia) is a bad sign.

The clinical symptoms that are more compatible with a good outcome are predominantly "positive" symptoms, especially delusions and catatonic behavior. Conversely, predominantly "negative" symptoms, such as withdrawal, apathy, and poverty of thoughts are bad. The presence of normal emotions is good, whereas flattening of emotions is bad. Obsessive and compulsive symptoms are also said to indicate a poor prognosis. If a diagnostic CT or MRI scan is done and it is normal, that is a good sign. If it shows enlargement of the ventricles in the brain and/or atrophy of brain tissue, that is a bad sign. The initial response of the person to antipsychotic medication is a strong indicator of prognosis: the better the response, the better the outcome is likely to be.

It should be emphasized again that each of these factors *by itself* has limited predictive value. It is only when they are all put together that an overall prognosis can be assigned. Many patients will, of course, have a mixture of good and poor outcome signs, whereas others will fall quite clearly into one category or the other.

It should also be remembered that *all predictors are only statisti-*

PREDICTORS OF OUTCOME

GOOD OUTCOME	POOR OUTCOME
Relatively normal childhood	Major problems in childhood
Female	Male
No family history of schizophrenia	Family history of schizophrenia
Older age at onset	Younger age at onset
Sudden onset	Slow onset
Paranoid or catatonic symptoms	Predominantly "negative" symptoms
Presence of normal emotions	Flattening of emotions
Good awareness of illness	Poor awareness of illness
Normal CT or MRI	Abnormal CT or MRI
Good initial response to medication	Poor initial response to medication

---

cal assertions of likelihood. There is nothing in the least binding about them. All of us who regularly care for patients with schizophrenia have seen enough exceptions to these guidelines to make us humble about any predictions. Thus, I have seen a patient with a normal childhood, no family history of the disease, a rapid onset at age twenty-two, and initial catatonic symptoms, who never recovered from even his initial illness and whose outcome was poor. More optimistically, I have seen patients with virtually every poor prognostic sign go on to almost complete recovery.

Male-Female Differences

Although older textbooks of psychiatry claimed that schizophrenia occurs in equal incidence among men and women, recent studies have clearly demonstrated that men are more commonly affected. Most striking is the earlier age of onset for men, which in the United States occurs three to four years earlier than in women. An analysis of a group of seventeen- or eighteen-year-old individuals with schizophrenia will reveal four or five males for every female.

Schizophrenia is also a more serious disease in men than it is in women. Men do not respond as well to antipsychotic drugs; they require higher doses of the drugs; they have a higher relapse rate; and their long-term adjustment—measured by such indices as social life, marriage, work record, suicide rate, and level of function—is not nearly so good as women's. There are, of course, many women with schizophrenia who have had a severe course and many men who have done well, but statistics clearly establish that schizophrenia occurs more commonly, earlier, and in a more severe form in men.

The reasons for such gender differences, still unknown, provide one of the many questions about schizophrenia needing to be researched. It should be noted that both infantile autism and childhood schizophrenia also have a strong predominance for males, and that male fetuses generally are known to be more susceptible to environmentally caused problems such as infections. The fact that males get schizophrenia both at a younger age and more severely, then, may simply be another reflection of Mother Nature's dictum that in many ways men are the weaker sex. Another speculation about why schizophrenia might be more severe in males is the possibility that female sex hormones (estrogens) may exert an antipsychotic effect and be protective. This possibility has led to some promising trials of estrogen as an add-on medication to treat women with schizophrenia (see chapter 7). It is also possible, although unlikely, that schizophrenia resembles diabetes in having two major subgroups: an early-onset, more severe variety that affects mostly men, and a later-onset, less severe variety more apt to afflict women.

Possible Courses: Ten Years Later

For individuals hospitalized with schizophrenia for the first time, the outlook at the end of one year is reasonably optimistic. Dr. Jeffrey Lieberman and his colleagues completed a study of seventy such patients, and at the end of one year 74 percent of them "were considered to be fully remitted" and 12 percent were "partially remitted." For those who went into remission, the mean time for those with a diagnosis of schizophrenia was forty-two weeks and for schizoaffective disorder twelve weeks.

The extended prognosis for schizophrenia is less optimistic than this one-year outcome. From the early years of this century, it has been said that there is a rule of thirds determining the possible courses in schizophrenia: a third recover, a third are improved, and a third are unimproved. Recent long-term follow-up studies of persons with schizophrenia both in Europe and in the United States suggest that this rule is simplistic and out-of-date. It is clear, for example, that the course of the disease over thirty years is better than it is over ten years. The use of medications has probably improved the long-term course for many patients, while the positive effect of deinstitutionalization has been to decrease dependency on the hospital and increase the number of patients able to live in the community. On the other hand, it is also clear that the mortality rate, especially by suicide, for persons with schizophrenia is very high and apparently increasing.

The Course of Schizophrenia

10 years later

25% completely recovered	25% much improved, relatively independent	25% improved, but requiring extensive support network	15% hospitalized, unimproved	10% dead (mostly suicide)

30 years later

25% completely recovered	35% much improved, relatively independent	15% improved, but requiring extensive support network	10% hospitalized, unimproved	15% dead (mostly suicide)

The best summary of possible courses of schizophrenia was done by J. H. Stephens, who analyzed twenty-five studies in which there was follow-up for at least ten years. The percentage of patients "recovered," "improved," or "unimproved" varied widely from study to study depending on the initial selection of patients, e.g., inclusion of large numbers with acute reactive psychosis increased the percentage of fully recovered. Utilizing all studies done to date, the ten-year course of schizophrenia can be seen in the chart and more nearly approximates a rule of "quarters" rather than a rule of "thirds."

Twenty-five Percent Recover Completely: This assumes that all patients with symptoms of schizophrenia are part of the analysis, including those who have been sick for less than six months with schizophreniform disorders. If only patients with narrowly defined schizophrenia are included (i.e., "continuous signs of the illness for at least six months"), then the percentage of completely recovered will be under 25 percent. Patients who recover completely do so whether they are treated with antipsychotic medication, wheat germ oil, Tibetan psychic healing, psychoanalysis, or yellow jellybeans, and all treatments for schizophrenia must show results better than this spontaneous recovery rate if they are to be accepted as truly effective. Those who recover also do so within the first two years of illness and usually have had no more than two discrete episodes of illness:

> Andrea became acutely psychotic during her second year of college and was hospitalized for six weeks. She recovered slowly, with medication and supportive psychotherapy over the following six months while living at home, and was able to resume college the following year. She has never had a recurrence. She believes she got sick because of a failed romance and her family, when they refer to the illness at all, talk vaguely of a "nervous breakdown."

Such families often deny that their family member had schizophrenia and rarely join family support groups such as NAMI (previously known as the National Alliance for the Mentally Ill).

Twenty-five Percent Are Much Improved: These patients usually have a good response to antipsychotic medication, and as long as they take it they continue to do well. They can live relatively independently, can have a social life, may marry, and often are capable of working part- or full-time:

> Peter had a normal childhood and successful high school career. He then married and joined the army to get training and travel. There was no family history of mental illness. At age 21, while assigned to Germany, he began to have strange feelings in his body and later to hear voices. He started drinking heavily, which seemed to relieve the voices, then turned to the use of hashish and cocaine. His condition deteriorated rapidly, and he was arrested for hitting an officer who he believed was trying to poison him. He was hospitalized and eventually discharged from the army with a full service-connected disability. Over the next three years he was hospitalized three more times.
>
> Peter responded slowly to very high doses of medication and was released from the hospital almost completely well. He returned faithfully for an injection of medicine every week, lived in his own apartment, and visited his family (including his divorced wife and children) and friends during the day. He clearly was capable of holding a job, but declined to do so for fear that it would jeopardize his monthly VA disability check. His only remaining symptoms were voices that he heard late in the day that he was able to ignore.

Twenty-five Percent Are Modestly Improved: These patients respond less well to medication, often have "negative" symptoms, and have a history of poorer adjustment prior to the onset of their illness. They require an extensive support network; in communities where this is available they may lead satisfactory lives, but where it is not they may be victimized and end up living on the streets or in public shelters:

> Frank was a loner as a child but had considerable musical ability and received a college scholarship. In his third year of college his grades slowly dropped as he complained of continuous auditory hallucinations. Hospitalization and medication produced a modest improvement so that he could eventually be placed in a halfway house in the community. He is supposed to attend a day program but usually walks the street talking to himself or composing music on scraps of

paper. He stays completely to himself and needs to be reminded to change his clothes, brush his teeth, and take his medicine.

Fifteen Percent Are Unimproved: These are the treatment-resistant patients for whom until recently we had little to offer. Some have responded to second-generation antipsychotic drugs such as clozapine (see chapter 7). Those who do not respond are candidates for long-term asylum care in a sheltered setting. When they are released into the community, often against their will, the results are frequently disastrous:

> Dorothy was known as a quiet child who attained straight As in school. Her mother was hospitalized for schizophrenia for two years during Dorothy's childhood, and a brother was in an institution for the mentally retarded. She was first hospitalized at age 15 for one month; information on this hospitalization was not obtainable except for a diagnosis of "transient situational reaction of adolescence." Following this, Dorothy dropped out of school, went to work as a domestic, married, and had three children. She apparently remained well until age 22, at which time she believed people were trying to kill her, believed people were talking about her, and heard airplanes flying overhead all day. She neglected her children and housework and simply sat in a corner with a fearful expression on her face. On examination she had a marked thinking disorder and catatonic rigidity and was noted to be very shy and withdrawn.
>
> Over the ensuing fifteen years Dorothy has been hospitalized most of the time and has responded minimally to medication. During the earlier years she was returned to her home for brief periods, with homemaker services, and in more recent years she lived for several months in a halfway house. There she was invariably victimized by men and was judged not to be capable of defending herself. She remains in the hospital, sitting quietly in a chair day after day. She answers politely but with absolutely no emotion and shows marked poverty of thought and of speech.

Ten Percent Are Dead: Almost all of these die by suicide or accident; other factors will be discussed at greater length on the following pages.

Possible Courses: Thirty Years Later

It has been clearly established in recent years that the thirty-year course of schizophrenia is more favorable for the average patient than the ten-year course. This directly contradicts a widespread stereotype about the disease that dates to Kraepelin's pessimistic belief that most patients slowly deteriorate. A major reason for this better long-term prognosis is that aging ameliorates the symptoms of schizophrenia in most people. Symptoms of this disease tend to be most severe when the person is in his/her twenties and thirties, then become somewhat less severe in the forties, and significantly less severe in the fifties and sixties. We do not understand why this is so and there are, of course, many exceptions, but schizophrenia represents one of the few conditions in life for which aging is an advantage.

The definitive work on the long-term course of schizophrenia has come from studies carried out by Dr. Manfred Bleuler, Dr. Luc Ciompi and his colleagues, and Dr. Gerd Huber and his colleagues in Europe, and by Dr. Courtenay Harding and her colleagues on patients deinstitutionalized from the Vermont State Hospital. Some patients followed up by these groups were as much as forty years older than when they became ill, and the agreement among the results of the different studies is impressive. As summarized by Ciompi for patients followed for an average of thirty-six years: "About three-fifths of the schizophrenic probands have a favorable outcome; that is, they recover or show definite improvement." And for patients with chronic schizophrenia in Vermont, followed up by Harding and her colleagues twenty to twenty-five years after leaving the hospital, "the current picture of the functioning of these subjects is a startling contrast to their previous levels described during their index hospitalization." Approximately three-quarters of the Vermont patients required little or no help in meeting their basic daily needs.

In most patients with schizophrenia, the "positive" symptoms of hallucinations, delusions, and thinking disorders decrease over the years. A person who was severely incapacitated at age twenty-five by these symptoms may have only residual traces of them at age fifty. It is almost as if the disease process has burned itself out over time and left behind only scars from its earlier activity. Patients also learn how to live with their symptoms, ignoring the voices and not responding to them in public.

The residual phases of schizophrenia are often referred to in psychiatric literature as a chronic defect state and are described as follows in a standard textbook:

> The patient, living in an institution or outside, has come to an *arrangement with his illness*. He has adapted himself to the world of his morbid ideas with more or less success, from his own point of view and from that of his environment. Compared with the experiences during the acute psychosis, his positive symptoms, such as delusions or hallucinations, have become colorless, repetitive, and formalized. They still have power over him but nothing is added and nothing new or unexpected happens. Negative symptoms, thought disorder, passivity, catatonic mannerisms and flattening of affect rule the picture, but even they grow habitual with the patient and appear always in the same inveterate pattern in the individual case. There is a robotlike fixity and petrification of attitude and reactions which are not only due to poverty of ideas but also to a very small choice of modes of behavior.

As with all rules, there are exceptions, so this final course can vary. Occasional patients retain their more florid symptoms all their lives. For example, I had under my care a seventy-five-year-old man who hallucinated all day every day and had been doing so for fifty years. His illness was virtually unaffected by medications. These kinds of patients are certainly exceptional, but they do exist.

It is currently popular among Scientologists and other antipsychiatry activists to attribute many of the symptoms of chronic schizophrenia to drug effects. The truth is that exactly the same clinical picture was described for fifty years before the drugs were introduced. Drugs used in schizophrenia may certainly produce some sedation, especially in older patients, but such effects account for a very small portion of the total clinical picture. Similarly, these late symptoms are often blamed on the effects of chronic institutionalization; this also accounts for only a small portion of the picture. The late symptoms may be attributed to depression and hopelessness in a patient who is chronically ill and sees no possibility of leaving the hospital; this too may account for a small portion. The vast majority of the late clinical symptoms seen in patients with chronic schizophrenia have been shown to be a direct consequence of the disease and its effects on the brain.

As seen in the chart, only 10 percent of patients with schizophrenia will require hospitalization (or a similar total-care facility such as a nursing home) thirty years later. The vast majority are able to live in the community, with about 15 percent of them requiring an extensive support network.

One of the mysteries that has perplexed mental illness professionals in recent years is where all the persons with schizophrenia have gone. Comparisons of past hospitalization rates with the number of patients receiving care as outpatients invariably find that approximately half of the expected number of patients are missing. The answer is that most of the missing patients are living in the community, usually taking no medication, with varying degrees of adjustment. A community survey in Baltimore, for example, found that half the persons with schizophrenia in the community were receiving no ongoing care or medication from any psychiatric clinic. An example of such a patient follows:

> A 72-year-old recluse was forcibly evicted from his rural decaying house by the police. He had been hospitalized for schizophrenia twice in his twenties, worked briefly as a clerk, then returned to live with his aging parents. After they died he had continued to live in the house for thirty years on Social Security disability checks. The house had no electricity or running water and the rooms were packed to the ceiling with piles of newspapers. He cooked over a sterno stove, did not bother anybody, and asked nothing except to be left alone.

The fierce independence and ability to live with his disease in such cases is commendable. The sad aspect, however, is how much better a life he might have led had he been on medication and had well-organized rehabilitation services been available. Many questions about the long-term course of schizophrenia are as yet unanswered. Do more episodes of schizophrenia cause progressively more damage to the brain? How much can the long-term course be affected by rehabilitation programs that provide jobs and social interaction?

Do People with Schizophrenia in Developing Countries Really Have a Better Outcome?

In the 1960s, the World Health Organization (WHO) undertook an ambitious nine-nation comparative prevalence study of schizophrenia, the International Pilot Study of Schizophrenia (IPSS). The initial findings, published in 1973, reported that patients with schizophrenia in the developing countries of Nigeria and India had a much more favorable outcome five years later than did patients in developed countries such as Denmark, England, Russia, and the United States. From those results came the idea, endlessly repeated in textbooks, that the outcome of schizophrenia in developing countries is much more benign. Various researchers have speculated why this may be, including factors such as more family and community support, less stigma, and fewer social demands on patients.

At the time of the original WHO publication, questions were raised about the validity of the data and the conclusions reached by the study. There were allegations that individuals with acute-onset schizophrenia, such as occurs in cases of viral encephalitis, were more common among the Indian and Nigerian samples; since patients with such organic causes usually go into complete remission, that was thought to account for the different outcomes. Over the years, other possible sources of selection bias have been proposed, such as the possibility that individuals with more severe forms of schizophrenia in developing countries died from famine and medical diseases, thus biasing the sample toward patients with better outcomes. Despite such reservations, the idea that schizophrenia has a better outcome in developing countries has often been repeated and was supported by a follow-up WHO study that had many of the same methodological problems as the original.

In recent years, several studies have been published that directly contradict the WHO claims. A 2007 study from Palau concluded that the outcome of schizophrenia in that country "is not consistent with the assumption that course or outcome is in any way more favorable in the Palauan setting than it is in others, 'developed' or otherwise." A 2008 report examined schizophrenia outcomes in twenty-three different studies from lower- and lower-middle-income countries and concluded that the outcomes were little different from outcomes in developed countries. A 2009 study from rural Ethiopia, methodologically probably the best study done to date, reported that only 6 percent of patients with schizophrenia there had achieved a complete remission of their symptoms, and one-third were continuously ill over a three-year period. It now seems clear that the original WHO claim is not valid. In all countries, some individuals with schizophrenia recover completely, some have a chronic and debilitating course, and the majority fall between these two extremes.

The Recovery Model

In the last decade, the recovery model of rehabilitation for individuals with schizophrenia has become very popular. Indeed, among some mental health officials at the federal and state levels, the recovery model has achieved the status of a psychiatric mantra. It has both positive and negative aspects, with the latter having been too often ignored.

On the plus side, the recovery model has been useful in encouraging individuals with schizophrenia to more actively participate in their treatment. It encourages assertiveness, empowerment, self-direction, setting personal goals, choices, self-fulfillment, and, most important of all, hope. It is the antithesis of being a chronic patient in a hospital setting, doing whatever the ward attendants tell you to do. The recovery movement focuses attention on the importance of psychoeducation, supported employment, social skills training, decent housing options, and all the other things necessary for successful rehabilitation. Finally, the recovery model has focused on the fact that some individuals with schizophrenia are able to achieve high levels of function and success in life.

On the minus side, many of the exhortations of the recovery movement are disingenuous, by implying that everyone with schizophrenia can "recover," without defining what is meant by "recover." Such claims are usually made by individuals who are among the one-quarter who do recover from their psychosis, as described above, or by individuals with milder forms of schizophrenia who are able to function at a comparatively high level. The implications of their statement are: "If I recovered, so can you." For an individual with schizophrenia with more severe symptoms and/or whose illness responds poorly to medications, such exhortations to "recover" are not helpful and may make individuals feel that it is their own fault for not recovering. When pressed, recovery movement advocates often claim that they did not mean that all people with schizophrenia can completely recover, but such qualifications are often lost in their message.

More seriously, the recovery movement is highly discriminatory. The first principle, as defined by the federal Substance Abuse and Mental Health Services Administration (see chapter 15), states: "By definition, the recovery process must be self-directed by the individual." This is fine for the half of people with schizophrenia who have some awareness of their illness, but 'it completely neglects the other half, who have varying degrees of anosognosia. Their brains are damaged by the schizophrenia disease process, so they are unable to appreciate their own illness, as described in chapter 1. If I asked my patients with anosognosia to define their goals, as recovery advocates suggest, they would have replied with such goals as "stopping the CIA from following me" or "making Army intelligence not send voices to the transmitter in my head." They would then remind me that there was nothing wrong with *them*, and they certainly did not need to take medication.

Thus, for approximately half of individuals with schizophrenia, the recovery movement has virtually no relevance. If a similar principle that neglected half of all patients with breast cancer, diabetes, or another disease was promulgated by a federal agency, there would be a major outcry by advocates for that disease.

Successful Schizophrenia

Those of us who work with people with schizophrenia often spend most of our time with those who have the more severe forms of the disease. We sometimes forget that there is another group of individuals who have schizophrenia who are doing quite well. As outlined above, the 30-year course of schizophrenia includes 35 percent who are much improved and relatively independent. Although they are still affected by the disease, the symptoms are under relatively good control, usually with medication, and these individuals are able to lead rewarding lives. Such individuals can be said to have successful schizophrenia.

The following are examples of such individuals.

Daniel Laitman

Daniel began hearing voices at age 15, followed by delusions and a diagnosis of schizophrenia. Following failed trials of other antipsychotics, he was stabilized on clozapine. He subsequently graduated from college with honors, moved to New York City, and is developing his career as a stand-up comedian. He is on Facebook and YouTube as "Any Time of Day with Laitman" and on Twitter as @skitzocomedy.

Recovery is a word that has been screamed at me for the past 10 years. Not literally of course, but as a quiet, subtle roar. It means something different for everyone. For some it means just being able to live through their day, for others to conquer the world and lay it at their feet. For me, of course, it's to be a working comedian, and so far it's working out pretty well. Though, it's a process. It has a beginning, middle, and hopefully no end in sight. I myself can say I am in recovery. I am living in the city with the aid of my parents. Nobody's perfect—close, but not perfect. The fact is that I'm able to live my life with the help of friends, family, and a hardy and wonderful handful of pills, including clozapine. Oh, and sleep, *way* too much sleep. But I have a life. I AM living with mental illness and I'm not sure it will ever go away. However it has allowed me to help people and to aid in their "recovery," and that strangely helps me out as well. It gives me life and purpose and friends. Recovery feeds recovery. It is so strange that helping me slowly helps others. So recovery means so many different things to so many different people. It's one of those ubiquitous words in the mental health community, but that's only because it's what everyone strives for. To one of my friends, it's that he gets to make movies. For another, it means she gets to talk about her experience to educate people. It's different and wonderful and hard. But it's recovery, and it was never meant to be easy or simple but worth it when you get to that mountain top and see the view.

Shannon Flynn

Shannon was 17 when she had her first psychotic break. She subsequently graduated from Georgetown University with a major in psychology, received a Master's degree in Art Therapy from George Washington University, and a Post-Masters Certificate in Counseling from Johns Hopkins University. She works full time and has been married for 15 years.

Haunted by delusions and deep depression as a late adolescent, I withdrew from the world into a maelstrom of psychosis. I was first hospitalized, given medication, and diagnosed with schizoaffective disorder. Despite my psychosis, the love and unwavering support of my family helped me recover over several months and successfully graduate from high school.

I went on to graduate from college with a Psychology major, then later attained graduate degrees in Art Therapy and Counseling. However, those years given to higher education were by no means continually marked by laughter and ease—indeed, I often rapid-cycled through black, agitated mixed manias and even blacker, lethargic depressions frequently marked by paranoid delusions that everyone around me, including strangers, were criticizing me constantly.

Over the years, although fortunately I've always complied with my psychotropic regimen and have avoided drug and alcohol abuse, I have fought a frustrating battle with medication side effects. I was once healthy and relatively thin; now I'm obese and deal with hypertension and hypercholesterolemia. Still, I continue to take my medications, knowing the higher cost that losing my hard-won sanity would bring.

Most importantly, I have a wonderful wellness tool, one that I can even pass along to others: creative art and art therapy. Since my first teenaged struggle I have endured many more episodes of psychosis, depression, and mania, yet my strong conviction that I have a calling to help my peers with similar challenges, as a therapist, has never died.

I have also drawn courage from the love of my husband of 15 years, and we own a house as well as a cat. I have a full-time job, in the Department of Schizophrenia Research, ironically for a government agency. And on weekends I pursue my dream of providing art therapy services to community members, which brings me great fulfillment. I've come to accept that there's no such thing as perfect, permanent recovery, but I have a rich and meaningful life regardless.

Frederick J. Frese

Fred was initially diagnosed with schizophrenia at the age of 25 when he was an officer in the US Marine Corps. He was subsequently voluntarily and involuntarily hospitalized 10 times and had a period of homelessness. After finally becoming stabilized on medication, he obtained a PhD in psychology, was the chief psychologist at an Ohio State hospital, married and raised a family, and has given over 2,000 lectures on what it is like to have schizophrenia. In July, 2018, Fred died at age 77 shortly after writing this.

In managing my disorder I can think of three things that have been particularly important. First, I feel it is important to have someone who can give you feedback as to how you are thinking. In my case, my wife does this very well. For others with this condition, a close friend, therapist, or other trusted person can serve a similar purpose.

Also, I find it helpful to be able to make some sort of contribution to society. In this regard, it is very important to be credentialed in some manner. This tends to make it easier to obtain and retain meaningful employment. Thus, I have found that working in a mental health setting has been very helpful. Co-workers in these settings tend to be more understanding about emerging symptoms.

Third, I study what I call "chronically normal persons," or CNPs, to see how my behavior differs. For example, CNPs look directly at you when they are talking, whereas we are easily distracted by their facial expressions, making it more difficult to focus on what they are saying. Also, I recommend not talking to your voices when CNPs can hear you since it makes them uncomfortable. Finally, I find it very helpful to retain a sense of humor. For example, I carry cards with me and hand them out to people who are unpleasant to me:

> Excuse me. I need to tell you that I am a person who suffers from Schizophrenia. When I am berated, belittled, insulted, or otherwise treated in an oppressive manner, I tend to become emotionally ill. Could I ask that you restate your concerns in a manner that does not tend to disable me?

Causes of Death:
Why Do People with Schizophrenia Die at a Younger Age?

It has been clearly established that individuals with schizophrenia die at a younger average age than do individuals who do not have schizophrenia. Between 1989 and 1991 three studies were published estimating the overall mortality in schizophrenia to be "about twice that of the general population," "nearly a threefold increase in overall mortality," and "5.05 times greater than expected" for males and "5.63 times greater" for females. A 1999 study in Massachusetts reported that men who are seriously mentally ill live 14.1 fewer years and women who are seriously mentally ill 5.7 fewer years than the general population. More recent studies have estimated that individuals with schizophrenia die from 15 to 25 years earlier than the general population.

Not only is the death rate for individuals with schizophrenia high, but there is also evidence that it is increasing. A 2005 study from Sweden reported that between 1960 and 2005, the death rate for individuals with schizophrenia *increased fivefold*. This dramatic increase precisely mirrored the decreasing number of psychiatric beds available; as the number of beds decreased, the death rate increased.

A major contributor to this excess mortality is suicide, which is ten to thirteen times higher in schizophrenia than in the general population, as will be discussed in chapter 10. In addition to suicide, however, there are other contributors to the excess mortality. These include accidents, diseases, unhealthy lifestyles, inadequate medical care, and homelessness.

- *Accidents:* Although individuals with schizophrenia do not drive as much as other people, studies have shown that they have double the rate of motor vehicle accidents per mile driven. A significant but unknown number of individuals with schizophrenia are also killed as pedestrians by motor vehicles; for example, one patient under my care accidentally stepped off a curb into the path of an oncoming bus. Confusion, delusions, and distraction by auditory hallucinations all contribute to such deaths. In 1995, for example, Margaret King, who had schizophrenia and believed that she was Jesus Christ, was mauled to death by lions after she climbed into their enclosure at the National Zoo in Washington, D.C. Deaths from accidental choking are also significantly increased in schizophrenia. An analysis of excess deaths in schizophrenia estimated that 12 percent of the excess was due to accidents.
- *Diseases:* There is some evidence that individuals with schizophrenia have more infections, heart disease, respiratory diseases (especially COPD), type II (adult onset) diabetes, and female breast cancer, all of which might increase their mortality rate. Partially offsetting this increased mortality rate is the likelihood that individuals with schizophrenia have a lower than expected incidence of prostate cancer, type I (juvenile onset) diabetes, and rheumatoid arthritis (to be discussed in chapter 5). The prostatic cancer data are especially interesting because one study found a relationship between having been treated with higher doses of antipsychotic medication and having a lower rate of prostate cancer, suggesting that the medication was in some way protective.
- *Unhealthy lifestyles:* It has long been known that individuals with schizophrenia smoke heavily (see chapter 10). A study in England of 102 individuals with schizophrenia also reported that they ate a diet higher in fat and lower in fiber than the general populations, and that they exercised very little.
- *Inadequate medical care:* Individuals with schizophrenia who become sick are less able to explain their symptoms

to medical personnel, and medical personnel are more likely to disregard their complaints and assume that the complaints are simply part of the illness. As noted in chapter 1, there is also evidence that some persons with schizophrenia have an elevated pain threshold, so that they may not complain of symptoms until a disease has progressed too far to be treatable. Even when diagnosed, individuals with schizophrenia are less likely to be offered standard medical or surgical care. For example, a study of cardiac catherizations for people who had had a heart attack reported that individuals diagnosed with schizophrenia were 41 percent less likely to undergo this procedure.

- *Homelessness:* Although it has not been well studied to date, it appears that homelessness increases the mortality rate of individuals with schizophrenia by making them even more susceptible to accidents and diseases. A study in England followed forty-eight homeless seriously mentally ill individuals for eighteen months; at the end of that time three had died of diseases (heart attack, suffocation during epileptic seizure, and ruptured aneurysm), one had been killed by a car, and three others had disappeared without taking their belongings with them. Scattered reports from around the United States suggest that homeless mentally ill individuals may have a very high mortality rate. For example, in Oklahoma a woman who was released from a psychiatric hospital in January sought shelter in an old chicken coop, where she froze to death and was not found for two years. In Houston, a homeless woman with schizophrenia and her young son were killed when a car hit them while she was pushing a shopping cart along a street. In Santa Ana, California, a woman with schizophrenia was killed by a train when the shopping cart she was pushing with her dog in it got stuck on the train tracks. It is likely that when we finally do a careful study of mortality rates among homeless individuals with schizophrenia in the United States, the results will show a shockingly high mortality rate.

Recommended Further Reading

Aleman, A., R. S. Kahn, J.-P. Selten. "Sex Differences in the Risk of Schizophrenia." *Archives of General Psychiatry* 60 (2003): 565–71.

Cannon, M., P. Jones, M. O. Huttunen, et al. "School Performance in Finnish Children and Later Development of Schizophrenia: A Population-Based Longitudinal Study." *Archives of General Psychiatry* 56 (1999): 457–63.

Ciompi, L. "Aging and Schizophrenic Psychosis." *Acta Psychiatrica Scandinavica*, Suppl. no. 319, 71 (1985): 93–105.

Frese, F. J., E. L. Knight and E. Saks. "Recovery from Schizophrenia: With Views of Psychiatrists, Psychologists, and Other Diagnosed With This Disorder." *Schizophrenia Bulletin* 35 (2009): 370–380.

Harding, C. M., J. Zubin, and J. S. Strauss. "Chronicity in Schizophrenia: Revisited." *British Journal of Psychiatry* (Suppl. 18), 161 (1992): 27–37.

Harris, A. E. "Physical Disease and Schizophrenia." *Schizophrenia Bulletin* 14 (1988): 85–96.

Harris, M. J., and D. V. Jeste. "Late-Onset Schizophrenia: An Overview." *Schizophrenia Bulletin* 14 (1988): 39–55.

Henry, L. P., G. P. Amminger, M. G. Harris, et al. "The EPPIC Follow-up Study of First-Episode Psychosis: Longer-Term Clinical and Functional Outcome 7 Years after Index Admission." *Journal of Clinical Psychiatry* 71 (2010): 716–28.

Howard, R., P. V. Rabins, M. V. Seeman, et al. "Late-Onset Schizophrenia and Very-Late-Onset Schizophrenia-like Psychosis: An International Consensus." *American Journal of Psychiatry* 157 (2000): 172–78.

Lewis, S. "Sex and Schizophrenia: Vive la Difference." *British Journal of Psychiatry* 161 (1992): 445–50.

Liberman, R. P., and A. Kopelowicz. "Recovery from Schizophrenia: A Concept in Search of Research." *Psychiatric Services* 56 (2005): 735–42.

Malmberg, A., G. Lewis, A. David, and P. Allebeck. "Premorbid Adjustment and Personality in People with Schizophrenia." *British Journal of Psychiatry* 172 (1998): 308–13.

Menezes, N. M., T. Arenovich, R. B. Zipursky. "A Systematic Review of Longitudinal Outcome Studies of First-Episode Psychosis." *Psychological Medicine* 36 (2006): 1349–62.

Olfson, M., T. Gerhard, C. Huang, et al., "Premature Mortality Among Adults with Schizophrenia in the United States." *JAMA Psychiatry* 72 (2015): 1–10.

Peschel, E., R. Peschel, C. W. Howe, and J. W. Howe, eds. *Neurobiological Disorders in Children and Adolescents*. San Francisco: Jossey-Bass, 1992.

Resnick, S. G., A. Fontana, A. F. Lehman, and R. A. Rosenheck. "An Empirical Conceptualization of the Recovery Orientation." *Schizophrenia Research* 75 (2005): 119–28.

Robling, S. A., E. S. Paykel, V. J. Dunn, et al. "Long-term Outcome of Severe Puerperal Psychiatric Illness: A 23 Year Follow-up Study." *Psychological Medicine* 30 (2000): 1263–71.

Shaner, A., G. Miller, J. Mintz. "Evidence of a Latitudinal Gradient in the Age of Onset of Schizophrenia." *Schizophrenia Research* 94 (2007): 58–63.

Torrey, E. F., A. E. Bowler, E. H. Taylor, et al. *Schizophrenia and Manic-Depressive Disorder.* New York: Basic Books, 1994.

Welham, J., M. Isohanni, P. Jones, et al. "The Antecedents of Schizophrenia: A Review of Birth Cohort Studies." *Schizophrenia Bulletin* 35 (2009): 603–23.

Wilson, L. *This Stranger, My Son.* New York: Putnam, 1968. Paperback by New American Library.

5

The Causes of Schizophrenia

Insanity in its various forms is now universally admitted to be a disease—differing, indeed, from ordinary disease as to its nature and phenomena—but a disease notwithstanding, and therefore to be viewed in the same light and treated on the same principles as those which regulate medical practice in other branches.

James F. Duncan, 1875

The idea that schizophrenia is a disease of the brain is not a new idea, as noted above. What *is* new is the outpouring of research that has conclusively proven this to be true. This research began in the 1980s; gathered momentum in the 1990s, the congressionally consecrated Decade of the Brain; and is continuing unabated in this century. In 2005 the biennial International Congress on Schizophrenia Research attracted more than 1,500 researchers; twenty years previously, it had attracted only 150.

This chapter will summarize research findings relevant to the causes of schizophrenia. The reader should keep in mind that research on schizophrenia is currently progressing so rapidly that anything written on it will be somewhat dated even as it is being published.

The Normal Brain

Before proceeding to a discussion of abnormalities in the brains of persons with schizophrenia, however, let us consider the normal brain—a three-pound, mushroom-like organ with a stem narrowing into the spinal cord, which runs down the back. The bulk of the brain consists of four arbitrarily defined lobes (frontal, parietal, temporal, and occipital), which are divided in half by a deep vertical cleft. At the bottom of the cleft is the corpus callosum, a thick band carrying nerve fibers back and forth between the two halves of the brain.

The entire brain is housed in the vaultlike bony skull and surrounded by a layer of cerebrospinal fluid for further protection. The fluid circulates around the brain and goes through the center of the brain by a series of canals that widen into ventricles. It is because the brain is so inaccessible and well protected that we understand comparatively little about it or its diseases. It has been facetiously suggested that if we could persuade the brain to change places with the liver we might then understand its functioning and what causes schizophrenia.

The actual work of the brain is performed by approximately 100 billion neurons and 10 times 100 billion glia. Another way to conceptualize the number of brain cells is to say that there are more neurons and glia in one brain than there are days since the world began. Until recently, it was assumed that schizophrenia was a disease of neurons, but glia are now prime suspects as well. The glia are divided into four types: astrocytes, oligodendroglia, microglia, and ependymal cells. The neurons are all interconnected, with an average neuron receiving input from at least 500 other neurons. Thus, the complex interrelatedness of the human brain is beyond comprehension. As one scholar astutely summarized it: "If the brain was so simple we could understand it, we would be so simple that we couldn't."

The primary way neurons communicate with each other is by neurotransmitters, which are chemical messengers sent from one neuron to another. The space between the arms (axons) of two adjacent neurons is called the synapse and is one-millionth of an inch wide. The neurotransmitter messengers cross the synapse at a rate of up to 600 per second. More than 100 different neurotransmitters have been identified, and there may be many more. Some of these neurotransmitters, such as dopamine, norepinephrine, serotonin, GABA (gamma-aminobutyric acid), and glutamate, are of great interest to schizophrenia researchers.

To understand the human brain, one must realize that it is the product of two hundred years of mammalian evolution. Some of its parts, such as the hippocampus and the cerebellum, are ancient structures, whereas other parts, such as the lateral prefrontal cortex and the inferior parietal area, apparently developed relatively recently. Schizophrenia affects many parts of the brain, as will be explained below, but appears to especially involve some of the newest brain areas. Schizophrenia researchers often speak about animal models of the disease, but this is wishful thinking. A rat or mouse, for example, does not have a brain area analogous to the human lateral prefrontal cortex or the inferior parietal area, both critical to the schizophrenia disease process. The fact that there is really no animal model for schizophrenia is another reason that research on this disease has progressed so slowly.

The other important fact for understanding the human brain is that it operates in networks for all higher brain functions. For basic brain functions, such as vision or controlling the muscles of your arms and legs, specific brain areas are dominant. But for all higher brain functions, such as thinking about yourself or planning for the future, many brain areas are tied together in an extraordinarily complex network. Thus there is no brain area for schizophrenia, but rather many brain areas, and connections among them. Practically, this means that the symptoms of the disease can be caused by damage to or malfunction of any one of the multiple areas and/or the connections among the areas. Increasingly, schizophrenia researchers are regarding it as a disease of connections, not just a disease of neurons or glia.

How Do We Know That Schizophrenia Is a Brain Disease?

Schizophrenia is a disease of the brain, just like Parkinson's disease, multiple sclerosis, and Alzheimer's disease. We know that they are diseases of the brain because we can measure abnormalities in the structure and function of the brain in individuals who are afflicted with these diseases. Such abnormalities were well described prior to the introduction of antipsychotic drugs in the 1950s, so cannot be attributed to the medication.

1. *Structural and Neuropathological Changes.* The most consistent structural changes in the brains of individuals with schizophrenia are enlargement of the ventricles and decreases in gray matter volume. Ventricular enlargement was clearly described two decades prior to the introduction of antipsychotics, using a research technique in which air replaced the fluid in the ventricles. In a 1933 study, 25 out of 60 individuals with schizophrenia had enlarged ventricles. Beginning in 1976 imaging techniques such as computerized axial tomography (CT) and magnetic resonance imaging (MRI) have confirmed the enlarged ventricles, averaging approximately 26 percent larger than unenlarged ventricles, and the reduced gray matter volume in well over 100 studies.

At the microscopic level, the structural changes in the brain of individuals with schizophrenia are subtler. Such research is difficult to do because of a shortage of well-characterized postmortem brains, and because it is very labor intensive. Most studies have focused on abnormalities in the frontal cortex and hippocampus, but there is also strong evidence for abnormalities in the insula, thalamus, and anterior cingulate. A 2015 review of this research concluded that, in addition to the above, there are also abnormalities in brain asymmetry; in the ridges on the brain's surface (gyrification); in the GABA-associated interneurons; and in the neuronal synapses. Similarly, a 2013 review of 33 studies involving 771 individuals with schizophrenia who had never been treated with antipsychotic medication reported that the consistent findings showed loss of volume in the thalamus and caudate nucleus. In all of these studies, white matter volume loss has also been

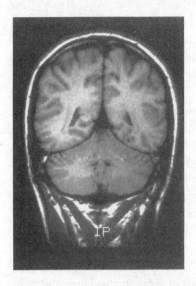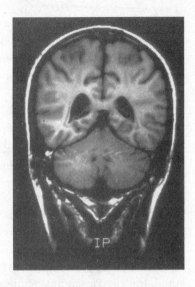

MRIs from twenty-eight-year-old identical male twins, in which the one with
schizophrenia has markedly enlarged posterior ventricles,
suggesting the loss of brain tissue associated with the disease.

observed, lending support to the increasing suspicion that the underlying pathology of schizophrenia may be in the connections of brain
areas.

2. *Neuropsychological Deficits.* The neuropsychological deficits of
schizophrenia are among the most impressive abnormalities found in
this disease and have been described in literally hundreds of studies.
In an early review of cognitive impairment, for example, it was found
that "three-quarters of the schizophrenic patients exhibited moderate
to severe dysfunction."

Four types of cognitive function are especially impaired in this
disease: attention, certain types of memory, executive function (planning, problem solving, abstracting, etc.), and awareness of illness. The
deficits in attention are demonstrable on tests that measure vigilance
and concentration. Individuals with schizophrenia are often distracted,
and in fact "distracted" was another commonly used term for insanity
in the early nineteenth century.

The memory deficits in schizophrenia are most prominent in

short-term, or "working," memory. For example, many patients have difficulty remembering three objects for five minutes. Long-term memory, on the other hand, is usually intact and the person's ability to recollect events from the period prior to the onset of his/her disease is often excellent.

Executive function deficits are apparent in tasks such as abstracting proverbs (see chapter 1). Another common way to measure executive function is by a test called the Wisconsin Card Sort, in which the person must match cards by shape or color at the same time that the rules for matching the cards are constantly changing; individuals with schizophrenia find it difficult to change how they are matching the cards to accommodate the changing rules.

The fourth type of neuropsychological deficit commonly found in schizophrenia is impaired awareness of illness, also called anosognosia. This was discussed in chapter 1 and, as was noted, can be measured. Impaired awareness of illness is of great practical importance in the treatment of this disease, as will be discussed in chapter 10 under "medication noncompliance."

The neuropsychological deficits in schizophrenia are inherent in the disease process itself and are not due to medication. Studies that have compared never-medicated patients with those on medication have reported very similar results. The neuropsychological deficits are mostly present at the time of the onset of the symptoms of schizophrenia and change surprisingly little in individuals with schizophrenia between when they are symptomatic and in remission.

It should be emphasized that the neuropsychological deficits in schizophrenia affect only selected brain functions. Many other brain functions are normal, or nearly normal, including such things as knowledge of commonplace information, verbal language skills, and visual spatial abilities.

3. *Neurological Abnormalities.* Neurological abnormalities in individuals with schizophrenia have been regularly noted since the middle of the nineteenth century. Since 1960 there have been more than sixty studies, and virtually all reported more neurological abnormalities in individuals with schizophrenia compared to normal controls.

Neurological abnormalities may be of two types. "Hard" neurological signs include things such as the patellar tendon reflex ("knee jerk") or the grasp reflex (found normally in infants) and usually indicate impaired function of a specific brain area. "Soft" neurological signs include such things as double simultaneous stimulation (being unable to feel two simultaneous touches), agraphesthesia (being unable to identify with your eyes closed numbers written on the palm of your hand), and confusion about the right and left sides of the body; these usually indicate impaired function of a neuron network. "Soft" sign abnormalities are much more common in schizophrenia than are "hard" sign abnormalities. A 1988 review of such studies concluded that between 50 and 60 percent of individuals with schizophrenia have neurological abnormalities.

Neurological abnormalities of the eye have also received much attention in schizophrenia research. The abnormality that has received the most attention is rapid eye movements, which are almost imperceptible to observers but can be measured by a special machine. Abnormal eye reflexes and abnormal blink rates (either frequent blinking or almost no blinking) have also been observed in some patients.

An important consideration in neurological studies of schizophrenia is the effect of antipsychotic medication. Since it is well known that these medications may cause tremors, movement disorders, and other neurological abnormalities in some patients, it has been assumed by some people that neurological abnormalities in individuals with schizophrenia are caused by medications. Against this belief is the finding in more than twenty studies that individuals who have never been treated with medication had just as many neurological abnormalities as those on medication. Thus, it is clear that the majority of neurological abnormalities seen in individuals with schizophrenia are inherent in the disease process, with the remainder being probable side effects of the medications.

4. *Electrical Abnormalities.* One method the brain uses to send information from one area to another is by electrical impulses, and these have been shown to be abnormal in many patients with schizophrenia. This is true when the electrical impulses are measured as evoked potentials, a special electrical impulse elicited by auditory, visual, or sensory input; abnormal evoked potentials (especially the P-300 component) have been reported in schizophrenia since the early 1970s. It

is also true when electrical activity is recorded on electroencephalograms (EEGs); approximately one-third of persons with schizophrenia have abnormal EEGs. Abnormal EEGs in schizophrenia are twice as common as among persons with mania, and four times as common as among persons with depression. A review article summarizing electrical abnormalities in schizophrenia concluded that "a broad interpretation of the EEG and EP [evoked potential] findings supports the presence of brain disease in many patients with this disorder."

5. *Known Risk Factors.* In addition to the clearly established structural, neuropsychological, neurological, and electrical abnormalities in the brains of individuals with schizophrenia, there are also known risk factors for developing the disease. Such factors often provide clues to the cause of the disease. In order to put these factors in proper perspective, they are listed in the accompanying table of Known Risk Factors for Schizophrenia. The chance of any young adult in the United States developing schizophrenia is approximately 1.0 in 100. As can be seen from the table, having a mother with schizophrenia increases your chance of getting the disease more than ninefold, from 1.0 in 100 to 9.3 in 100. Having particular genes, in contrast, increases your chance only slightly, from 1.0 in 100 to 1.2 in 100 (or, to put it another way, from 10 in 1,000 to 12 in 1,000).

Immigration is clearly established as a risk factor for developing schizophrenia, but only when the immigrant goes from specific countries (Jamaica, Morocco) to other specific countries (England, the Netherlands). Of great interest is the finding that the children of immigrants who are born in the new country have a higher risk of developing schizophrenia than do their parents. Many theories have been proposed to explain this risk pattern, including psychosocial theories and exposure to infectious agents. Also of interest is a report that individuals who immigrate as young children have a greater risk of developing schizophrenia than do individuals who immigrate when they are older.

Being born to an elderly father, especially if he was fifty-five or older at the time of birth, is a modest risk factor for developing schizophrenia. Being born or raised in an urban area, compared to being born or raised in a rural area, is a modest risk factor. So is being infected with *Toxoplasma gondii*, discussed below; using marijuana, as discussed

TABLE 5.1. KNOWN RISK FACTORS FOR SCHIZOPHRENIA

The chance of any young adult in the United States being diagnosed with schizophrenia is about 1.0 in 100. Table 5.1 shows how much various risk factors change these odds.

RISK FACTOR	CHANCE OF BEING DIAGNOSED WITH SCHIZOPHRENIA
Person's mother was diagnosed with schizophrenia	9.3 in 100
Person's father was diagnosed with schizophrenia	7.2 in 100
Person's brother or sister was diagnosed with schizophrenia	7.0 in 100
Person immigrated from a specific country (e.g. Jamaica, Morocco) to another specific country (e.g. England, the Netherlands)	2.3 in 100
Child of person above was born in the new country	4.5 in 100
Person's father was fifty-five or older at time of person's birth	2.2–5.9 in 100
Person's father was forty-five or older at time of person's birth	1.2–1.7 in 100
Person uses marijuana	2.1–2.9 in 100
Person was born or raised in an urban area	2.2–2.8 in 100
Person has antibodies to *Toxoplasma gondii*, indicating past infection	2.7 in 100
Person has minor physical anomalies	2.2 in 100
Person has a history of traumatic brain injury	1.7 in 100
Person was sexually abused in childhood	1.5 in 100
Person's mother had complications during pregnancy or delivery	1.3–1.4 in 100
Person has specific genetic polymorphisms thought to predispose to schizophrenia	1.1–1.2 in 100
Person was born in the winter or spring	1.1 in 100
Person's mother was pregnant during an influenza epidemic	1.1 in 100

in chapter 3; and having minor physical anomalies, such as an arched palate, an indicator of developmental problems in utero.

The lowest-level risk factors for developing schizophrenia, other than having specific genes, are having a history of traumatic brain injury in childhood; having been sexually abused in childhood; the mother having had complications during the pregnancy or delivery; being born in the winter or spring; or having a mother who was exposed to influenza during the pregnancy. All of these are statistical factors, but the risk is so small that they are not very important. The cause-and-effect relationship for some of them is also not clear. For example, if the person was sexually abused, was it by a parent who had schizo-phrenia? In that case the risk might not be the sexual abuse itself, but rather having a parent with schizophrenia.

Finally, there is one other clearly established but curious fact about schizophrenia. Individuals with schizophrenia almost never get rheumatoid arthritis, and individuals with rheumatoid arthritis almost never get schizophrenia. Thus rheumatoid arthritis would appear to be a protective factor against schizophrenia. Since 1936, eighteen studies of this association have been done, with fourteen of them reporting a lower-than-expected incidence of rheumatoid arthritis in individuals with schizophrenia. Among the three studies that were methodolog-ically the best, no individuals with rheumatoid arthritis were found among 111 and 301 inpatients with schizophrenia in two of the studies, and a very low incidence was found in the third.

There are many similarities between schizophrenia and rheuma-toid arthritis that make this inverse correlation even more interesting. Neither disease was clearly described until the beginning of the nine-teenth century. Both diseases have a lifetime incidence of approxi-mately 1 percent and a pairwise concordance rate in identical twins of approximately 30 percent (i.e., when one twin gets it, the second twin also gets it approximately 30 percent of the time). Both diseases are said to be more common in urban than in rural areas. A major differ-ence between the diseases is that rheumatoid arthritis is more common in women than in men by a ratio of three to one.

Several theories have been proposed to explain this inverse cor-relation, but none has been proven. It is possible that there are ge-netic factors that render a person susceptible to schizophrenia and at the same time resistant to rheumatoid arthritis. Biochemical factors, including prostaglandins, essential fatty acids, beta-endorphins, and tryptophan, have all been hypothesized as playing a role by some re-searchers. Viruses could explain it if both diseases were caused by closely related types; becoming infected with one virus might confer immunity to the second virus. The most intriguing challenge is that if we are able to understand the causes of one of these diseases, then it may help us to understand the other as well.

In summary, what can be said about the brains of individuals with schizophrenia? It can be said that schizophrenia is firmly and unequiv-ocally established to be a brain disease, just as surely as multiple scle-rosis, Parkinson's disease, and Alzheimer's disease are established as brain diseases. As Dr. Henry Griesinger said more than one hundred years ago: "Psychiatry and neuropathology are not merely two closely related fields; they are but one field in which only one language is spo-ken and the same laws rule." The dichotomy used in the past, whereby schizophrenia was classified as a "functional" disorder as distinct from an "organic" disorder, is now known to be inaccurate; schizophrenia has impeccable credentials for admission to the organic category.

Brain Disease Deniers

Despite the overwhelming evidence that schizophrenia is a disease of the brain, a few small groups deny that it is. For individuals who have schizophrenia, such denial is somewhat understandable; schizophre-nia is an unpleasant disease and it would be nice if it did not exist. Mental health professionals who deny that schizophrenia is a brain dis-ease probably also believe that the earth is flat.

Thomas Szasz was probably the best-known denier of schizo-phrenia as a brain disease, as reasoned in his books such as *The Myth of Mental Illness* (1961) and *Schizophrenia: The Sacred Symbol of Psychiatry* (1976). He claimed that schizophrenia and other mental illnesses were merely metaphors for human problems of living. Szasz acknowledged that brain diseases, such as Alzheimer's disease, are real and agreed that if schizophrenia could be shown to have a neurological basis, it too would be a brain disease. Even though many of us presented him with such evidence, he refused to publicly change his position until his death in 2012. A major reason why Szasz had difficulty in understanding schizophrenia is because he apparently never treated any patient with this disease. He trained in psychiatry at the Chicago Institute for Psychoanalysis and later proudly claimed that he had never prescribed medication for any patient he had ever treated.

Ronald Laing, a British psychoanalyst, had one of the most bizarre reasons for denying the reality of schizophrenia. He promoted the idea that schizophrenia was a sane response to an insane world and may even be a growth experience, a romantic if nonsensical idea that appealed to many 1960s radicals. Laing's ideas grew out of Freudian and family interaction theories. Laing's ideas about schizophrenia take on a poignant air when it is realized that his eldest daughter was diagnosed with schizophrenia and was hospitalized for many years. Laing became increasingly disillusioned and an alcoholic as he grew older. In 1982 he commented to an interviewer: "I was looked to as one who had the answers but I never had them."

Scientologists as a group deny the reality of schizophrenia as a brain disease. They direct their animosity to psychiatry through their Citizens' Commission on Human Rights, which is part of Scientology. Their beliefs about schizophrenia are based on the writings of their founder, L. Ron Hubbard. According to one account, "Hubbard taught that the psychotic person is a 'potential trouble source' who is connected to forces opposed to Scientology. People who behave as psychotics are 'unethical' and 'immoral.'" Hubbard also taught that the "forces" behind psychiatry are extraterrestrial. According to a recent published account, Hubbard claimed that "Earthlings are the pawns of aliens," and that "the psychiatric establishment—which always looked askance at his theories—was not just a present day evil but a timeless one. In a distant galaxy, alien 'psychs' [as Hubbard called them] devised implants that would ultimately wreck the spiritual progress of human beings." Thus, psychiatrists were the Darth Vaders of Hubbard's universe.

All of this sounds like harmless nonsense until one realizes that many Scientologists actually believe it. In addition to the scientologists, many of the individuals who call themselves "consumer-survivors" deny that schizophrenia is a brain disease. Most such individuals have been diagnosed with some form of mental illness and hospitalized, then adopt an opposition to psychiatry as their goal in life. Many members of the Hearing Voices Network (see chapter 8) also count themselves among the deniers of schizophrenia as a brain disease.

What Parts of the Brain Are Affected?

Researchers argue endlessly about what parts of the brain are primarily affected in schizophrenia. In the past, each research group had its favorite region, such as the anterior cingulate or the lateral prefrontal cortex, and would focus its research efforts on that region. This has changed, largely because of the availability of neuroimaging techniques whereby many brain areas can be studied simultaneously. Another factor that has led to a better understanding of the part of the brain affected is the greater availability of postmortem schizophrenia brain tissue from brain banks, such as that created in 1995 by the Stanley Medical Research Institute. Since that time, there has been an outpouring of neuropathological studies.

What is now abundantly clear, as mentioned above, is that schizophrenia is a brain disease involving a widespread network of multiple brain areas. There is no schizophrenia brain area; rather, there is a schizophrenia-affected brain network. The disease process almost certainly involves both neurons and glia in the multiple areas affected and also involves the white-matter connections between the areas.

The schizophrenia-affected network includes medial aspects of the prefrontal cortex, including the anterior cingulate, as well as the lateral prefrontal cortex, which evolved much later. These are highly connected to the insula, lying between the frontal and temporal lobes, and to the superior temporal gyrus. The last includes an important center for hearing, and it is presumably this involvement that results in the high prevalence of auditory hallucinations in schizophrenia. The superior temporal gyrus is immediately adjacent to the inferior parietal lobule, also thought to play a central role in causing anosognosia and other symptoms of schizophrenia. The junction between the superior temporal gyrus and the inferior parietal lobule is known as the temperoparietal junction (TPJ), and has been prominent in many neuroimaging studies of this disease.

The hippocampus and adjacent parahippocampal gyrus, evolutionarily older brain areas, are also involved in the schizophrenia disease process. Many of the microscopic studies of schizophrenia brain tissue have shown consistent abnormalities in the hippocampus. The pulvinar, which is the posterior portion of the thalamus, is also thought to play a central role in causing many symptoms. Other areas thought to be involved, although their roles are less clear, are the posterior cingulate and the medial aspects of the cerebellum. The connections between most of the brain areas cited above are very well developed.

Neuroimaging studies have demonstrated that many of these brain regions can produce symptoms of schizophrenia. For example, in a woman undergoing brain surgery to correct her epilepsy, it was found that stimulation of the left temperoparietal junction produced "a feeling of the presence of another person" and "the impression that somebody was behind her." Activation of the regions of the inferior parietal lobule can produce feelings that your actions are being controlled by another person. Activation of the medial frontal area and inferior parietal lobule can produce distortions of body image and sense of self. In short, it is now clear that all the symptoms experienced by people with schizophrenia are associated with the abnormal functioning of specific areas in the schizophrenia-affected brain network.

There is one other curious fact about the anatomical location of schizophrenia. In recent years there have been several studies suggesting that the left side of the brain is primarily affected in schizophrenia much more often than the right side of the brain. Patients with temporal lobe epilepsy, for example, are more likely to have schizophrenia-like symptoms if the epilepsy is in the left temporal lobe. Similarly, studies of visual evoked potentials, abnormal EEGs, lateral eye movements, auditory discrimination, galvanic skin response, information processing, and neurological signs all suggest that the major problem may lie in the left hemisphere.

When Does the Disease Process Begin?

The question of when the disease process of schizophrenia begins has provoked lively controversy among researchers in recent years and has led to development theories (see below). It is an important question, because it has implications for the prevention of the disease.

What is increasingly clear is that, at least for one-quarter of cases of schizophrenia, the brain changes leading to the disease begin early in life, even though the actual symptoms of the disease do not begin until the person's late teenage years or twenties. The evidence pointing toward early brain changes include the studies of pregnancy and birth complications, minor physical anomalies, the winter and spring excess of births, the urban risk factor for birth or early rearing, and, finally, some microscopic changes found in some brains postmortem that suggest changes that took place during the brain's development.

Do all individuals with schizophrenia have brain changes that date to early in life, or is that true merely for a subgroup? We do not yet know the answer to this. What we do know is that the early brain changes occur in approximately one-quarter of individuals with schizophrenia. This was shown, for example, by our study of identical twins in which one had schizophrenia and the other did not. When we looked for neurological or behavioral diferences between the twins before the age of five, in 7 out of 27 pairs (26 percent), there clearly were differences even though the symptoms of schizophrenia in the affected twin did not begin until many years later.

It remains to be ascertained whether this group of individuals with early changes is a clinical subgroup; that is, do they have a different cause for their disease? Or do all individuals with schizophrenia have a disease process that dates to early in life but cannot be measured yet? This is one of the most important research questions currently facing schizophrenia researchers.

The known facts about schizophrenia, as outlined above, are reasonably well established and not in dispute. What is in dispute is how to link these facts to schizophrenia in a coherent theory of causation.

Theories About the Causes of Schizophrenia

One of the most remarkable facts about schizophrenia is that researchers in the mid-nineteenth century were closer to the truth regarding its causes than were researchers in the mid-twentieth century. By the

1830s, in both England and the United States, there was a consensus among most mental illness professionals that insanity was a brain disease. In England, for example, William A. F. Browne stated that, "insanity, then, is . . . produced by an organic change in the brain." Researchers, looking for abnormalities, assiduously examined the post-mortem brains of insane individuals, but the results were contradictory since the available techniques were inadequate to find them. In 1867 Henry Maudsley recognized that the "important molecular or chemical changes may take place in those inner recesses to which we have not yet gained access . . . [and] to conclude from the non-appearance of change to the non-existence thereof would be just as if the blind man were to maintain that there were no colors, or the deaf man to assert that there was no sound."

Incredibly, one hundred years after Browne, Maudsley, and their colleagues were discussing insanity as a brain disease, their psychiatric offspring were investigating insanity as a product of bad mothering or mislabeling. In no other area of medicine—perhaps in all of science—did research go backward for as far or as long as it did in psychiatry.

Beginning in the last quarter of the twentieth century, research on schizophrenia finally got back on track. The present challenge is to synthesize the rapidly accumulating data into a coherent theory and then prove them to be correct. One is reminded of Edna St. Vincent Millay's sonnet that described "a meteoric shower of facts" that "lie unquestioned, uncombined":

> Wisdom enough to leech of our ill
> Is daily spun, but there exists no loom
> To weave it into fabric.

A major impediment to weaving the facts about schizophrenia into a coherent theory is the question of heterogeneity: Is schizophrenia one disease or many diseases? Most researchers have assumed the latter, but that is not established as fact. A case can be made for the opposite approach—that most cases of schizophrenia may turn out to have a single major cause. Dr. Lewis Thomas pointed out that syphilis, tuberculosis, and pernicious anemia were all conditions with a bewildering variety of manifestations that few scientists thought could constitute a single illness, yet in each case a single cause (spirochete, tubercle bacillus, and vitamin deficiency) was eventually found to be the primary cause. That this may be true for schizophrenia (and possibly for bipolar disorder as well) is certainly possible.

This section will summarize theories about the cause of schizophrenia. The reader should keep in mind that many of these theories are not mutually exclusive, and the final answer may involve some combination of them. The reader should also be aware that my own research is on infectious causes of schizophrenia, so I may not be completely objective regarding competing theories.

Genetic Theories

Genetic theories regarding schizophrenia have been prominent since the 1960s, when biological researchers promoted them as an alternative to psychoanalytic theories. Initially, many geneticists believed that schizophrenia was caused by a dominant or recessive gene. Blood samples were collected from families with more than one affected family member, and attempts were made to identify the putative genes. By the 1990s, candidate genes had been identified on every one of the twenty-three chromosomes but none of them turned out to be associated with schizophrenia. Researchers then decided that schizophrenia must be caused by many genes of small effect rather than a few genes of large effect. The decoding of the human genome in the 1990s made it possible to look for such genes across the entire genome in what were called genome-wide association studies (GWAS). An outpouring of GWAS studies identified single nucleotide polymorphisms (SNPs) in hundreds of genes, all with a very small effect. It seemed clear that if schizophrenia was indeed a genetic disease, it was much more complex than anyone had previously thought.

Most current genetic theories of schizophrenia assume that genes by themselves do not cause the disease, but rather make the person more susceptible to developing the disease if the person is also exposed to specific environmental factors. The identity of these environmental factors is widely debated, but may include birth trauma, infectious agents, nutritional factors, immune deficiency, etc. Attempts are now under way to try and link the suspected susceptibility genes to specific environmental factors in what is called a gene-environment interaction. Despite the expenditure of approximately $100 million dollars a year (as of 2016) on such genetic research by the National Institute of Mental Health, the results to date have been very disappointing.

In retrospect, there are plenty of reasons to doubt whether genetics plays a major role in the cause of schizophrenia. The theory rests in large measure on the fact that schizophrenia runs in families and the assumption that this means it is transmitted genetically. However, tuberculosis also runs in families, not because it is transmitted genetically, but rather because family members transmit it to each other. Infectious agents could theoretically cause schizophrenia and give the appearance of being a genetic disease. For example, *Toxoplasma gondii*, an infectious parasite carried by cats and which will be discussed below, has been documented as having caused human toxoplasmosis in family clusters because of the family's exposure to a toxoplasma-infected common water source, infected food (goat's milk), and exposure to infected family cats. It is also known that the parasite can be transmitted from infected pregnant mothers to their fetus. More disturbingly, in animals it has been shown that the parasite can be transmitted sexually in male sperm, and in mice it can be transmitted from mother to offspring over five generations. Whether this can happen in humans is unknown, but it clearly illustrates that everything that is familial is not necessarily genetic.

Twin studies have been the other bedrock of genetic theories of schizophrenia, especially the schizophrenia prevalence rate among identical (monozygotic) twins versus familial (dizygotic) twins. Geneticists have frequently claimed that the schizophrenia concordance rate among identical twins is about 50 percent. However, when the research is confined to unselected twin samples, such as the Scandinavian national twin registers, the pairwise concordance rate is only 28%. By using dubious assumptions and questionable statistical methods, geneticists have often claimed that the heritability of schizophrenia is 80 percent or more. Such estimates have no foundation in fact.

There are additional reasons for doubting that schizophrenia is primarily a genetic disease. One of the strongest is what is often referred to as the "schizophrenia paradox—the continuing existence of

schizophrenia despite a low fertility rate and a high mortality rate."
Indeed, between about 1830 and 1950 the vast majority of individuals
with severe schizophrenia were confined to mental hospitals, unable to
procreate. Yet during those same years the prevalence of schizophrenia
appeared to increase.

In summary, genes almost certainly play some role in the causation
of schizophrenia, but it is a much more modest role than previously
thought. Most likely there are susceptibility genes that make it more
likely that you will get the disease if you are exposed to specific environmental agents, infectious or otherwise. The fact that schizophrenia
is not primarily a genetic disease should also be regarded as good news,
since we couldn't do much about it if it was. Non-genetic causative
factors are more susceptible to alteration.

Inflammatory, Infectious, and Immunological Theories

The last decade has seen the emergence of inflammatory, infectious,
and immunological theories as the most promising theories regarding
the cause of schizophrenia. The three theories are discussed together
because they are interrelated; for example, an infectious agent may
activate the immune system and cause inflammation. A major reason
for the striking increase in interest in these theories in recent years
has been a genetic finding. Among all the genetic research into schizophrenia that has been carried out over the past two decades, the single
strongest finding has been the activation of genes on a region of chro-
mosome 6 that controls the body's inflammatory and immune response
to infection.

Evidence linking inflammation to the schizophrenia disease process is strong. It consists of elevations of inflammation-related proteins
in the blood, spinal fluid, and postmortem brain tissue of individuals
with schizophrenia, especially those who have been sick for several
years. Such elevations have been found in individuals being treated
with antipsychotics as well as in those never treated. The most prominent inflammatory-related protein is C-reactive protein, which has
been found to be elevated in 28 percent of individuals with schizophrenia. Other inflammatory-related proteins are called cytokines.

Additional evidence of inflammation in the brains of individuals with schizophrenia includes studies reporting the activation of microglia cells, the cells that respond to inflammation.

Immunological abnormalities in schizophrenia have been described for almost a century, including various measurements of the immune response and lymphocyte function. The majority of this research took place in Europe, especially Eastern Europe, and had a limited influence on American researchers. As part of the recent interest in inflammation, immunological research is undergoing a revival.

Regarding specific infectious agents that might be causing some cases of schizophrenia, published studies have reported elevated antibodies to a wide array of viruses including herpes simplex virus 1 and 2, cytomegalovirus, Epstein-Barr virus, influenza, Coxsackie virus, polio, rubella, measles, and mumps. Some of these studies have been done on individuals with schizophrenia and others on pregnant women who gave birth to individuals who later developed schizophrenia. The main center for such infectious research for the last two decades has been the Stanley Laboratory of Developmental Neurovirology at the Johns Hopkins University Medical Center in Baltimore and the associated research unit at Sheppard Pratt hospital.

The infectious agent that is currently of greatest interest as a possible cause of some cases of schizophrenia is not a virus but rather a parasite, *Toxoplasma gondii,* that is carried by cats. More than 80 studies have reported that individuals with schizophrenia and related psychoses have increased antibodies to *T. gondii.* Four studies have reported that individuals who have schizophrenia were more likely, compared to controls, to have lived during childhood in a house with a cat but two other studies failed to find this. *T. gondii* is known to make dopamine, which is of interest since people with schizophrenia are thought to have elevated levels of dopamine. Epidemiologically there are many similarities between toxoplasmosis and schizophrenia, and some antipsychotics have been shown to suppress *T. gondii.* Finally, a study in China reported that having antibodies to *T. gondii* at the time students entered university made it significantly more likely that the student would be diagnosed with psychosis during the next four years.

A recent new aspect of the inflammatory-infectious-immunological theory of schizophrenia is the possibility that the person's intestine is involved in the disease process. It has become increasingly clear that the huge number of bacteria, viruses, and other infectious agents, collectively referred to as the microbiome, play an important role in regulating our immune system, including the immune system of the brain. This gut-brain axis, as it is called, is poorly understood but thought to operate by a direct connection to the vagus nerve, by the release of chemicals by the microbiome, and/or by immune system activation of the brain. Such research is giving rise to therapeutic attempts to affect the microbiome using probiotics as described in chapter 7. This is merely one of the new approaches to the treatment of schizophrenia that is being generated by research on the inflammatory, infectious, and immune aspect of the disease.

Neurochemical Theories

Along with genetic theories, neurochemical theories dominated schizophrenia research from the 1960s until recently. Neurotransmitters, chemicals that carry messages between brain cells, have been especially prominent. Among the neurotransmitters, dopamine has been a favorite of researchers because amphetamine, which releases dopamine, causes schizophrenia-like symptoms. In addition, the earlier antipsychotics were found to block dopamine, so it became widely assumed that an excess of dopamine causes schizophrenia and that antipsychotic drugs work by blocking dopamine. Alas, four decades of research on this theory have yielded little supporting evidence, and some newer antipsychotics appear to work without blocking dopamine.

Glutamate, another neurotransmitter, has been regarded as a promising candidate in recent years. Much of the interest stems from the fact that the street drug PCP (phencyclidine) causes schizophrenia-like symptoms and also blocks glutamate. Glutamate is a major excitatory neurotransmitter in the brain and is often paired with GABA (gamma-aminobutyric acid), a major inhibitory neurotransmitter. In contrast to dopamine, there is considerable evidence that both glutamate and GABA are somehow involved in the causation of schizophrenia.

There are, however, over one hundred known neurotransmitters, and it is increasingly apparent that they interact with each other in a complex manner. Thus, when one becomes abnormal, it affects the next, and then the next, and so on. Other neurochemicals are also being studied by schizophrenia researchers. A group of considerable interest are neuropeptides, some of which also act as neurotransmitters. Endorphins are one type of neuropeptide. Another group of neurochemicals that has generated considerable interest are those involved in sending messages within cells (intracellular signaling).

There is no question that there are some neurotransmitter and other neurochemical abnormalities in individuals with schizophrenia, but many questions remain regarding whether such abnormalities are the cause or the effect of the disease process. And if they are the cause, what causes the abnormalities themselves? Some researchers combine genetic theories with neurochemical theories in an attempt to fill the gaps, but the validity of this approach remains to be seen.

Developmental Theories

Developmental theories of schizophrenia are elegant and currently fashionable. They are based on the hypothesis that something goes wrong during the period of brain development. During fetal life, neurons are being made at a rate of 250,000 per minute. They then have to migrate to the part of the brain where they belong and differentiate into a particular type of neuron. Finally, a pruning process of excess neurons begins during fetal life and continues until at least three years after birth. Clearly, there are many chances for something to go wrong in this extended and complex process.

Developmental theories of schizophrenia do not focus on *what* causes schizophrenia but rather *when* the disease begins. According to developmental researchers, any one of a number of agents could theoretically cause developmental problems. Such agents might include genes, infectious agents, alcohol, chemicals, medications, radiation, malnutrition, or very stressful experiences. As summarized by one proponent of developmental theories, possible agents include "a hereditary encephalopathy or predilection to environmental injury, an infection or postinfectious state, damage from an immunologic disorder, perinatal trauma or encephalopathy, toxin exposure early in development, a primary metabolic disease, or other early developmental events." Once the original insult has taken place at a critical stage of brain development, the damage is done. In most cases, however, its effects are not immediately noticeable, except perhaps for nonspecific signs such as lack of coordination or behavioral problems in childhood. Once the brain matures, according to the developmental theory, the signs and symptoms of schizophrenia appear.

Developmental theories of schizophrenia are consistent with findings such as minor physical anomalies, pregnancy and birth complications, and an excess of winter and spring births, as described above. Developmental theorists also point to animal models wherein damage is intentionally done to vital brain structures (e.g., hippocampus, prefrontal cortex) while the animal is still a fetus and then the animal is found to behave abnormally when it reaches puberty. In one animal model, the hippocampal-damaged rat is also said to respond abnormally to chemicals that increase dopamine, thus tying a developmental theory to the dopamine theory. The most important evidence supporting developmental theories, however, are occasional reports of neuronal disorganization in schizophrenia, which could have taken place only during fetal development.

Despite their elegance, developmental theories have many limitations. Evidence to support the cornerstone of those theories, neuronal disorganization, is relatively rare. The animal models have also been criticized as not relevant; what, for example, are equivalent symptoms of schizophrenia in rats? It can also be argued that if the disease process of schizophrenia really begins during fetal life in most cases, why don't we see more minor physical anomalies, seizures, and mental retardation? Finally, developmental theories, like neurochemical theories, are theories of the pathophysiology, or *process* of the disease, and leave the identity of the original cause unanswered.

Nutritional Theories

Nutritional theories of schizophrenia have had adherents since it was discovered that beriberi, pellagra, and pernicious anemia, all of which may have psychiatric symptoms, were vitamin deficiency diseases. Researchers searched for a wide variety of nutritional deficiencies and food allergies with relatively little success, although it must be acknowledged that most of the studies were methodologically poor. In the 1950s Drs. Humphrey Osmond and Abram Hoffer began treating patients with schizophrenia with high doses of niacin, other vitamins, and minerals and claimed remarkable success. Their claims were not substantiated.

In recent years there has been a modest revival of interest in nutritional theories of schizophrenia. One area of interest is possible abnormalities in lipid metabolism, specifically in the fatty acids that are important components of brain cells. Another area of interest is possible abnormalities in protein metabolism, specifically in the amino acids, such as methionine, tryptophan, glycine, and serine, which are the building blocks of protein. In contrast to the earlier orthomolecular claims, most current research is being done more carefully and uses controls.

Interest in nutritional theories of schizophrenia has also been stimulated by recent studies reporting that women who were subjected to relative starvation during pregnancy were more likely to give birth to offspring who later developed schizophrenia. A 1992 study from the Netherlands reported that pregnant women subjected to hunger during the winter of 1944–1945, when Nazi Germany cut off food to the region, were twice as likely to give birth to offspring who later developed schizophrenia if their pregnancy was in its first three months during the height of the hunger. A 2005 study from China similarly reported that women who were pregnant during a 1959–1961 famine in Anhui province were twice as likely to give birth to offspring who later developed schizophrenia.

There are multiple possible explanations for these results. First, nutritional deprivation may alter brain development in the developing fetus and make the brain more liable to later develop schizophrenia.

Alternatively, famine conditions may cause pregnant women to eat foods they would not ordinarily eat. In the Dutch study, this included tulip bulbs, and in the Chinese study, many women ate the bark from trees. Finally, nutritional deprivation weakens the body's immune system, thereby making it more susceptible to infections that may affect the brain.

Some of the most promising evidence for a nutritional cause of schizophrenia comes from the studies of Dr. John McGrath et al. in Australia on vitamin D deficiency. In a 2010 study, they reported that children who later develop schizophrenia tend to have abnormal vitamin D levels at birth. The vitamin D theory might also explain some of the epidemiological findings, such as seasonal births, higher risk for individuals born or raised in an urban setting, and higher prevalence among some immigrant groups.

Another novel approach to nutritional research on schizophrenia is being carried out by Dr. Emily Severance et al., in The Stanley Laboratory at the Johns Hopkins University Medical Center. It has been long known that some individuals with schizophrenia have a sensitivity to proteins found in milk and wheat. It may be that an immunological reaction to these protein triggers an inflammatory reaction. Studies are exploring whether such inflammation causes the entry into the circulation of different types of gut-based products, including bacteria. In turn, the body responds with its own inflammatory molecules. This research thus combines nutritional with inflammatory theories. It is not yet clear what these observations mean, and additional research is under way.

Endocrine Theories

Interest in endocrine dysfunction as a possible cause of schizophrenia is linked to observations that severe hypothyroidism, hyperthyroidism, and hyperfunction of the adrenal gland (Cushing's syndrome) may all produce psychiatric symptoms that resemble schizophrenia. A related observation is that maternal psychosis following childbirth is thought to be triggered by massive hormonal changes that occur postpartum. Such observations have led some researchers to question whether more subtle endocrine dysfunction may contribute to the causation of schizophrenia.

One finding that points in this direction is the occurrence of compulsive water drinking (polydypsia) among some individuals with schizophrenia. Water intake is related to hormones in the posterior pituitary gland. The anterior pituitary has also been provisionally linked to schizophrenia in some patients who show altered response to growth hormone when given apomorphine, a dopamine-stimulating drug. There have also been claims that reproductive hormones (FSH and LH), which come from the anterior pituitary, are abnormal in individuals with schizophrenia. The interruption of menstrual periods in some female patients is well known.

The fact that insulin coma produced brief remissions in some individuals with schizophrenia led to interest in insulin metabolism, and there have been claims that schizophrenia is less common than expected in type I (insulin-dependent) diabetics and more common than expected in type II (noninsulin-dependent) diabetics. There has been renewed interest in recent years in the relationship between schizophrenia and diabetes because second-generation antipsychotics, especially olanzapine and clozapine, markedly increase blood glucose levels in some patients. There has also been extensive research on melatonin and the pineal gland in schizophrenia, although the current consensus is that these are not abnormal.

The precise meaning of endocrine dysfunction in schizophrenia is unclear. It could represent an endocrine response to the stress of the illness or an effect of antipsychotic drugs. The endocrine dysfunction may also be another aspect of the disease process.

Childhood Trauma and Stress Theories

Childhood trauma and stress theories of schizophrenia have a long and disreputable scientific history. Throughout the 19th century, stressors such as "disappointment in a love affair" were regularly invoked to explain the cause of insanity. In the 1960s such theories were revived, and became the stimulus for claims that "schizophrenogenic mothers" were the cause of schizophrenia in their children. By the mid-1980s such theories had been discarded, and it was stated categorically that "there is no good evidence that life stress is causally related to episodes of schizophrenia."

At the turn of the 21st century, the "schizophrenogenic mothers" rose from the dead in the form of childhood trauma. Dozens of papers have been published claiming to prove that various traumatic experiences of childhood cause schizophrenia. Some studies have been picked up by the media, leading to headlines such as "Child Sex Abuse Linked to Schizophrenia." Traumatic events of childhood can unquestionably leave lasting psychic scars. Sexual abuse of children in particular has been plausibly linked to later depression, dissociative disorder, PTSD, and substance abuse. However, there are major problems with the childhood trauma studies and no credible evidence to support the linkage of such trauma to the causes of schizophrenia.

Scientifically, most of the childhood trauma studies are very weak. One review examined 46 such studies for scientific merit and found that only six had used an appropriate control group. Childhood trauma theorists often summarize many such studies together and claim merit by numbers, but piling 100 scientifically questionable studies on top of each other does not improve their scientific credibility. Another problem is the variety of childhood traumas used by these researchers, often in the same study. These include everything from sexual abuse, physical abuse, and emotional abuse to parental death, parental poverty, witnessing parental violence, neglect, and bullying. Another major problem with these studies is that most of them collected data on abuse retrospectively. As one critique of childhood trauma studies correctly notes, "an extensive literature has cast doubt on the validity of retrospective reports about child rearing, family conflicts and psychological states in childhood." Indeed, it appears that many of the childhood trauma researchers have learned nothing from the scandals associated with the false memory syndrome.

A handful of the scientifically sound childhood trauma studies do report a correlation between such trauma and the development of schizophrenia, but correlation is not causation. One explanation may be reverse causality, especially when the study includes adolescents. In other words, an adolescent who is in the earliest stages of schizophrenia, not yet diagnosed, may behave in such a way as to elicit traumatic behavior from others. Retrospectively, it may then appear that the trauma caused the schizophrenia when in fact it was the reverse. The possibility of reverse causality was perceptively noted by Dr. Eugen Bleuler in his classic 1911 book *Dementia Praecox:*

> In cases in which we have excellent anamneses [histories], one regularly notes that signs of disease existed before the suspected psychic trauma so that it becomes difficult to impute to such trauma any causal significance. In the majority of cases, it is also quite evident without much searching that the unfortunate love affair, demotion from office, etc are consequences and not causes of the disease if there was any connection between them at all.

Still another possible reason why one may observe a correlation between child abuse and the later development of schizophrenia is that schizophrenia is a familial disease, as explained earlier in this chapter. Thus, a child who grew up in a family with seriously mentally ill parents is more likely to have experienced abuse and also more likely to develop schizophrenia, not caused by the abuse but rather by exposure to the common environmental factor, infectious or otherwise.

A final problem with the childhood trauma and schizophrenia research is that much of it has been carried out and summarized by a small number of overtly anti-psychiatry British and Dutch mental health professionals. They acknowledge being firmly opposed to the biomedical model of schizophrenia, believing rather that the disease has predominantly psychological, not medical, roots. Such overt bias impairs their credibility in interpreting the studies that have been carried out.

Obsolete Theories

As knowledge evolves in every field of scientific inquiry, new theories arise to explain these observations. At the same time, older theories that no longer fit the facts are set aside and eventually discarded. All areas of science have dusty shelves full of discarded theories, and schizophrenia research is no exception. Some of the more unusual prominent theories are as follows:

Freudian Theory: For the first half of the twentieth century, Freud's psychoanalytic theories were prominent in the United States. Freud taught that bad mothering causes schizophrenia. Freud himself knew almost nothing about the disease and avoided seeing patients who had it. In a 1907 letter, he acknowledged: "I seldom see dements [dementia praecox, or schizophrenia] and hardly ever see other severe types of psychosis." Four years later, he wrote: "I do not like these patients [with schizophrenia]. . . . I feel them to be so far distant from me and from everything human." Any mental health professional who still professes Freudian beliefs about schizophrenia should be regarded as incompetent.

Bad Families: In addition to Freudian theories about bad mothers, in the 1950s a series of theories about bad families was put forward to explain the cause of schizophrenia. Individuals associated with these theories included Theodore Lidz, Gregory Bateson, and Don Jackson. These family interaction theories were tested in controlled studies and found to be wrong, and have been discarded. An offshoot of the bad families theories was what was called "expressed emotion." It postulated that families who were overly critical, hostile, and overinvolved, and who overidentified with the family member with schizophrenia, caused the person to relapse. Dozens of papers and even a few books were published on expressed emotion in the 1980s and 1990s, but the theory faded away when careful studies showed that it had no scientific basis.

Although the concept of expressed emotion has quietly passed away, does it have anything useful to teach us? People with schizophrenia do best in situations where people are calm and communicate clearly and directly. The attributes of the right attitude (sense of perspective, acceptance of the illness, family balance, and expectations that are realistic), discussed in chapter 11, are the antithesis of high expressed emotions; insofar as families are striving to achieve these, they should not worry about expressed emotion.

In addition to lacking any scientific basis, both the bad mothers and bad families theories of schizophrenia fell victim to common sense. Any parent who has raised a child knows that parents are not powerful enough to cause a disease like schizophrenia simply by favoring one child over another or giving the child inconsistent messages. Furthermore, families in which one child had developed schizophrenia usually contained one or more other children who were perfectly normal; they stood as the final refutation of these theories.

Bad Cultures: In addition to bad mothers and bad families, a few individuals have proposed that bad cultures may cause schizophrenia. This idea was first developed by anthropologists Margaret Mead and Ruth Benedict in the 1930s. In more recent years it has found expression among some intellectuals, most of whom have become enamored with sociology, socialism, or both.

One such writer was Christopher Lasch, who in his 1979 book, *The Culture of Narcissism,* claimed that psychoses are "in some sense the characteristic expression of a given culture." He also quoted Jule Henry, who wrote that "psychosis is the final outcome of all that is wrong with a culture." Another example of this theory is included in the 1984 book *Not in Our Genes* by R. C. Lewontin, Steven Rose, and Leon Kamin who, in the Preface, claim that "we share a commitment to the prospect of the creation of a more socially just—a socialist— society." After disparaging biological research on schizophrenia, the authors write: "An adequate theory of schizophrenia must understand what it is about the social and cultural environment that pushes some categories of people toward manifesting schizophrenic symptoms." The social and cultural environment, they believe, produce biological changes in the brain that "might be the reflections or correspondents of that schizophrenia with the brain." Such theorizing, atavistic in view of contemporary knowledge, is now heard only rarely.

Recommended Further Reading

Bakhshi, K., and S. A. Chance. "The Neuropathology of Schizophrenia: A Selective Review of Past Studies and Emerging Themes in Brain Structure and Cytoarchitecture." *Neuroscience* 303 (2015): 82-102.

Carlson, A. "The Dopamine Theory Revisited." In S. R. Hirsch and D. R. Weinberger, eds. *Schizophrenia.* Oxford: Blackwell Science, 1995.

Dickerson, F. B., C. Stallings, A. Origoni, et al. "Markers of Gluten Sensitivity and Celiac Disease in Recent-onset Psychosis and Multi-episode Schizophrenia." *Biological Psychiatry* 68 (2010): 100–104.

Dickerson, F. B., J. J. Boronow, C. Stallings, et al. "Association of Serum Antibodies to Herpes Simplex Virus 1 with Cognitive Deficits in Individuals with Schizophrenia." *Archives of General Psychiatry* 60 (2003): 466–72.

Dickerson, F., Stallings, C., Origoni, A. et al. "Inflammatory Markers in Recent Onset Psychosis and Chronic Schizophrenia." *Schizophrenia Bulletin* 42 (2016): 134-141.

Ellison-Wright, I., and E. Bullmore. "Anatomy of Bipolar Disorder and Schizophrenia: A Meta-Analysis." *Schizophrenia Research* 117 (2010): 1–12.

English, J. A., K. Pennington, M. J. Dunn, et al. "The Neuroproteomics of Schizophrenia." *Biological Psychiatry* 69 (2011): 163–72.

Garver, D. L. "Neuroendocrine Findings in the Schizophrenias." *Endocrinology of Neuropsychiatric Disorders* 17 (1988): 103–9.

Haijma, S. V., N. Van Haren, W. Cahn, et al. "Brain Volumes in Schizophrenia: A Meta-Analysis in Over 18,000 Subjects." *Schizophrenia Bulletin* 39 (2013): 1129-1138.

Harrison, P. J., and D. R. Weinberger. "Schizophrenia Genes, Gene Expression, and Neuropathology: On the Matter of Their Convergence." *Molecular Psychiatry* 10 (2005): 40–68.

Kirkpatrick, B. and B.J. Miller, "Inflammation and Schizophrenia," *Schizophrenia Bulletin* 39 (2013): 1174-1179.

Knable, M. B., J. E. Kleinman, and D. R. Weinberger. "Neurobiology of Schizophrenia." In A. F. Schatzberg and C. B. Nemoroff, eds., *Textbook of Psychopharmacology*, 2nd ed., Washington, D.C.: American Psychiatric Association Press, 1998, pp. 589–607.

Lieberman, J., and R. Murray, eds. *Comprehensive Care of Schizophrenia*. London: Martin Dunitz Publishers, 2000.

McGrath, J. J., T. H. Burne, F. Féron, et al. "Developmental Vitamin D Deficiency and Risk of Schizophrenia: A 10-Year Update." *Schizophrenia Bulletin* 36 (2010): 1073–78.

Mesholam-Gately, R. I., A. J. Giuliano, K. P. Goff, et al. "Neurocognition in First-Episode Schizophrenia: A Meta-Analytic Review." *Neuropsychology* 23 (2009): 315–36.

Mortensen, P. B., C. B. Pedersen, T. Westergaard, et al. "Effects of Family History and Place and Season of Birth on the Risk of Schizophrenia." *New England Journal of Medicine* 340 (1999): 603–8:44:973–982.

Muller N., M. Schwarz, "Immune System and Schizophrenia," *Current Immunology Review* 6 (2010): 213–220.

Muller, N. "Inflammation in Schizophrenia: Pathogenetic Aspects and Therapeutic Considerations," *Schizophrenia Bulletin* (2018): 44:973–982.

Oken, R. J., and M. Schulzer. "At Issue: Schizophrenia and Rheumatoid

Arthritis: The Negative Association Revisited." *Schizophrenia Bulletin* 25 (1999): 625–38.

Owen, F., and M. D. C. Simpson. "The Neurochemistry of Schizophrenia." In S. R. Hirsch and D. R. Weinberger, eds. *Schizophrenia*. Oxford: Blackwell Science, 1995.

Torrey, E. F. "Are We Overestimating the Genetic Contribution to Schizophrenia?" *Schizophrenia Bulletin* 18 (1992): 159–70.

Torrey, E. F. "Studies of Individuals with Schizophrenia Never Treated with Antipsychotic Medications: A Review." *Schizophrenia Bulletin* 58 (2002): 101–15.

Torrey, E. F., and R. H. Yolken. "Familial and Genetic Mechanisms in Schizophrenia." *Brain Research Reviews* 31 (2000): 113–17.

Torrey, E. F., B. M. Barci, M. J. Webster, et al. "Neurochemical Markers for Schizophrenia, Bipolar Disorder, and Major Depression in Postmortem Brains." *Biological Psychiatry* 57 (2005): 252–60.

Torrey, E. F., J. J. Bartko, and R. H. Yolken. "*Toxoplasma gondii* and Other Risk Factors for Schizophrenia: An Update." *Schizophrenia Bulletin* 38 (2012): 642–47.

Torrey, E. F., J. Miller, R. Rawlings, et al. "Seasonality of Births in Schizophrenia and Bipolar Disorder: A Review of the Literature." *Schizophrenia Research* 28 (1997): 1–38.

Torrey, E. F. and R. H. Yolken, "Schizophrenia and Infections: The Eyes Have It." *Schizophrenia Bulletin* 43 (2017): 247–252.

Weinberger, D. R. "Schizophrenia as a Neurodevelopment Disorder." In S. R. Hirsch and D. R. Weinberger, eds. *Schizophrenia*. Oxford: Blackwell Science, 1995.

Weinberger, D. R., "Future of Days Past: Neurodevelopment and Schizophrenia." *Schizophrenia Bulletin* 43 (2017): 1164–1168.

Yolken, R. H., and E. F. Torrey, "Are Some Cases of Psychosis Caused by Microbial Agents? A Review of the Evidence." *Molecular Psychiatry* 13 (2008): 470–79.

Yolken, R. H., F. B. Dickerson, and E. F. Torrey. "Toxoplasma and Schizophrenia." *Parasite Immunology* 31 (2009): 706–15.

Yolken, R. H., H. Karlsson, F. Yee, et al. "Endogenous Retroviruses and Schizophrenia." *Brain Research Reviews* 31 (2000): 193–99.

6

The Treatment of Schizophrenia: Getting Started

To lighten the affliction of insanity by all human means is not to restore the greatest of the divine gifts; and those who devote themselves to the task do not pretend that it is. They find their sustainment and reward in the substitution of humanity for brutality, kindness for maltreatment, peace for raging fury; in the acquisition of love instead of hatred; and in the acknowledgment that, from such treatment improvement, and hope of final restoration, will come if hope be possible.

Charles Dickens, Household Words, *1852*

Contrary to the popular stereotype, schizophrenia is an eminently treatable disease. That is not to say it is a curable disease, and the two should not be confused. Successful treatment means the control of symptoms, whereas cure means the permanent removal of their causes. Curing schizophrenia will not become possible until we understand its causes; in the meantime we must continue improving its treatment.

The best disease model to explain schizophrenia is diabetes, a disease that has many similarities. Both schizophrenia and diabetes have childhood and adult forms, both probably have more than one cause; both have relapses and remissions in a course that often lasts over many years; and both can usually be well controlled, but not cured, by drugs. Just as we don't talk of curing diabetes but rather of controlling its symptoms and allowing the person with diabetes to lead a comparatively normal life, so we should also do with schizophrenia.

How to Find a Good Doctor

There is no easy solution to the problem of finding a good doctor, a task that usually falls to the friends and relatives of the person with schizophrenia. There are relatively few doctors in the United States who either know anything about, or have any interest in, treating schizophrenia. This is both shocking and sad, since it is one of the most important chronic diseases in the world. In Europe it is somewhat easier to find a good doctor.

Since schizophrenia is a true biological disease, and since drugs are the mainstay of treatment, there is no avoiding the doctor-finding issue. If schizophrenia is to be properly treated, sooner or later a doctor will need to be involved. He or she will be needed not only to prescribe the proper drugs but also to do an initial diagnostic workup, including laboratory tests, in order to rule out other diseases that may be masquerading as schizophrenia. Before the schizophrenia is treated, one had better be certain that it is not really a brain tumor or herpes encephalitis in disguise. Only a doctor can ascertain this.

The best way to find a good doctor for schizophrenia or any other disease is to ask others in the medical profession whom they would send their own family to if they had a similar problem. Doctors and nurses know who the good doctors are and pass the information freely among themselves; often they will tell you if you ask. If your brother-in-law has a sister who is a nurse, all the better. Use every contact and every relative you have, however distant, to locate and identify competent doctors who may know something about schizophrenia. It is an appropriate time to cash in all your IOUs, for the information is invaluable and may save you months of searching.

Another way to find a good doctor is through other families who have a family member with schizophrenia. They can often provide a quick rundown of the local resources and save weeks of hunting and false starts. Sharing this information is one of the most valuable assets of local chapters of NAMI and is an important reason to join. (Local and state chapters of NAMI can be contacted through NAMI, as listed in appendix B.)

Distinctly *un*helpful in searching for a good doctor are referral lists maintained by local medical societies or the local chapters of the American Psychiatric Association. Anyone can call these organizations and obtain three names. The names, however, are taken from a rotating list of those doctors who are looking for additional patients. Since any doctor who wishes to pay the annual dues can belong to these organizations, there is no screening or ascertainment of quality of any kind. Even those doctors who are under investigation for malpractice will continue to be listed by such organizations until they are specifically removed from membership, which is an all-too-rare occurrence. Thus, referral lists from medical and psychiatric societies are really no better than picking a name at random from the physicians' list in the Yellow Pages.

What should one look for in a good doctor who can treat schizophrenia? Ideally he/she should combine technical competence with an interest in the disease and empathy with its sufferers. Training in psychiatry or neurology is helpful but not mandatory; there are some internists and family practitioners who have an interest in schizophrenia and can treat it very competently. As a general rule younger physicians who have been trained recently are more likely to view schizophrenia as a biological disease. However, there are major exceptions to this rule: some older practitioners who will tell you, "I've said all along it was a real disease," and a few younger practitioners who still know remarkably little about it.

Another important quality possessed by doctors who are good in treating schizophrenia is an ability to work with the patient, the family, and other members of the treatment team. Psychologists, psychiatric nurses, social workers, case managers, rehabilitation specialists, and other members of the team are all part of the therapeutic process. Physicians who are reluctant to work with the family or as team members are not good doctors for treating schizophrenia no matter how skilled they may be in psychopharmacology.

In trying to find a good doctor it is perfectly legitimate to ask questions such as "What do you think causes schizophrenia?" "What has been your experience with clozapine?" "What do you think about risperidone (or any other drug)?" "How important is psychotherapy in treating schizophrenia?" Such open-ended questions will quickly elicit the relative biological orientation of the doctor as well as some sense of how well the person is keeping up with new treatments. As families and patients become increasingly knowledgeable and sophisticated about the treatment of schizophrenia, it is becoming common to find that they know as much (or more) than some of the treating doctors. The ultimate goal in looking for a good doctor, then, is to find one who is knowledgeable and who also views individuals with schizophrenia, in the words of one psychiatrist, "as a suffering patient, not a defective creation of abstruse, mystical, psychic body parts."

How important is it for the physician to be "board eligible" or "board certified" in his/her specialty? "Board eligible" means that the physician has completed an approved residency program in that specialty. "Board certified" means that the physician has taken and passed an examination in the specialty. Such board examinations are completely optional and are not required for licensure or for membership in any professional organization. They simply mean that the doctor had the theoretical knowledge required to be competent in that specialty at the time he/she took the examination. They do not indicate whether or not the doctor has kept up-to-date since the examination, and for that reason there is relatively little relationship between board certification and competency. All medical specialists should be required to become recertified by examination every five years. Until that time comes, families should give relatively little weight to selecting a "board certified" psychiatrist over a "board eligible" one unless all other things are equal.

What about international medical graduates? Psychiatry has attracted more international medical graduates than any other medical specialty in the United States, and in many states these psychiatrists constitute a majority of all psychiatrists in mental health centers and state hospitals. A 1996 survey reported that international medical graduates were almost twice as likely as American medical graduates to work in public psychiatric settings (42 percent vs. 22 percent) and that they saw almost twice as many patients with psychosis (20 percent vs. 11 percent). International medical graduates are therefore the backbone of American public psychiatry, and without them the disaster of deinstitutionalization would have been even worse than it has been.

On the plus side, some international medical graduates are among the most caring and competent psychiatrists I have known. On the minus side, other international medical graduates range from being mediocre to incompetent. The two foreign medical schools that contributed the greatest number of psychiatrists to American state hospitals both have had very low pass rates on the Education Council for Foreign Medical Graduates (ECFMG) examination. Some of the international graduates who cannot pass basic licensing exams are given special exemptions by the state to practice only in the state institutions. In essence, the state is saying that it does not consider them competent to treat the "worried well" in private practice but will accept them if they treat the truly sick in the state hospitals.

The most disturbing aspect of utilizing large numbers of international medical graduates to treat patients with schizophrenia is the inevitable difficulty in communication. Verbal language skill is only one part of this; beyond it are many other levels of communication that involve nonverbal language, shared ideals and values, and other components of what is called culture. Communication between a psychiatrist and a person with schizophrenia is difficult enough even when they share a common language and culture; when they do not share these things, communication becomes almost impossible. Delusions must be assessed in the context of the patient's culture. Affect that may appear appropriate within one culture context may be inappropriate within another. The evaluation of subtle disorders of thinking assumes a complete command of the idioms and metaphors of a language. One psychiatrist, for example, argued for an increase in medication for a patient who complained about "butterflies in her stomach." Another used as evidence of a patient's delusions the fact that she had talked of "babies coming from birds." "Do you mean storks?" asked the psychologist present. "Yes, that's the one," exclaimed the psychiatrist. "Isn't that crazy!" Still another foreign-trained psychiatrist was observed asking a patient the following proverb during a diagnostic interview: "What does it mean, a stitch in time gathers no moss?" That kind of question inspires neither confidence nor clarity of thought in a person with schizophrenia.

What about using nonphysicians to treat schizophrenia? In fact psychologists, nurses, social workers, case managers, rehabilitation specialists, and other nonphysicians treat people with schizophrenia regularly and are often the primary contact on the treatment team. It is not uncommon to have the physician on the team merely be the manager of medication and play a relatively small role in the overall treatment plan.

The other aspect of using nonphysicians to treat schizophrenia is using them to prescribe medication. In many states physician assistants and nurse practitioners are already licensed to prescribe medications. Psychologists are now licensed to prescribe medication in Hawaii, New Mexico, and Louisiana and are lobbying for similar privileges in other states; this, not surprisingly, is being vigorously opposed by psychiatrists. With proper training in the use of medications and appropriate supervision, any one of these nonphysician groups can competently treat routine cases of schizophrenia while referring difficult diagnostic or therapeutic problems on to a supervising psychiatrist. It is extremely difficult to attract psychiatrists to work in state mental hospitals or public clinics, or in rural areas. Utilizing these nonphysician groups is one reasonable solution to the chronic shortage of psychiatrists in these settings.

To those looking for a good doctor to treat schizophrenia, one final word of caution. Doctors are human beings and, as such, run a wide range of personality types. Throughout the medical profession can be found some physicians who are dishonest, mentally ill, addicted to alcohol or drugs, or sociopathic, or who have some combination of the above. I have a sense that psychiatry attracts more than its share of such physicians, often because the physician has become interested in his/her own mental aberrations. Thus, one should not make an absolute assumption that physicians who treat persons with schizophrenia are themselves beyond question. If the physician seems strange to you, move on quickly to another. There *are* occasionally strange birds in the psychiatric aviary.

What Is an Adequate Diagnostic Workup?

In its full-blown stages, most cases of schizophrenia are not difficult to diagnose. Auditory hallucinations and/or delusional thinking are among the commonest and most prominent symptoms, and more than three-quarters of all patients will have one or the other. Various kinds of thinking disorders become evident in simple conversation (e.g., thought blocking) or on asking the patient to give the meaning of proverbs (e.g., inability to think abstractly). Emotions may be blunted or inappropriate, and the individual's behavior may vary from unusual to catatonic to bizarre.

For a person with the symptoms of schizophrenia who has become ill for the first time, what kind of diagnostic tests and procedures are appropriate? Most public psychiatric hospitals, and many private ones as well, offer cursory diagnostic workups, and there is no question that some patients are diagnosed with schizophrenia who have the diseases described in chapter 3. Given this fact, what should be done diagnostically to maximize the chances of uncovering all potentially reversible diseases masquerading as schizophrenia? The following diagnostic workup is what I would personally want to happen if I or a member of my family were admitted to a hospital with symptoms of schizophrenia for the first time.

History and Mental Status Examination: These are routinely done for all psychiatric admissions but often incompletely so. Visual hallucinations, headaches, and recent head injury should be specifically asked about. A general review of organ systems other than the central nervous system may turn up diseases masquerading as schizophrenia (e.g., abdominal pains suggesting acute intermittent porphyria; urinary incontinence suggesting normal pressure hydrocephalus). Perhaps the single most important question the examining physician can ask is:

"What drugs are you using?" It is a two-pronged question intended to elicit information about street drug use, which may be producing or exacerbating the psychiatric symptoms, as well as prescription drug use, which may be producing psychiatric symptoms as a side effect (see chapter 3). Since acutely psychotic patients often cannot give a coherent history, family members and friends play an essential role in providing the needed information.

Physical and Neurological Examinations: These are also often done superficially, with the consequence that many medical and neurological diseases are missed. A careful neurological examination of patients with schizophrenia will elicit abnormal findings in a significant number of them (see chapter 5). A useful part of the neurological exam, which can be taught to nonphysicians who must screen psychiatric patients, is a series of pencil-and-paper tests such as write-a-sentence and draw-a-clock; as Dr. Robert Taylor described in *Psychological Masquerade: Distinguishing Psychological from Organic Disorders,* such tests can help identify patients with other brain diseases, such as brain tumors or Huntington's disease, who may initially present with schizophrenia-like symptoms.

Basic Laboratory Work: Blood Count, Blood Chemical Screen, and Urinalysis: These are also routine everywhere, but abnormal results are sometimes not noticed or followed up. The blood count may elicit unexpected findings suggesting such diseases as pernicious anemia, AIDS, or lead intoxication. Blood chemical screens have become widespread and do many different tests on a single sample of blood. These normally include tests that may screen endocrine or metabolic imbalances. If a thyroid function test is not included in the routine blood chemical screen, it should be ordered separately. A routine test to screen for syphilis should also be included. Urinalysis should include screening tests to detect street drugs in the urine. A useful and cost-effective diagnostic algorithm for detecting physical disease in psychiatric patients has been developed by Dr. Harold Sox and colleagues. It is also useful at this time to get a baseline electrocardiogram (EKG); since some drugs used to treat schizophrenia affect the heart, having a baseline EKG done prior to starting medication may be helpful in future assessments of such side effects.

Psychological Tests: The choice of psychological tests varies from hospital to hospital and depends on the psychologist. Such tests can be extremely useful in making the diagnosis of schizophrenia in early or borderline cases and can also point the examiner away from schizophrenia and toward other brain diseases. Acutely agitated patients frequently are unable to concentrate long enough to do psychological tests.

MRI Scan: Magnetic resonance imaging (MRI) scans are now widely available and, with improving technology, should become less expensive. Computerized tomography (CT) scans can also be used if MRI scans are not available, but they are much less sensitive for detecting most brain pathology. Many, but not all psychiatrists, believe that an MRI scan should be done on every individual who presents with psychosis for the first time. Diseases that mimic schizophrenia and that may be detected by MRI scans include brain tumors, Huntington's disease, Wilson's disease, metachromatic leukodystrophy, sarcoidosis, subdural hematomas, Kuf's disease, viral encephalitis, and aqueductal stenosis. For a person who has had symptoms of schizophrenia for many years, a scan probably is not justified diagnostically, for the diseases the procedure is capable of detecting would have become evident over the years because of other signs or symptoms.

Lumbar Puncture: Despite the stereotype to the contrary, lumbar punctures are simple procedures producing little more discomfort than the drawing of blood. Cerebrospinal fluid is withdrawn by a needle from a sac in the lower back; since the sac is connected to fluid channels in the brain, examination of the cerebrospinal fluid often provides clues (e.g., antibodies to viruses) about events in the brain. Lumbar punctures are routinely used in the diagnosis of brain diseases, such as multiple sclerosis, and probably will become routine for schizophrenia in the future. They are capable of detecting a variety of diseases, especially viral diseases of the central nervous system. Indications for their use in patients admitted for a first episode of schizophrenia include the following:

INDICATIONS FOR LUMBAR PUNCTURE IN FIRST-EPISODE SCHIZOPHRENIA

1. Patient complains of headache (20 percent do) or stiff neck with nausea or a fever
2. Rapid onset of psychotic symptoms
3. Fluctuations in patient's orientation (e.g., patient knows where he is one day but does not know the next day)
4. Visual or olfactory (smell) hallucinations
5. Neurological signs or symptoms suggesting central nervous system disease other than schizophrenia (e.g., nystagmus of the eyes in which the gaze moves rapidly from side to side)
6. Concurrent or recent history of flu or fever

Lumbar punctures in patients with schizophrenia are relatively free of side effects, since persons with schizophrenia are especially immune to getting post–lumbar puncture headaches that occur in approximately one-third of people who do not have schizophrenia. The utility of routine diagnostic use of lumbar puncture and CT scans was illustrated by a German study of one hundred thirty newly admitted patients with symptoms of schizophrenia; twelve cases of neurological diseases were found among the one hundred thirty patients, including three cases of AIDS encephalitis, two cases of encephalitis caused by other viruses, two cases of cerebral syphilis, one case of Lyme disease, and one case of multiple sclerosis.

Electroencephalogram (EEG): The indications for an EEG are almost identical to those for lumbar puncture, and in fact the two are often ordered together. I personally believe that both the lumbar puncture and the EEG should be routinely included in the diagnostic workup of any young adult presenting with symptoms of psychosis for the first time. An EEG should always be ordered if there is a history of meningitis or encephalitis, birth complications, or severe head injury; it should be mandatory for any patient who has had episodic attacks of psychosis with a sudden onset. An EEG may detect temporal-lobe epilepsy, which sometimes mimics schizophrenia.

To be most useful, an EEG should be done using nasopharyngeal leads (electrodes are put into the mouth as well as on the scalp) and be done after the person has been kept up all night (sleep-deprived); the diagnostic rewards for doing this more sophisticated type of EEG are appreciable. EEGs are completely harmless procedures that simply measure electrical impulses in the brain; there are no known side effects or harmful effects of any kind.

Other Tests: Other diagnostic tests may be indicated by specific findings but are not routine. Newer brain scans can be done in a variety of ways (e.g., functional MRI scans, PET scans), but their use is still mostly for research purposes. The dexamethasone suppression test (DST) was at one time thought to be useful to differentiate certain kinds of patients, but it has not proven to be so. As technology improves, the diagnostic workup of schizophrenia will become increasingly complex and sophisticated.

Markers of Inflammation: The most recent addition to a complete diagnostic work-up for schizophrenia is markers of inflammation. As discussed in chapter 5, evidence has accumulated that many individuals with schizophrenia and other types of psychoses have elevated markers of inflammation in their blood and cerebrospinal fluid. Since blood is already being collected from the patient for other diagnostic tests, it seems reasonable to use it to also assess for inflammation. At this time, the easiest inflammatory marker to assess is the C-reactive protein (CRP) since it is also used by physicians to assess inflammation in cardiac and other conditions. Thus, it is available in most laboratories and provides a measure of general inflammation at the time of assessment. If the CRP is significantly elevated, it might suggest the addition of an anti-inflammatory medication, as described in chapter 7. It is likely in the near future that a battery of inflammatory markers will routinely be measured in individuals with first-onset psychosis, including some cytokines, but the identification of the most useful markers is not yet known.

Hospitalization: Voluntary and Involuntary

In most cases, persons *acutely* ill with schizophrenia need to be hospitalized. Such hospitalization accomplishes several things. Most important, it enables mental health professionals to observe the person in a controlled setting. Laboratory tests can be performed to rule out other medical illnesses that may be causing the symptoms, psychological testing can be done, and medication can be started in an environment in which trained staff can watch for side effects. In addition, the hospitalization often provides the family with a respite from what have often been harrowing days and nights leading up to the acute illness.

Hospitalization is also frequently necessary to protect patients. Some will try to injure themselves or others because of their illness (e.g., their voices tell them to do so). Ben Silcock, a young man with schizophrenia, who while acutely psychotic jumped into the London zoo's lion enclosure and was almost killed, stated it as follows: "The hospital becomes a good place to be; for after being so shaken up it's vital to be in a situation where there is some protection." For this reason most hospitals utilize a locked ward for acutely agitated patients, and its use is often needed. Even in a locked setting the person occasionally may be dangerous and require additional restraints. These may include wrist or ankle restraints (usually made of leather), a special jacket that keeps the arms next to the body (the famous straitjacket of popular lore), or a seclusion room. None of these measures should be necessary for more than a few hours if the person is being properly medicated. It is currently fashionable to condemn locked wards and all use of restraints as "barbaric" and antiquated; the people who make such statements have usually never been faced with the task of providing care for persons with acute schizophrenia. Someday we will arrive at the point where medications are instantly effective in acutely disturbed patients and restraint is not necessary, but we have not reached that nirvana yet.

There are ancillary benefits of hospitalization for persons with schizophrenia. Well-functioning psychiatric units have group meetings for the patients; this often allows each of them to see that his or her experience is not unique. Occupational therapy, recreational activities, and other forms of group interaction often accomplish the same thing. For someone who has been acutely ill and who has experienced many of the disturbances described in chapter 1, it is usually a relief to learn that other people have experienced them too. None of the above activities are likely to be of much benefit, however, unless the person is also being properly medicated to relieve his or her acute symptoms.

There are several different types of hospitals available in which people can be treated for schizophrenia. State psychiatric hospitals were used most commonly in the past, but that has changed dramatically. The driving force behind the phasing-out of state psychiatric hospitals, as will be discussed in chapter 14, has been the federal Institution for Mental Disease (IMD) Medicaid exclusion, whereby states are not eligible for federal reimbursement for most state hospital patients. The states therefore shut down state hospitals and force the patients to seek admission in general hospitals and other "semihospital" facilities that are eligible for federal Medicaid reimbursement. This effectively shifts the fiscal burden from the state government to the federal government.

This game of musical psychiatric beds may be good for states economically, but it is not necessarily good for patients clinically. Many general hospitals are not staffed to be able to care for individuals acutely ill with schizophrenia, and there are predictable untoward consequences. Care in private hospitals also runs a broad gamut, from very good to abysmal; many private hospitals run by for-profit hospital chains are notorious for keeping patients for whatever length of time their insurance benefits permit, then declaring them well and summarily discharging them. A 2002 study comparing nonprofit and for-profit psychiatric inpatient units found that the nonprofit units were superior in almost all aspects of psychiatric care.

In looking for a hospital for someone with schizophrenia, then, shop carefully. The most important factor by far is the competence of the treating psychiatrist. State hospitals, Veterans Administration (VA) hospitals, general hospitals, university hospitals, and private hospitals all may vary from very good to very bad. In contrast to most other diseases, paying more money does not necessarily buy you better care for schizophrenia.

A measure of hospital quality that previously was considered to be useful was accreditation by the Joint Commission on Accreditation of Healthcare Organizations (JCAHO). At the invitation of a hospital, JCAHO sends a survey team to evaluate it, as well as provide consultation and education. The survey focuses on patient care and services but also includes such related issues as the therapeutic environment, safety of the patient, quality of staffing, and administration of the hospital. The survey team then recommends that the hospital receive full three-year accreditation, full accreditation with a contingency (which may necessitate a follow-up inspection to ensure that the contingency has been corrected), or no accreditation. Full accreditation by JCAHO at one time was thought to signify that the hospital was a good one, although since the accreditation was for the hospital as a whole, individual wards in an accredited hospital still may have been below standard. In more recent years JCAHO accreditation has itself been discredited because of what one federal report labeled the "cozy relationship" between the hospitals and the privately run JCAHO. Hospitals pay many thousands of dollars for the survey and they expect to be accredited; JCAHO consequently accredits many hospitals despite evidence of poor patient care. JCAHO accreditation can therefore no longer be relied on as a measure of quality.

One aspect of hospitalization that has changed markedly in recent years is the length of hospitalizations. In the past, hospitalizations for schizophrenia were usually measured in weeks or even months. However, with the pressure of managed care and insurance companies, the average length of stay has decreased dramatically and is now measured in days. In 1993 the average hospital stay for acute psychiatric care was thirteen days, but by 2009 it had decreased to nine days. This has become a tremendous problem for both patients and their families because the patients are often being discharged prematurely.

Ideally, people with schizophrenia will recognize when they are becoming sick and then voluntarily seek treatment for their sickness. Unfortunately, as described in chapter 1, this is not often the case. Schizophrenia is a disease of the brain, the body organ charged with the responsibility of recognizing sickness and the need for treatment—the same organ that is sick. Out of this unfortunate circumstance arises the frequent need for persons to be committed to psychiatric treatment settings against their will. Inpatient commitment will be discussed here, and outpatient commitment, another and less restrictive form of assisted treatment, in chapter 10.

All laws governing commitment of psychiatric patients are state laws, not federal laws. Therefore commitment laws vary from state to state, especially those governing long-term commitment. Between 1970 and 1980 there was a broad shift in the United States to change state laws to make it more difficult to involuntarily hospitalize individuals with psychiatric illnesses. The effect of this shift was to make it practically impossible in many states to hospitalize an individual with schizophrenia unless that person was shown to be an immediate danger to self or others. Because of the problems produced by these stringent laws, there is growing sentiment to modify the laws so that such persons can be involuntarily hospitalized and treated.

Legally there are two rationales for the commitment of mental patients. The first is referred to as *parens patriae*, which is the right of the state to act as parent and protect a disabled person; it arose from the belief that the king was the father of all his subjects. This may be invoked when people are so disabled that they do not recognize their own need for treatment or cannot provide for their own basic needs because of the symptoms of their illness. The second legal justification for commitment is the right of the state to protect other people from a person who is dangerous. This is used when persons, because of their mental illness, are dangerous to others.

There are also two kinds of commitment—emergency and long-term. The basic purpose of commitment laws is to, when appropriate, place persons who are psychiatrically ill in treatment in order to provide them with needed care and to prevent harm to themselves or others. State laws vary, but generally this can be done as follows:

1. A petition for emergency commitment of the person thought to be psychiatrically ill must be initiated. In most states this can be done by one of several persons; for example, Tennessee allows petitions to be filed by "[t]he parent, legal guardian, legal custodian, conservator, spouse, or a responsible relative of the person alleged to be in need of care and treatment, a licensed physician, a licensed psychologist who meets [certain requirements], a health or public welfare officer, an of-

ficer authorized to make arrests in the state, or the chief officer of a facility that the person is in[.]" In many states, any person can initiate a petition for emergency commitment.

2. The person initiating the petition asks a physician (not necessarily a psychiatrist) to examine the person for whom commitment is sought. Some states require two physicians to be examiners, whereas others allow psychologists. If the examiner(s) concludes that the person is mentally ill and meets the grounds for commitment in that state, then the examiner's report is attached to the petition and it is filed. In many states, an affidavit from a physician who has recently examined the person may be substituted for this examination.

3. The examination may take place in a doctor's office, mental health facility, or other location.

4. If the person for whom commitment is sought refuses to be examined, many states have a provision for the petitioner to file a sworn written statement or petition. In Nevada, for example, this says, there is "probable cause to believe that the person has a mental illness, and because of that illness, is likely to harm himself or herself or others if allowed his or her liberty."

5. Once the petition has been filed, the person must appear for examination by a physician. If the person refuses, a law enforcement official can bring him or her to a hospital for the examination.

6. Alternatively, if a person appears to be mentally ill and is acting strangely or dangerously in public, a police officer, sheriff, mental health crisis team, etc., can bring the person to the hospital for examination by a physician.

7. The examining physician at the hospital decides on the basis of his/her examination whether the person meets the criteria for commitment in that state. If the person does, emergency commitment is effected and the person is kept at the hospital. If not, the person is released.

8. An emergency commitment lasts for seventy-two hours in most states, not including weekends and holidays. At the end of that period the person must be released unless either the director of the hospital or the family has filed a petition with the court asking for longer-term commitment. If this has been filed, then the person can be held until the hearing.

9. The hearing for long-term commitment may be held in a room in the hospital or in a courtroom. In most states, the person alleged to be mentally ill is expected to be present unless a physician testifies that the person's presence would be detrimental to his/her mental state. The person is represented by a lawyer appointed by the state if necessary; normal judicial rules of evidence and due process apply, although such hearings are often less formal than other court proceedings. Testimony may be taken from the examining physician, from family members, and from the person alleged to be mentally ill.

10. The hearing is held before a mental health commission, judge, or similar judicial authority depending on the state. In some states the person has the right to a jury trial if he/she so wishes.

The major differences in commitment procedures among states are the grounds that are used for commitment and the standard of proof. In states that utilize only dangerousness to self or others and define dangerousness stringently, it is generally more difficult to get a commitment than in states that define dangerousness vaguely (for example, Texas law previously said a mentally ill person could be committed "for his own welfare and protection or the protection of others"). Similarly, in states in which "gravely disabled" or "in need of treatment" are grounds for commitment by themselves, it should be easier to get a person with a severe mental illness committed for treatment.

All states have a provision for the involuntary commitment of someone who is "gravely disabled" except for Alabama, Maryland, New York, and the District of Columbia. The following 17 states also allow the commitment of a person who is in "need of treatment": Alaska, Arizona, Arkansas, Colorado, Idaho, Illinois, Indiana, Michigan, Mississippi, Missouri, New Hampshire, North Carolina, North Dakota, Oklahoma, South Carolina, Washington and Wisconsin.

Probably the most important variables in determining how easy or difficult it is to obtain a legal commitment to get a mentally ill person into treatment are the specific judge involved and the local community standards. As lawyers well know, laws are written one way but can be interpreted in many ways, and this is especially true for laws concerning psychiatric commitment. Thus, in the same state one judge may interpret dangerousness much more stringently than another. Similarly, what for one judge is "clear and convincing evidence" might not be at all persuasive for another. Community standards vary as well, with some localities more inclined to "lock up all those crazies," whereas others in the same state may be reluctant to commit people unless they have completed a dangerous act. Also important is the current local milieu. For example, if the local paper reports that a former psychiatric patient has recently been accused of murder, the tendency may be to commit everyone with acute symptoms. If, on the other hand, the local newspaper is doing an exposé on the poor conditions in the state hospital, the tendency may be to not commit anybody unless absolutely necessary.

Individual horror stories abound of clearly psychotic persons who could not be involuntarily placed in treatment because of the stringent interpretation given to "dangerousness to self or others" by law enforcement and judicial officials. In 1984 in the District of Columbia, I personally examined a homeless woman who was blatantly hallucinating and had been carrying an axe around town; the police refused to take her to a hospital for possible commitment because they said she had not *yet* done anything to demonstrate dangerousness. In Wisconsin "a man barricaded himself in his house and sat with a rifle in his lap muttering 'Kill, kill, kill.' A judge ruled that the man was not demonstrably violent enough to qualify for involuntary commitment."

At another commitment hearing in Wisconsin, a man with schizophrenia, already mute and refusing to eat food or to bathe, was observed to be eating feces while being held in jail. He was released because such behavior did not qualify as dangerous. The dialogue at the commitment hearing included the following:

Public defender: "Doctor, would the eating of fecal material on one occasion by an individual pose a serious risk of harm to that person?"

Doctor: "It is certainly not edible material. . . . It contains elements that are considered harmful or unnecessary."

Public defender: "But, Doctor, you cannot state whether the consumption of such material on one occasion would invariably harm a person?"

Doctor: "Certainly not on one occasion."

The public defender then moved to dismiss the action on the grounds that the patient was in no imminent danger of physical injury or dying, and the case was dismissed.

It is such absurd and inhumane legal decisions as these that spurred a continuing movement toward broadening grounds for commitment. The State of Washington was one of the first to move in this direction in 1979, and since then several others have followed. Currently, about one-half of the states have incorporated some form of need for treatment or deteriorating clinical condition as criteria for involuntary treatment.

In 1983 the American Psychiatric Association proposed a model commitment statute that would allow psychiatrically ill persons to be placed in treatment if their behavior indicated "significant deterioration" of their psychiatric state and they were clearly in need of treatment. I believe it is a good model for state laws. It permits the treatment of a relapsing patient *before* the person has had to demonstrate dangerousness. Waiting to treat those afflicted with severe mental illnesses until they become dangerous to themselves or others ensures that many will become exactly that. Even courts have recognized the importance and validity of these criteria. In 1998 the Washington Supreme Court noted that the state has a legitimate interest in "protecting the community from the dangerously mentally ill and providing care to those who are unable to protect themselves." Likewise, in 2002 Wisconsin upheld the need for treatment criteria in its "Fifth Standard."

What does all this mean for a family with a member who is in need of treatment and who refuses to go to the hospital? It means that the family must first learn the commitment procedures and criteria that apply in their state. The quickest way is to go on the website of the Treatment Advocacy Center (see below) and contact the admission unit of the nearest psychiatric hospital or the clerk of the local court, whose personnel are usually experts in this area. Other potential resources for this information are the Treatment Advocacy Center, the local or state chapter of NAMI, psychiatrists in your area, the local or state Department of Mental Health, the public defender, or the police. A good state-by-state summary of standards for commitment and assisted treatment can be found at the Treatment Advocacy Center website, www.treatmentadvocacycenter.org. The family must also learn what kinds of evidence are necessary and admissible to prove dangerousness. For instance, are threats to other people sufficient, or does the person actually have to have injured someone? The answer depends on what your state law is and how it is applied. Families who wish to can usually testify at the commitment hearing. Their knowledge of what proof is necessary often determines whether a person with schizophrenia gets the treatment he or she needs. Even in states with the most humane and progressive treatment laws, families need to be tenacious and demand that their loved ones receive all the care to which their state entitles them. Indeed, many family members of people with schizophrenia end up becoming amateur lawyers in order to survive!

The long-term consequences of involuntarily hospitalizing a person with schizophrenia are quite variable. On one end of the spectrum are individuals who, following an involuntary hospitalization, refuse to have anything to do with their families. Some may even run away from home. The more radical consumer groups of so-called "psychiatric survivors" appear to be primarily made up of individuals who were once involuntarily hospitalized and who then decided to turn their resentment into a career. Such individuals adopt their illness as their identity.

On the other end of the spectrum are those who retrospectively regard their involuntary hospitalization very positively because it got them into treatment. In one of the few studies done on this question, Dr. John Kane and his colleagues in New York interviewed thirty-five involuntarily admitted patients shortly after their admission and again just prior to discharge approximately two months later. They found that most patients had "significant changes toward recognition of the original need for involuntary treatment." Most other studies have reported similar results. I have personally participated in an involuntary commitment hearing in which a woman with schizophrenia told her daughter, who was testifying for the commitment, that she would never speak to her again; a year later, on medication and in complete remission, the woman expressed profound thanks to her daughter for being the only family member who had had the courage to get her the treatment she needed.

Alternatives to Hospitalization

Hospitalization is usually necessary for patients with schizophrenia who are sick for the first time, for the reasons described above. For those who have already been clearly diagnosed and who have relapsed (often because they have stopped taking their medicine), hospitalization can sometimes be avoided. There are several possible alternatives.

One such alternative is the use of drugs given by injection in an emergency room or clinic. A skilled physician can dramatically reduce the psychotic symptoms in approximately half of patients with schizophrenia within six to eight hours, thereby allowing the person to return home. One problem with this technique, however, is that frequently the family members are so worn out by the person's recent behavior that *they* need the rest and understandably are not prepared to accept the person home again immediately.

Another increasingly popular alternative to hospitalization is the use of mobile treatment teams that go to the individual's home, assess the situation, and frequently begin treatment on the spot. This can effectively decrease the use of hospitalization but is effective only where there is also skilled and coordinated follow-up.

Another recent development is the increasing use by states and counties of psychiatric beds for short-term hospitalization in institutions other than hospitals, primarily because such beds are less expensive. These institutions, referred to in chapter 14 as "semihospitals," have different names in different places, such as IMDs (Institutions for Mental Diseases) or crisis homes. Some IMDs in California have over two hundred beds and are similar to state mental hospitals in everything except name.

Another alternative is the treatment of the patient at home, using public health nurses or, rarely, physicians to make home visits. This technique is used much more often in England, with apparent success.

It was also demonstrated to be feasible in a 1967 study done in Louisville, Kentucky, by Dr. Benjamin Pasamanick and his colleagues, who concluded that "the combination of drug therapy and public health nurses' home visitation is *effective* in preventing hospitalization, and that home care is at least as good a method of treatment as hospitalization by any or all criteria, and probably superior by most." I personally utilized this method once when practicing in a rural village, when the family expressed a wish to keep the person at home if possible; it required home visits for injections twice a day for a week, but it was successful.

The use of partial hospitalization is another good alternative. Day hospitals, in which the patient goes to the hospital for the day and returns home at night, and night hospitals, in which the patient goes to the hospital only to sleep, can both be effective in selected cases. Since both cost less than full hospitalization, they may be useful in communities in which they are available. They are usually affiliated with a full-time institution. Unfortunately, both are much less available than they should be in the United States, primarily because of restrictions on how federal Medicaid funds can be used.

Payment for Treatment, Insurance Parity, and Health Care Reform

Selecting the optimal place for hospitalization and follow-up psychiatric care is usually constrained by the reality of costs. These can be astronomical, and even the wealthiest individuals have learned to sit down before opening bills for psychiatric care.

Like other Americans, a large number of individuals with schizophrenia have no medical insurance. A 1998 study of 525 individuals with psychosis being admitted to hospitals for the first time reported that 44 percent had no insurance, 39 percent had private insurance, 15 percent had Medicaid or Medicare, and 2 percent were covered by the Veterans Administration. For those with private insurance, there are often stricter limits on number of hospital days and outpatient visits allowed for psychiatric diagnoses than there are for other medical or surgical diagnoses. This has led to a major push for insurance parity for psychiatric coverage, and since 1990 the majority of states have passed legislation mandating parity.

Resistance to insurance parity for psychiatric conditions has come primarily from insurance companies, who have to pay the bills. This resistance is based on the fact that psychiatrists have a reputation for gaming the insurance system and inflating costs. A 1985 study reported that "psychiatrists form a disproportionately large segment of the total" physicians who were suspended from the Medicaid and Medicare programs because of fraud and abuse. And psychiatrists played major roles in the private psychiatric hospital insurance scams of the early 1990s (see Joe Sharkey's description of this in *Bedlam: Greed, Profiteering, and Fraud in a Mental Health System Gone Crazy*).

Resistance to insurance parity for psychiatric conditions also arises from the vague outer limits of psychiatric diagnoses as defined by the American Psychiatric Association. Almost anybody can qualify for one or another diagnosis and therefore theoretically become eligible for insurance benefits for psychotherapy or hospitalization. This problem was summarized in December 1999 in an editorial in the *Wall Street Journal:*

> The reason "parity" doesn't exist is that, beyond treatment of obvious disorders, "mental health" is a vague and open-ended term. The difficulty has been abuse of mental-health insurance by both individuals and the "provider network" who gamed insurance plans to make endless payments for dubious benefits of apparently marginal problems, all the while lobbying to gain coverage for an ever-expanding definition of mental illness.

In 2008, after years of efforts by advocates, legislation mandating insurance parity was finally passed by Congress. Under these laws, coverage for psychiatric disorders under Medicare and private insurance plans must provide the same level of benefits as that available for general medical and surgical services, including deductibles and co-payments. Since most individuals with schizophrenia do not have private insurance, the insurance parity laws by themselves will not have much effect on these individuals.

America spends more on health care than any other country but gets a relatively poor product for such a huge expense. Proposals to improve the system will ultimately benefit individuals with schizophrenia. In the meantime, for individuals with schizophrenia who are not covered by private insurance, establishing eligibility for Medicaid benefits is the most important thing to do. The easiest way to do this is to become eligible for Supplemental Security Insurance (SSI), since recipients of SSI are automatically eligible for Medicaid. Applying for SSI is discussed in chapter 8.

Recommended Further Reading

Cadet, J. L., K. C. Rickler, and D. R. Weinberger. "The Clinical Neurologic Examination in Schizophrenia." In H. M. Nasrallah and D. R. Weinberger, eds. *The Neurology of Schizophrenia*. Amsterdam: Elsevier, 1986.

Garfield, R. L., S. H. Zuvekas, J. R. Lave, et al. "The Impact of National Health Care Reform on Adults with Severe Mental Disorders." *American Journal of Psychiatry* 168 (2011): 486–94.

Goldman, H. H. "Will Health Insurance Reform in the United States Help People with Schizophrenia?" *Schizophrenia Bulletin* 36 (2010): 893–94.

Stevens, A., N. Doidge, D. Goldbloom, et al. "Pilot Study of Televideo Psychiatric Assessments in an Underserviced Community." *American Journal of Psychiatry* 156 (1999): 783–85.

Taylor, R. *Psychological Masquerade: Distinguishing Psychological from Organic Disorders*. New York: Springer Publishing, 2007.

7
The Treatment of Schizophrenia: Medication and Other

"Lunacy, like the rain, falls upon the evil and the good, and although it must forever remain a fearful misfortune, yet there may be no more sin or shame in it than there is in an ague fit or a fever."

Inmate of the Glasgow Royal Asylum, 1860

Drugs are the most important treatment for schizophrenia, just as they are the most important treatment for many physical diseases. Drugs do not *cure*, but rather they *control*, the symptoms of schizophrenia—as they do those of diabetes. The drugs we now use to treat schizophrenia are far from perfect, but they work for most people with the disease if they are actually taken and used correctly.

The main drugs used to treat schizophrenia are usually called antipsychotics. They have also been called neuroleptics and major tranquilizers, but the best term is antipsychotics, because it describes their purpose. The first antipsychotic was chlorpromazine (its generic name), with the trade names of Thorazine, Largactil, and others.

(Hereafter the trade names will be capitalized and in parentheses.) Chlorpromazine was discovered serendipitously in France in 1952.

Do Antipsychotics Work?

The efficacy of antipsychotics has been well established. They are especially effective against the so-called positive symptoms of schizophrenia, but minimally effective against the negative and cognitive symptoms. On average, for patients experiencing their first episode of psychosis, 70 percent of patients on antipsychotics improve significantly, 20 percent improve minimally, and 10 percent do not improve at all. It should be remembered that, before antipsychotics were discovered, many patients with schizophrenia spent most of their life in a hospital. If antipsychotics are taken regularly, they markedly reduce the chances of relapse and rehospitalization. For example, as early as 1975, Dr. John Davis reviewed twenty-four studies of individuals taking antipsychotics and reported that those who took their medication regularly had only half the risk of relapse of those who did not. In 2012 Stefan Leucht et al. reviewed sixty-five studies and reported that at the end of one year, 27 percent of individuals with schizophrenia taking antipsychotics and 64 percent not taking antipsychotics had relapsed. What this means is that taking the drugs does not guarantee that the person will *not* get sick again, and *not* taking the drugs does not guarantee that the person *will* get sick, but taking the drugs does markedly improve the odds that the person will not relapse. The efficacy of antipsychotics is about the same as the efficacy of most drugs used in internal medicine. There is also some evidence that antipsychotics improve the neurological symptoms that often accompany the disease, as described in chapter 5.

Of course antipsychotics only work if people with schizophrenia take them. Studies in the United States indicate that "approximately 40% of the respondents with schizophrenia report that they have not received any mental health treatments in the preceding 6–12 months." Two large studies in Europe recently reported that individuals with schizophrenia who do not take antipsychotic drugs die earlier than those who do. Thus our failure to treat individuals with this disease may be one explanation for the high premature mortality observed for schizophrenia, as discussed in chapter 4.

Although we know that antipsychotics work, we don't know precisely how they work. We know that antipsychotic drugs primarily target the brain's neurotransmitter receptors, especially dopamine. It later became clear that some antipsychotics target other receptors, such as serotonin, glutamate, GABA, norepinephrine, and histamine. However, we still do not understand the relationship between these neurotransmitters and schizophrenia. Knowing which receptor is targeted by a specific antipsychotic can tell you what side effects to expect, but does not tell you much about the efficacy of the drug. It is now known that some antipsychotics are also effective against infective agents and have effects on the immune system, so this may be how they work. The bottom line is that we really don't know how they work. But then, we don't yet know how aspirin works, either.

Whose Information Can You Trust?

Antipsychotics are big business. Before it became generic, olanzapine (Zyprexa) was the pharmaceutical company Eli Lilly's bestselling drug, with sales of almost $3 billion a year. In 2010 sales of all antipsychotics totaled $16 billion. In 2014 aripiprazole (Abilify) was the single most profitable drug in the U.S. Because treating schizophrenia is big business, major pharmaceutical companies have given money to many leading schizophrenia researchers to try to influence them to support their drug. The researchers, in turn, write papers and give talks to clinicians, recommending the use of that particular drug. For this reason, you cannot believe much of what is written by mental health professionals about these drugs. In addition, the pharmaceutical industry pays for the vast majority of studies done on these drugs. In the past they only published studies with positive results, although more recently some companies have also published negative studies. There should be a requirement that all studies be made publicly available.

I personally have never taken any money from drug companies and have based my recommendations in this chapter on the opinions of colleagues I know to be independent of the companies, especially John Davis and his research colleagues. I have also relied on *Worst Pills, Best Pills News*, the *Medical Letter*, and the 2009 recommendations of the Schizophrenia Patients Outcome Research Team (PORT), a group funded by the National Institute of Mental Health, not drug companies. I believe these are the most reliable recommendations. Some other sets of guidelines, such as the Texas Medication Algorithm Project (TMAP), have been funded mostly by drug companies and are thus highly biased.

Which Antipsychotic Should You Use?

Currently in the United States there are 20 antipsychotics available in pill form for oral administration and six antipsychotics available in long-acting injectable form (Tables 7.1 and 7.2). Additional antipsychotics are available in other countries but only one of them, amisulpride, is highly regarded and would be a useful addition. Unfortunately, the French company that makes it, Sanofi, has never sought FDA approval. One other antipsychotic, molindone (Moban), previously was available in the U.S. but was withdrawn in 2010; this was unfortunate since it was one of the drugs causing the least weight gain.

Given the number of antipsychotics available, deciding which antipsychotic to use can be bewildering. The following general principles can be helpful.

1. Clozapine is the single most effective antipsychotic, significantly better than the others. It is the only one that has been shown to have effects on violent and suicidal behavior. It has its own set of side effects and problems (see section on clozapine, below), but nobody with schizophrenia should be labeled as treatment resistant unless they have been given a trial of clozapine.

2. Except for clozapine, first-generation antipsychotics (introduced before 1990) are, as a group, just as effective as second-generation antipsychotics (introduced after 1990). The two groups differ on side

TABLE 7.1. ANTIPSYCHOTICS AVAILABLE IN THE US IN PILL FORM

FIRST-GENERATION

Antipsychotic	Trade name	Usual daily dosage (mg.)	Generic?
chlorpromazine	Thorazine	400–600	yes
fluphenazine	Prolixin	5–15	yes
haloperidol	Haldol	5–15	yes
loxapine	Loxitane	60–100	yes
perphenazine	Trilafon	12–24	yes
thioridazine	Mellaril	400–500	yes
thiothixene	Navane	15–30	yes
trifluoperazine	Stelazine	10–20	yes

SECOND-GENERATION

Antipsychotic	Trade name	Usual daily dosage (mg.)	Generic?
aripiprazole	Abilify	10–30	yes
asenapine	Saphris	5–15	no
brexpiprazole	Rexulti	2–4	no
cariprazine	Vraylar	1.5–6	no
clozapine	Clozaril	400–800	yes
Iloperidone	Fanapt	12–24	yes
lurasidone	Latuda	40–80	no
olanzapine	Zyprexa	15–20	yes
paliperiodone	Invega	6–12	yes
quetiapine	Seroquel	400–800	yes
risperidone	Risperdal	4–6	yes
ziprasidone	Geodon	120–200	yes

effects but not on overall efficacy, although there are differences among the individual drugs. Large studies in both the United States and Europe have confirmed the equal efficacy.

3. The largest study comparing the effectiveness of antipsychotics assessed 15 drugs in 212 trials; 12 of the antipsychotics are available in the U.S. Each drug received a score based on the effect size of being

TABLE 7.2. ANTIPSYCHOTICS AVAILABLE IN
THE US AS LONG-ACTING INJECTABLES

Antipsychotic	Trade name	Usual daily dosage (mg.)	Generic?
fluphenazine decanoate	Prolixin	12.5–25 mg. IM every 2–3 weeks	yes
haloperidol decanoate	Haldol	10–15 times previous daily oral dose, given IM once/month	yes
aripiprazole	Abilify Maintena	400 mg. IM once a month	yes
aripiprazole lauroxil	Aristada	882 mg. IM every 6 weeks	yes
olanzapine pamoate	Zyprexa Relprevv	300–405 mg. IM once a month	no
risperidone	Risperdol Consta	25–50 mg IM every 2 weeks	soon
paliperidone palmitate	Invega Sustenna	117–234 mg. IM once a month	no
	Invega Trinza	410–819 mg. IM every 3 months	no

superior to placebo, as shown in Table 7.3. As expected, clozapine scored significantly higher than all other antipsychotics, followed by olanzapine, risperidone, and paliperidone. The last two are chemically very similar.

TABLE 7.3. COMPARATIVE EFFICACY OF 12 ANTIPSYCHOTICS

Antipsychotic	Effectiveness score
clozapine	88
olanzapine	59
risperidone	56
paliperidone	50
haloperidol	45
quetiapine	44
aripiprazole	43
ziprasidone	39
chlorpromazine	38
asenapine	38
lurasidone	33
iloperidone	33

4. In selecting an antipsychotic, the four most recently introduced drugs can be safely ignored: lurasidone (Latuda); asenapine (Saphris); brexpiprazole (Rexulti); and cariprazine (Vraylar). All are still patent protected and thus very expensive. Preliminary studies suggest that all four are merely me-too drugs with nothing special to recommend them. Brexpiprazole is just a chemically slightly altered version of aripiprazole. It should be remembered that to market a new antipsychotic in the United States the FDA merely requires that it be shown to be better than a placebo, not that it is as good as or better than existing drugs. Thus many of the newer drugs are not as good as the older drugs.

5. It is now widely accepted that the primary consideration in selecting antipsychotics should be side effects. Weight gain, often accompanied by increased blood sugar and increased blood lipids, is a major side effect and is a risk factor for heart attacks and strokes. Increased blood sugar may occur even in individuals who have had no previous problems with blood sugar, and may happen quickly, although it is uncommon in patients who have not gained significant weight. If blood sugar increases to a very high level, ketoacidosis occurs, which can be fatal. There is apparently a genetic predisposition to this problem, and it occurs more commonly among African-Americans. Both of these side effects occur much more commonly in individuals taking second-generation antipsychotics, especially clozapine (Clozaril) and olanzapine (Zyprexa). Chlorpromazine (Thorazine), thioridazine (Mellaril), quetiapine (Seroquel), risperidone (Risperdal), and paliperidone (Invega) may also cause weight gain. Haloperidol (Haldol), fluphenazine (Prolixin), loxapine (Loxitane), perphenazine (Trilafon), thiothixene (Navane), trifluoperazine (Stelazine), ziprasidone (Geodon), and aripiprazole (Abilify) are least likely to cause these problems, but any antipsychotic, first- or second-generation, may do so. Therefore, it is good practice for the treating psychiatrist to get a baseline weight on any patient being started on antipsychotics, and for those taking clozapine (Clozaril) and olanzapine (Zyprexa), a baseline blood sugar and hemoglobin Ac as well. During the first year on these drugs, weight and blood sugar should be checked periodically. For those taking clozapine, the blood sugar can be checked using the same blood drawn to check the white blood cell count (see section on clozapine). Individuals taking drugs that cause weight gain should also be referred to a dietician for

assistance with their diets and should markedly increase their exercise to help with weight control. Weight gain occurs most rapidly in the first few months after starting these drugs, and that is when the diet and exercise are most important.

6. Another set of side effects that should be considered are various movement disorders, often called extrapyramidal symptoms (EPS). These include stiffness; tremor; slowed movements; acute stiffening of the muscles of the neck and/or eyes (called an acute dystonic reaction); and restlessness (akathisia), causing the person to pace constantly. These are common and very unpleasant side effects of antipsychotics. Acute dystonic reactions are especially frightening to the patient, although they do not cause any permanent damage and can be reversed within minutes with an anticholinergic drug such as benztropine (Cogentin). For this reason, many psychiatrists give a preventative anticholinergic to patients taking the antipsychotics most likely to cause EPS. These are haloperidol (Haldol), fluphenazine (Prolixin), thiothixene (Navane) and, to a lesser extent, risperidone (Risperdal), and paliperidone (Invega). All of the other antipsychotics may do so, but they are less likely to than the drugs listed above. Clozapine (Clozaril), quetiapine (Seroquel), olanzapine (Zyprexa), and thioridazine (Mellanil) are the least likely to cause EPS. It should be added that stiffness and tremor may also occur as neurological symptoms of schizophrenia and can be seen in some individuals who have never been treated with antipsychotic medication. EPS can be treated using anticholinergics. Beta blockers and benzodiazepines are also commonly used but are less effective and, of course, these drugs have their own side effects.

The most serious movement disorder that may develop as a side effect of antipsychotic usage is tardive dyskinesia. It usually does not appear until months or years after starting the drug. It consists of involuntary movements of the tongue and mouth, such as chewing movements, sucking movements, pushing the cheek out with the tongue, and smacking the lips. Occasionally these are accompanied by jerky, purposeless movements of the arms or legs or, rarely, the whole body. It usually begins while the patient is taking the drug but may begin shortly after the drug has been stopped. Occasionally it persists indefinitely.

The incidence of tardive dyskinesia is difficult to ascertain because it may occur as part of the disease process as well as being a side effect of medication. A study of the records of more than six hundred patients admitted to an asylum in England between 1845 and 1890, before the discovery of antipsychotics, found an "extraordinary prevalence of abnormal movements and postures. . . . Movement disorder, often equivalent to tardive dyskinesia, was noted in nearly one-third of schizophrenics." A study of spontaneous dyskinesia in individuals with schizophrenia who had never been treated with antipsychotic medication reported it to be present in 12 percent of individuals below age thirty and in 25 percent of individuals ages thirty to fifty. Most estimates of the incidence of tardive dyskinesia have assumed that all such cases are drug-related, when in fact a substantial percentage are not. In a study of this problem aptly titled "Not All That Moves Is Tardive Dyskinesia," Khot and Wyatt concluded that the true incidence of drug-related tardive dyskinesia was less than 20 percent. This also falls within the 10 to 20 percent range estimated by the American Psychiatric Association's 1980 task force on the subject.

First-generation antipsychotics seem more likely to cause tardive dyskinesia than second-generation antipsychotics, although it may occur with any of them. Women appear to be more susceptible to tardive dyskinesia than men. Patients, families, and treating mental health professionals should be on the lookout for the early signs of tardive dyskinesia, especially the person's tongue pushing against the cheek. If the symptoms begin, the patient can be switched to a second-generation antipsychotic and/or tried on various treatments that have been reported to be effective in some cases: ondansetron, valbenzine, tetrabenazine, or ECT. If there is no additional treatment, tardive dyskinesia will not necessarily get worse. In one ten-year follow-up of forty-four patients, 30 percent got worse, 50 percent remained the same, and 20 percent actually improved despite continuing use of the antipsychotic.

7. Some antipsychotics may also cause sexual side effects by increasing a hormone called prolactin. Prolactin can also be increased as part of the schizophrenia disease process. This increase can cause breast discharge (galactorrhoea), slight enlargement of the breast (gynaecomastia), menstrual irregularities, and sexual dysfunction.

There are also suggestions that chronic elevation of prolactin may cause osteoporosis. The antipsychotics most likely to increase prolactin are risperidone (Risperdal) and paliperidone (Invega). Intermediate in risk are ziprasidone (Geodon) and all first-generation antipsychotics. Least likely to increase prolactin are aripiprazole (Abilify), quetiapine (Seroquel), olanzapine (Zyprexa), and clozapine (Clozaril).

Note that increased prolactin is a two-edged sword. At the same time that it may cause unwanted side effects, it also markedly decreases the chances of women becoming pregnant, by interfering with the menstrual cycle. Thus in the 1990s, when many women with schizophrenia were being switched from first-generation antipsychotics, which caused increased prolactin, to olanzapine or clozapine, which did not, many unexpected and unwanted pregnancies resulted.

8. Sedation can be a troublesome side effect, especially for individuals with schizophrenia who are employed. The sedation is most severe when starting the antipsychotic, then becomes less severe. Clozapine (Clozaril) is the antipsychotic that causes the most sedation; others that cause sedation are quetiapine (Seroquel), ziprasidone (Geodon), chlorpromazine (Thorazine), and thioridazine (Mellaril). Least likely to cause sedation are aripiprazole (Abilify), iloperidone (Fanapt) or paliperidone (Invega). The sedation risk of the other antipsychotics appears to be intermediate. Sedation can be minimized by taking the medication at bedtime. Sedating antipsychotics can also be used to help individuals with schizophrenia sleep better.

9. If the person has conduction problems of their heart such as certain arrhythmias, some antipsychotics should not be used, especially thioridazine and ziprasidone but also asenapine, chlorpromazine, and iloperidone. Aripiprazole, paliperidone, or other first-generation antipsychotics are safer.

10. The only antipsychotic that is known to be abused to get high is quetiapine (Seroquel). It can be crushed and inhaled or taken IV and can be sold on the street.

11. The cost of antipsychotics varies widely, as noted in the section on costs below. If you or your family are going to be paying for the antipsychotic you may wish to use one of the least expensive ones. According to *The Medical Letter* (December 19, 2016), olanzapine and risperidone are the least expensive oral antipsychotics with a cost to

wholesalers for a 30-day supply of less than $20 per month, although retail prices vary widely. Haloperidol, loxapine, quetiapine, thioridazine, and ziprasidone are also comparatively inexpensive. Drug costs are also a major consideration for jails and prisons that need to medicate many prisoners with serious mental illness but have very limited funds to do so.

12. What is the role of genetic testing in helping to select an antipsychotic? Pharmacogenetics, as it is called, has been widely promised to lead to "personalized medicine" by the geneticists. For rare genetic diseases and for some cancers it has great promise but not for schizophrenia. In the future, genetic testing may play a modest role in helping to predict side effects of antipsychotics but at this point in time genetic testing for schizophrenia is mostly hype.

13. Women with schizophrenia who become pregnant pose special problems. In general, antipsychotic drugs are considered to be relatively safe for the growing fetus and have not been associated with causing fetal abnormalities such as have been seen with drugs like lithium and valproate. One study showed that olanzapine (Zyprexa) and haloperidol (Haldol) cross the placenta more readily than some other antipsychotics, but the consequences are unknown. A recent review of all published studies reported that the use of second-generation antipsychotics, which are associated with metabolic abnormalities, leads to babies being heavier at birth and thus suggests that first-generation antipsychotics may be preferred. See chapter 10 for a discussion of this problem.

A Treatment Plan for First-Break Psychosis

Given these principles, how do they translate into the actual treatment of patients? For a person who develops a psychotic disorder for the first time, how should the choice of drug be made? *Whenever possible, the choice should be made jointly by the patient and patient's family with the psychiatrist.* Such shared decision making not only shows respect for the patient and family but also leads to a better engagement in treatment and better medication compliance. As described in a useful article on the subject, joint decision making also "provides a model for [the patient and family] to assess a treatment's advantages and disadvantages within the context of recovering a life after a diagnosis of a major mental disorder." I have treated some patients with excellent awareness of their illness who were able to independently increase and decrease their antipsychotic medication dose within a specified range depending on how they were feeling. Unfortunately, shared decision making is possible for only approximately half of individuals with schizophrenia. The other half has varying degrees of anosognosia and therefore denies that anything is wrong with them. Such patients often need to be treated involuntarily, as described in chapter 10.

A possible treatment plan for an individual with first-break psychosis is shown by figure 7.1. If the person is violent or suicidal that should be the primary consideration. Clozapine is the antipsychotic of choice for such patients but often cannot be used immediately since it must be started at a low dose and increased gradually. Therefore it is often necessary to stabilize such patients on another antipsychotic and then switch them to clozapine a few weeks later. The treatment plan also suggests raising the cost issue early in the treatment planning process and starting with the least expensive antipsychotics if the individual with psychosis or family will be responsible for the costs. As of 2016, generic olanzapine and risperidone were the least expensive antipsychotics but haloperidol, loxapine, quetiapine, thioridazine, and ziprasidone were also affordable compared to the cost of other antipsychotics. Starting people on antipsychotics that they cannot afford is a prescription for failure. If there is a high likelihood that the person with psychosis will not voluntarily take medication, it may be wise to begin with one of the antipsychotics that can be given if necessary by long-acting injection.

The treatment plan then suggests addressing the weight gain issue which, with its accompanying increased blood sugar and/or increased blood lipids, has emerged as the single most troublesome side effect of antipsychotic drug treatment. If the person is already overweight or prediabetic or if weight gain is likely to be viewed as a major disaster by the person, then it makes sense to begin antipsychotic treatment with those drugs least likely to cause weight gain, as listed in figure 7.1.

For all other individuals it is suggested that either olanzapine or risperidone be used for an initial course of therapy since these anti-

Figure 7.1 Treatment Plan for First-Break Psychosis

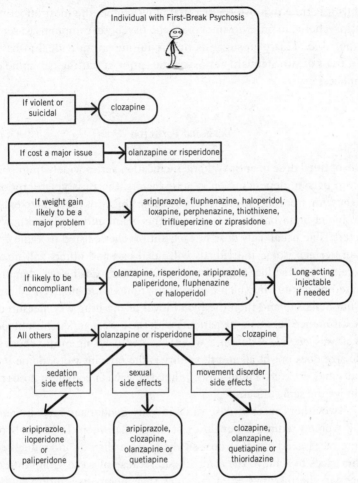

psychotics have been rated highest for efficacy, except for clozapine, as described above. During the course of this initial treatment trial, if sedation, sexual side effects, or movement disorders emerge, figure 7.1 lists alternative antipsychotics that can be used. If the person does not respond to an adequate trial of one standard antipsychotic, a second one can be tried or a trial of clozapine started. A recent European study suggested that the chances of responding to a second standard antipsychotic are not high if the person has not responded to the first. Thus it is time to move on to a trial of clozapine, the most effective antipsychotic, in order to ameliorate the psychotic symptoms as soon as possible. This plan suggests that requiring an individual to have had trials of two standard antipsychotics prior to starting clozapine is unnecessary.

Dose and Duration

The optimal dose of antipsychotic medication varies widely from person to person, depending on genetic factors, the variable absorption of the drug from the intestine, the variable ability of the drug to cross the blood-brain barrier and get into the brain, and other unknown factors. The usual daily dose of each antipsychotic listed in Table 7.1 is an average; some individuals will need less and others will need more. The individual variability of antipsychotic dosing was demonstrated by a study in which a group of patients were all given 20 mg. of fluphenazine and then the blood level of the drug was measured; the difference between the patients with the lowest and highest blood levels was *fortyfold*. Therefore, when it comes to dosing antipsychotics, one size does not fit all and flexibility is the operant word. Some patients may do well on mini-doses, while a few may need mega doses to achieve the same effect.

Two other causes of dose variability are gender and race. In general, women require lower doses of drugs than men. Individuals of some races need a higher dose of medication than do individuals of other races to achieve the same effect because of racial group differences in the distribution of enzymes that metabolize antipsychotic drugs. Studies suggest that whites and African-Americans require approximately the same dose, while Hispanic patients require a lower dose, and Asian-Americans need the lowest dose of these four groups. These are merely statistical generalizations, of course, and are not predictive of the needs of any given individual, because of interindividual variation in enzyme levels. It is also generally agreed that it is best to start patients on a low dose of the antipsychotic and increase slowly; however, if they are violent or suicidal they may need to be started on a higher dose. Similarly, when stopping an antipsychotic, the dose should be tapered slowly.

When a person is being treated for their first episode of schizophrenia, how long should an antipsychotic be tried before declaring the trial a failure? Given the wide variation in antipsychotic blood levels for patients taking the same dose of the same medication, it is not surprising to find that response rates vary widely. Some individuals with acute schizophrenia may respond in three days, while others may take three weeks or even three months. As a general rule, it has been recommended that if the person has shown no improvement in symptoms by the end of two weeks, another antipsychotic should be tried. If they have had some improvement, the antipsychotic should be continued for at least eight weeks, as improvement may increase for sixteen weeks or longer. As summarized by one study, "Many first-episode patients respond between weeks 8 and 16 of treatment with a single antipsychotic medication."

Once started, how long should an antipsychotic be continued following a first episode of psychosis? This is a controversial question that should be answered jointly by the individual affected, his/her family, and the treating physician. On one hand, we know that one quarter of individuals who experience an episode of psychosis are unlikely to get sick again; however, we have no sure way to identify them. On the other hand, there are recent studies reporting that the individuals who continue the antipsychotic medication for longer periods do better in both the short run and also the long (10 year) run. In making a decision, the predictors of outcome (see chapter 4) should be seriously considered. Assuming the predictors are reasonably good and the person has had a good response to mediation, I would suggest very slowly tapering down the antipsychotic and eventually stopping it after several months. If there is any recurrence of symptoms, the antipsychotic should be restarted immediately.

When individuals with schizophrenia relapse, they do so at a variable rate. Some will have a significant increase in symptoms within days of stopping medication, whereas others may remain symptom-free for months. The recurrence of symptoms may occur abruptly or very slowly.

Once a person has had two or more episodes of schizophrenia, it is likely they will have to continue medication for years. I encourage them to think of themselves as having diabetes, with the medication needed to remain relatively symptom-free. At times they may need a higher dose, and at other times a lower dose. Efforts should always be made to keep the antipsychotic dose as low as possible while still preventing recurrence of symptoms; this dose will vary widely from patient to patient. In the past, studies were done with intermittent dosing, giving the antipsychotic when the patient was symptomatic but stopping it during remission of symptoms. Such studies showed that intermittent dosing did not work for most people. As individuals with schizophrenia age, they often need a lower dose of their antipsychotic medication, and some older people can stop their medication altogether.

In view of the variable response to antipsychotic medications, *it is incumbent on individuals with schizophrenia and their families to keep records of their treatment.* This should include the drug, dosage, response, side effects, and length of time it was given. This can be extremely helpful in preventing duplicate failed trials and save weeks of trial-and-error medications in future treatments. The variable response to treatment is another reason that continuous treatment teams (see chapter 9) are so important. Having a single psychiatrist and treatment team care for an individual with schizophrenia over many years makes a good outcome much more likely.

Clozapine: The Most Effective Antipsychotic

Clozapine (Clozaril) is the gold standard for the treatment of schizophrenia, the one antipsychotic that has been proven in multiple studies to be more effective than all the others. In 1993 it even made the cover of *Time* magazine. It is the only antipsychotic that has been demonstrated to decrease violent behavior and suicidal ideation and has been approved for those uses by the Food and Drug Administration. Studies have reported that clozapine also decreases the arrest rate and emergency room utilization of individuals with schizophrenia and, most important, decreases their premature mortality. Clozapine also saves money by decreasing hospitalization; a 2016 study reported that the Veterans Health Administration would save $80 million a year if clozapine was properly used.

Despite this enviable record, it is infrequently used in the United States. Presently, only 4 percent of individuals with schizophrenia in the United States receive clozapine, compared with 20 percent in Germany, 35 percent in Australia, and 25 to 60 percent in various parts of China. Why is clozapine so underutilized in the United States? The most important reason is clozapine's reputation for causing a decrease in white blood cells (agranulocytosis), as described below. Another reason is that it is generic, so no pharmaceutical company promotes it. Instead, companies spend millions of dollars to convince mental health professionals to prescribe the latest antipsychotics, which are less effective and much more expensive.

Clozapine is also under prescribed because it has significant side effects. Sedation is a big problem, mitigated somewhat by taking clozapine at bedtime. Weight gain is a major problem, as it is with olanzapine (Zyprexa). Patients taking clozapine also may complain of excess salivation, constipation, and occasionally urinary incontinence. But the most important side effect is that in 8 out of 1,000 individuals, clozapine causes a decrease in white blood cells, a condition called agranulocytosis; if allowed to continue, it can be fatal. For this reason, it is necessary to get a blood test every week for the first six months after starting clozapine, then every two weeks for the second six months, then every month thereafter. The blood test will show if the white blood count (WBC) goes below 3,500/mm or the absolute neutrophil count (ANC) goes below 2,000/mm. As long as blood tests are done as prescribed, clozapine is safe, but if the testing is not done, the decrease in white blood cells can be fatal. Since the blood testing is now mandatory, clozapine should be considered as safe as other antipsychotics. In 2007 a genetic test was put on the market that offers some help in predicting which patients are more likely to develop agranulocytosis. However, because it does not provide an absolute answer but merely divides the patients into lower-risk and higher-risk groups, it is of limited usefulness.

Because of the risk of agranulocytosis, clozapine is not usually used as a first-choice drug. *No individual with schizophrenia should be called treatment-resistant until they have been tried on clozapine.* Clozapine is also the drug of choice for individuals with schizophrenia for whom aggression, suicidal thoughts, or tardive dyskinesia are significant problems. An adequate trial of clozapine should last for twelve weeks at a dose of up to 500 to 800 mg. per day, although some patients will respond at a lower dose. Many clinicians assess the level of clozapine in the blood to make sure it is at a therapeutic level and recommend that the blood level be at least 350 ng/ml. There is evidence that higher blood levels of clozapine are more effective than lower levels, although patients vary widely on the dose they need because of individual variation in how clozapine is metabolized. In 2017 a useful book on clozapine was published by the late Lewis Opler, et al. (see Recommended Further Reading). The CURESZ Foundation, founded by a patient for whom it was helpful, also promotes the use of clozapine (www.curesz.org).

Monitoring: Is the Person Taking the Antipsychotic?

Medication noncompliance by individuals with schizophrenia is the single biggest cause of relapse and rehospitalization, as described in chapter 10. There are many reasons why such individuals do not take their medication but the most common reason is that they do not think they are sick; they have anosognosia, as described in chapter 1.

There are several options for ensuring that people with schizophrenia really take their antipsychotic medication. For individuals who hide the pills in their cheek ("cheeking") or under their tongue and later spit them out, a few antipsychotics are available in a form that rapidly disintegrates and are absorbed as they are held in the mouth. The medications for which this form of tablet is available are risperidone (Risperdal M-Tab), aripiprazole (Abilify Discmelt), olanzapine (Zyprexa Zydis), and clozapine (Clozaril FazaClo).

Many antipsychotics are also available orally in liquid form. This can be useful for individuals who have a problem swallowing pills as well as those who "cheek" their pills. The disadvantage of using liquid formulations of antipsychotics is the greater risk of mistakes in measuring the dose as well as the significantly greater cost. The liquid antipsychotic is usually added to juice (but not grapefruit juice) and in most cases should not be taken with coffee, tea, or cola, since caffeine is thought to increase the absorption rate of the drug and thus increase the serum level. Liquid formulations are available for chlorpromazine (Thorazine), fluphenazine (Prolixin), haloperidol (Haldol), loxapine (Loxitane), thioridazine (Mellaril), trifluoperazine (Stelazine), aripiprazole (Abilify), and risperidone (Risperdal).

Another option for ensuring that the person is taking their antipsychotic medication is to check their blood level. This is done routinely for clozapine and can be done for other antipsychotics although it may require a more specialized laboratory. Checking blood levels can also be useful in determining whether the person should be tried on a higher dose of the antipsychotic; for example, some individuals have a poor intestinal absorption of antipsychotics and/or higher rates of metabolizing them and need higher doses than normal in order to reach a therapeutic blood level.

Another option for ensuring that people take their antipsychotic medication became available in 2017. The Food and Drug Administration approved the use of a pill with a built-in sensor. When the pill reaches the person's stomach and disintegrates the sensor sends a signal to a band-aid style device worn by the person. These devices, in turn, can be programmed to send a message that the medication was taken to any remote computer or mobile device. Thus it could be used by individuals who have problems in remembering to take their medication, and also used in situations where individuals are required to take their medication. In this regard such pills have been tried for individuals with tuberculosis and found to improve medication compliance. For schizophrenia the antipsychotic that was approved by the FDA in 2017 was for aripiprazole (Abilify) and will be sold as Abilify MyCite. In 2018 the cost for one month was $1,650.

Long-Acting Antipsychotic Injections

Among all the possibilities for ensuring that an individual is taking antipsychotic medication, the surest method is to give the medication by a long-acting injection. Table 7.2 lists those that are available and includes two first-generation (fluphenzine and haloperidol) and four second-generation (aripiprazole, olanzapine, risperidone and paliperidone) antipsychotics. Most are given by injection every two to four weeks although aripiprazole (Aristade) can be given every six weeks and paliperidone (InvegaTrinza) can be given every three months. Injections can be given either in the upper arm (deltoid) or rear end (gluteal) and are equally effective. It is very important to first establish the individual on that medication using pills and to assess any side effects before giving a long-acting injection.

The effectiveness of long-acting antipsychotics has been well established. Several studies have reported that the long-acting injections reduce relapses by 30 percent compared to oral antipsychotics. In one study long-acting injections also significantly reduced episodes of violence by individuals with schizophrenia. Of great interest was a 2017 study from Sweden reporting that "among patients with schizophrenia, LAI [long-acting injectable] use is associated with an approximately 30% lower risk of death compared to oral agents." Despite this track record, long-acting injection antipsychotics are used for individuals with schizophrenia in the United States only about half as frequently as they are used in most European countries.

Medications to Try When All Else Fails

Many individuals with schizophrenia respond only partially to existing antipsychotics, including clozapine (Clozaril). What are the treatment options for such people? They include combining two or more antipsychotics or adding an adjunct medication to the existing antipsychotic. Such options are referred to as polypharmacy, which is a common practice in treating other diseases, such as hypertension, diabetes, and epilepsy. It is a relatively new strategy for treating schizophrenia.

Polypharmacy may well be worth trying for some patients, but it carries with it increased expense as well as definite risks of drug interactions. Interactions between an antipsychotic and another drug may affect the antipsychotic by decreasing the serum level (thus making it less effective) or by increasing it (thus making side effects more likely). Other drug interactions have little or no effect on the antipsychotic drug but instead cause generalized effects (e.g., the combination of an antipsychotic and a barbiturate may cause severe sedation).

Still other interactions have no effect on the antipsychotic but instead cause changes in the effects of the other drug, e.g., some antipsychotics taken with the blood thinner Coumadin may cause a further increase in the clotting time of blood. Individuals with schizophrenia and their families should thus ask the treating psychiatrist about drug interactions. Most pharmacists can also access this information in computerized drug databases.

Combining antipsychotics is common. Studies have reported that in the United States "33 percent of patients may receive two antipsychotics and almost 10 percent receive three." Although antipsychotic combinations are widely used, no study to date has reported that a combination is any more effective than one antipsychotic alone. The combination usually consists of one first-generation and one second-generation antipsychotic, or two second-generation antipsychotics. It is important that the treating physician know enough about the drugs to select combinations wisely. It would make no sense to combine antipsychotics that are very similar. Risperidone (Risperdal) and paliperidone (Invega), for example, are virtually identical. Fluphenazine (Prolixin), perphenazine (Trilafon), and trifluoperazine (Stelazine) are all piperazine phenothiazines, so there is little advantage in combining them.

Many medications have been tried as adjunct medications to existing antipsychotics. The most common are drugs used to treat epilepsy (anticonvulsants), because some of them are effective in treating bipolar disorder. These include valproic acid (Depakene), valproate (Depakote), carbamazepine (Tegretol), lamotrigine (Lamictal), and topirimate (Topamax). Carbamazepine should definitely not be combined with clozapine, since it can also decrease white blood cell count. Despite numerous studies, there is no evidence that these drugs are effective in treating schizophrenia, although they may be effective in some cases of schizoaffective disorder. The same can be said of lithium, a standard treatment for bipolar disorder that affords little benefit for schizophrenia except in rare cases.

Benzodiazepines such as diazepam (Valium), lorazepam (Ativan), and clonazepam (Klonopin) are sometimes used as adjunct medications for schizophrenia to decrease anxiety and agitation or to help with sleep. Evidence for their effectiveness is modest. Benzodiazapines should not be given simultaneously with clozapine except under strict medical supervision, because of the danger of a severe, even fatal, drug interaction. Benzodiazepines also have the disadvantage of being addictive if taken over several months and of causing withdrawal symptoms such as seizures if stopped abruptly.

Antidepressant medications are frequently used as adjunct medications for individuals with schizophrenia who are depressed or who have predominantly negative symptoms. Most commonly used are selective serotonin reuptake inhibitors (SSRIs), such as fluoxetine (Prozac), sertraline (Zoloft), paroxetine (Paxil), fluvoxamine (Luvox), and citalopram (Celexa). Some clinicians have claimed that these drugs improve negative symptoms other than depression, but the results of treatment trials have not been consistent. SSRIs increase the blood level of many antipsychotics, so that could also be their mechanism of effectiveness. Other antidepressants such as trazadone (Desyrel) and mirtazapine (Remeron) are sometimes used to help patients who have insomnia.

When combining a second medication with an antipsychotic, one must always be careful about adding a medication with the same problematic side effects as the antipsychotic has. The most significant consideration here is adding a medication that has weight gain or other metabolic side effects to a second-generation antipsychotic that has these same properties. Examples include valproic acid (Depakene), valproate (Depakote), and mirtazapine (Remeron). That is not to say it should not be done—it often is—but that one needs to be aware of cumulative side effects.

In recent years, medications that are useful in treating other diseases have been increasingly tested as adjunct medications for schizophrenia. Some of these appear to be promising, although additional studies are needed to verify their effectiveness. Especially interesting are anti-inflammatory medications, since it is known that inflammation is part of the schizophrenia disease process (see chapter 5). Positive studies have been reported for aspirin, celecoxib, and minocycline. For women with schizophrenia, estrogen and raloxifene have also shown promise as adjunct medications. There has been much interest in using omega-3 fatty acids (fish oil) in the early stages of schizophrenia. Folate, a naturally occurring B vitamin, has shown some promise for individuals with schizophrenia who have a low folate level. Details of these potential adjunct medications can be found in the 2012 publication "Adjunct Treatments for Schizophrenia and Bipolar Disorder: What to Try When You Are Out of Ideas," in the list of recommended reading at the end of this chapter.

Drug Costs and the Use of Generics

The cost of medication in the United States is a scandal. For example, before it became generic, olanzapine (Zyprexa) cost one-fourth as much in Spain and one-half as much in Finland and Canada as it did in the United States. The reason for these gross discrepancies is simple: other countries either cap the profit margin of the pharmaceutical companies (England allows a 20 percent profit) or they negotiate the price by buying in bulk for their national health service. In the United States, there is no limit to how much pharmaceutical companies can mark up drugs. Consequently, according to a 1999 report, "*Fortune* magazine ranked the pharmaceutical business as the most profitable of all industries . . . measured on returns on equity, sales and assets." American pharmaceutical companies rationalize their profits by claiming that the profits are needed to develop new drugs. However, many antipsychotics were developed primarily in Europe, and a large proportion of expenditures by American pharmaceutical companies are spent on advertising, not on drug development.

The most useful way to control antipsychotic drug costs is to use generic brands. Fortunately, most of the commonly used antipsychotics can be purchased as generics (Table 7.1), so their cost is significantly lower. Generic medications are regulated by the Food and Drug Administration. The strength (bio equivalency) of generic medications may legally vary by as much as 20 percent, although in most cases the variation is only 2 to 3 percent. Manufacturers of brand-name drugs want patients and families to believe that switching to generic drugs is risky; they have an economic interest in promoting such misinformation. The only generic medication used to treat schizophrenia for which problems of efficacy have been reported is carbamazepine, but similar problems of efficacy have been reported for Tegretol, its brand-name version.

The biggest problem in switching to generic formulations of antipsychotic drugs is confusion for patients. If a person has been taking a tablet of a particular color and shape for many months, it may take much explanation to help the person understand that a tablet of another color and shape is the same drug.

Antipsychotic medications can also be purchased less expensively in other countries. Americans have increasingly been using online Canadian pharmacies to save money. In order to do so, you need to obtain a prescription from a physician, then mail or fax the prescription to the Canadian pharmacy, which will then send you the medication. Buying from online pharmacies in other countries may be risky as there have been reports of counterfeit or contaminated products. Using the Internet to shop for better prices in your own city is also useful; prices sometimes vary widely.

Still another way to save money on medications is to buy larger-sized tablets and split them in half. For many medications, the cost of a 5 mg. and a 10 mg. tablet is very similar. For a person taking olanzapine 5 mg. per day, buying 10 mg. tablets and cutting them in half can yield remarkable savings. Most pharmacies sell inexpensive plastic tablet cutters, but a sharp knife can also be used. Tablets are easier to cut if they are scored (i.e., have a groove), but do not worry if the two halves are not exactly the same size; blood levels of most antipsychotics will remain stable if the person ingests both halves, even if they are of uneven size, over two days.

Criticism of Antipsychotics

Antipsychotics are far from perfect, given their side effects and lack of efficacy against many symptoms of schizophrenia. But they are the best we have and are probably comparable in terms of side effects and efficacy to the medications available to treat heart disease and rheumatoid arthritis, for example.

Antipsychotic medications have been criticized from the time they were first introduced, initially by psychoanalysts who believed that schizophrenia was caused by faulty parental relationships. In the 1980s, the main source of criticism of antipsychotics shifted to Scientologists, who are rabidly anti-psychiatry, viewing it as a competitor to their own purported healing methods. Over the years, Scientologist criticisms have been complemented by a few fellow travelers, such as Peter Breggin, who published books such as *Toxic Psychiatry* and *Psychiatric Drugs: Hazards to the Brain.*

All such criticisms were largely ignored until recently, when Robert Whitaker, a respected science writer, elaborated on many previous criticisms in *Anatomy of an Epidemic: Magic Bullets, Psychiatric Drugs, and the Astonishing Rise of Mental Illness in America.* He correctly attacked the pharmaceutical industry for greed and American psychiatrists for allowing themselves to be seduced by drug representatives. However, regarding schizophrenia, Whitaker maintained that antipsychotic drugs largely *cause* the disease and that patients have a better outcome if they are treated only briefly or not at all.

These are extraordinary claims and would never be made by anyone who had spent time in a facility with people with schizophrenia who were not being treated. Indeed, from the early 1800s until the 1950s, before we had antipsychotic medications, we had the opportunity to observe the outcome of not treating individuals with schizophrenia, and the results were not pretty. During those years, the number of patients with schizophrenia appears to have increased sharply (see chapter 14), and the number who spent much of their life in state hospitals grew steadily larger as the population increased. Whitaker argues that the increased incidence has been a more recent consequence of treatment. He cites outcome studies in which some individuals with schizophrenia do well without antipsychotic medications. As detailed in chapter 4, it is well known that approximately one-quarter of individuals initially diagnosed with a schizophrenia-like psychosis recover spontaneously and do not need medication. Finally, Whitaker relies heavily on the claim that individuals with schizophrenia in third-world countries, especially those not being treated, have a much better outcome than those in first-world countries. This claim was criticized as being untrue thirty years ago, when it was initially made by the World Health Organization, and several recent studies have substantiated its fallaciousness (see the section on developing countries in chapter 4).

Whitaker is correct that much more research needs to be carried out on antipsychotic drugs to better understand how they work and their long-term consequences. Such research should be supported by the National Institute of Mental Health (NIMH), since the pharmaceutical industry is unlikely to do so. Whitaker raises the issue of supersensitivity psychosis, the possibility that antipsychotics sensitize the brain's neurotransmitter receptors so that psychotic symptoms get worse when an antipsychotic drug is withdrawn, especially abruptly. This has been shown in rats, but there is no evidence that it occurs in humans.

Finally, some people have criticized the use of antipsychotics because they are said to cause changes in the brain. Of course they cause changes in the brain—that is why they are effective. Medications used to treat epilepsy and Parkinson's disease also cause changes in the brain. Antipsychotics are known, for example, to increase the density of glial cells in the frontal lobe and to increase the connections between neurons (synapses). In monkeys, antipsychotics have also been observed to decrease gray matter volume. We need much more research to understand the relationships between medications and these brain changes.

Electroconvulsive Therapy (ECT) and Repetitive Transcranial Magnetic Stimulation (rTMS)

Electroconvulsive therapy (ECT), most commonly used to treat severe depression, has a modest but definite role to play in the treatment of schizophrenia despite the adverse publicity it has received. It is a favorite whipping boy for Scientologists and anti-psychiatry advocates and was even banned from use in Berkeley, California, in 1982 by a local referendum. In European countries it has been used more widely for the treatment of schizophrenia than in the United States.

The use of ECT for treating acute schizophrenia is now rare. The *New England Journal of Medicine* summarizes the indications for its use as "when the onset is acute and confusion and mood disturbance are present; and [for] catatonia from almost any underlying cause." It is useful in some treatment-resistant cases, especially those with mood symptoms, violent or suicidal thoughts, and is definitely worth trying if clozapine does not work. It produces some clinical improvement in about half the cases. Modern ECT is done using unilateral electrodes over the nondominant lobe to minimize memory loss. Some memory loss may nevertheless occur and is the major side effect of the procedure. Despite Scientologist claims to the contrary, there is no evidence that ECT causes any damage to the brain. Some patients respond to as few as twelve ECT treatments, whereas others need twenty or more. For individuals who respond well to ECT but then rapidly relapse, it is possible to use monthly maintenance treatments; this is occasionally done in the U.S. but is more common in some European countries.

Transcranial magnetic stimulation (TMS) was introduced in the 1990s as a treatment for depression. It consists of the application of an electromagnetic coil to the outside of the skull and is both painless and noninvasive. Applications differ regarding precisely where the magnet is applied (e.g., frontal or temporal areas, left or right), how frequently it is applied, and the strength of the electromagnet. If the frequency of the electromagnetic wave is greater than one per second, it is called repetitive TMS, usually written rTMS.

TMS has been tried as a treatment for depression, bipolar disorder, obsessive-compulsive disorder, anxiety disorders, and post-traumatic stress disorder as well as for schizophrenia. Like ECT, it is not known precisely how TMS works. Initial trials have shown some modest effect in temporarily reducing auditory hallucinations in some patients, with the improvement lasting as long as twelve weeks. For individuals whose auditory hallucinations do not respond to drug treatment, rTMS may be worth trying. Of greater interest are reports that rTMS may alleviate some of the negative symptoms of schizophrenia; studies to date suggest a modest effect.

Herbal Treatments

Herbal treatments have become increasingly popular in the United States in recent years. This popularity has been fueled in part by rapid distribution of information on the Internet and in part by dissatisfaction with existing medications. Herbal treatments are attractive to many individuals because they are thought to be natural; advocates also point out that one-quarter of all existing medications, including digitalis and morphine, are derived from plants. Herbal treatments are widely available in health food stores and over the Internet. As long as the product is not advertised to treat a specific disease, there is essentially no regulation in the manufacture or testing of the compounds, a fact many consumers do not realize. It is therefore difficult to ascertain what is actually in the herbal remedy, and instances of adulteration have been documented.

Almost no studies have been done on the use of herbal treatments by individuals with schizophrenia. One survey reported that 22 percent of individuals with "mania or psychosis" had used some form of alternative medicine, including herbal treatments, within the previous twelve months. The herb most likely to be taken for schizophrenia is evening primrose oil, which contains omega-6 fatty acids and is also used by women for premenstrual symptoms. Its efficacy has not been scientifically studied, but it is thought to interact adversely with phenothiazine antipsychotics and to occasionally exacerbate mania. Ginkgo biloba, an herb used in the treatment of Alzheimer's disease, has also been used to treat cognitive symptoms in schizophrenia.

Many herbal therapies have been documented to have serious side effects, which many individuals who take them are not aware of. Kava, widely used for anxiety, has caused fatal liver failure and is banned in Canada and some European countries. Some herbal treatments may also exacerbate the symptoms of psychosis or cause psychotic symptoms in individuals who have not previously had them: yohimbine, ephedra (also known as ma huang), and Metabolife are examples. Still other herbal treatments may interfere with the other psychiatric medications the person is taking; a woman taking lithium, for example, experienced severe lithium toxicity (4.5 mml/liter) when she began to also take an herbal mixture for fluid retention. Individuals with schizophrenia should be cautious in taking herbal treatments and should report what they are taking to their treating physician.

Psychotherapy and Cognitive-Behavioral Therapy

Supportive psychotherapy, if used in combination with antipsychotics, can be very helpful for a person with schizophrenia, just as it is for anyone with a chronic disease. It may provide friendship, encouragement, and practical advice such as access to community resources or help developing a more active social life, vocational advice, suggestions for minimizing friction with family members, and, above all, hope that the person's life may be improved. Discussions focus on the here and now, not the past, and on problems of living encountered by the patient as he or she tries to meet the exigencies of life despite a handicapping brain disease. The opening approach I took with my own patients was something like the following: "Look, I'm sorry you have this lousy brain disease, which is not your fault; let's see what we can do to help you live better with it." It is the same approach one might take with a patient with multiple sclerosis, polio, chronic kidney disease, severe diabetes, or any other long-term disease. The person who provides counseling or supportive psychotherapy can be the physician who is overseeing the medication, or it can be any other mental illness professional or paraprofessional on the care team.

There is some evidence that supportive psychotherapy, when used in conjunction with antipsychotic medications, decreases rehospitalization. In one study, patients with schizophrenia were provided with supportive psychotherapy alone, antipsychotic medication alone, or both together. The rehospitalization rates after one year were, respectively, 63 percent, 33 percent, and 26 percent. The supportive psychotherapy in this study included social services and vocational counseling.

In contrast to supportive psychotherapy, psychoanalysis and insight-oriented psychotherapy have no place in the treatment of schizophrenia. Studies done in the 1960s and 1970s, when psychoanalysis was still commonly practiced in the United States, reported that even two years of psychoanalysis with skilled therapists had no effect on the symptoms of schizophrenia. More alarming was the finding that in many cases the psychoanalysis even made the patient's symptoms worse.

Given what we now know about the brains of people with schizophrenia, it should not be surprising to find that insight-oriented psychotherapy makes them sicker. Such people are overwhelmed by external and internal stimuli and are trying to impose some order on the chaos. In the midst of this, an insight-oriented psychotherapist asks them to probe their unconscious motivations, a difficult enough task even when one's brain is functioning perfectly. The inevitable consequence is to unleash a cacophony of repressed thoughts and wishes into the existing internal maelstrom. To do insight-oriented psychotherapy on persons with schizophrenia is analogous to directing a flood into a town already ravaged by a tornado.

The publication in 2007 of Elyn Saks best-selling book, *The Center Cannot Hold: My Journey through Madness*, revived some interest in the use of psychoanalysis in schizophrenia. Saks, who has had a very successful legal and academic career despite being diagnosed with a schizoaffective disorder, credits her extensive psychoanalysis with her success. A careful reading of the book, however, suggests that whenever Saks relied on psychoanalysis without taking antipsychotics, she relapsed. The most striking thing, in fact, is how long it took Saks, who is otherwise clearly very bright, to realize that antipsychotic medication was the key to remaining well and able to function at a high intellectual level.

Cognitive-behavioral therapy (CBT) is a special form of psychotherapy that has received much attention in recent years. It was originally developed to treat depression and anxiety but has become popular for treating the positive symptoms (delusions and hallucinations) of schizophrenia. In this approach, the therapist helps the patient develop coping methods for specific symptoms. The therapist may have the patient explore the rationale behind delusional beliefs or discuss the possible source of auditory hallucinations.

Many randomized trials have been carried out on cognitive-behavioral therapy and suggest that it is modestly effective in helping patients cope with delusions and hallucinations. It appears to be most helpful to individuals with longstanding symptoms who have not responded well to antipsychotic medications and who are distressed about their symptoms. It can, of course, only be used with those patients who have an awareness of their illness and are willing to undergo therapy sessions over several months. Whether it is more useful than supportive psychotherapy is unclear. As with all forms of psychotherapy, the most important determinant of its effectiveness is the therapeutic alliance between the therapist and the patient, and this is in large measure determined by the personality characteristics of the therapist, such as genuineness, empathy, and warmth.

Family therapy is an important component in the treatment of schizophrenia. A supportive family is crucial in the successful rehabilitation and continuing functioning of a patient. It is important for family members to understand the symptoms of the illness, and particularly that the perceived "laziness" is a negative symptom of the disease. Family members can be very helpful in ensuring that patients are compliant with their medication. Patients should be encouraged to see that they need their families support.

RAISE and the Early Treatment of Schizophrenia

One of the most striking changes in the treatment of schizophrenia in recent years has been an increased interest in treating patients as early as possible. This approach began in the 1990s, when a number of studies were published claiming that long delays in beginning treatment lead to a more serious disease and a poorer long-term outcome. Most, but not all, recent studies have supported this claim. A study in Ireland, for example, reported that "a longer duration of untreated psychosis was associated with a significantly poorer functional and symptomatic outcome four years later." A Norwegian study similarly asserted that "reducing the DUP [duration of untreated psychosis] has effects on the course of symptoms and functioning, including negative symptoms." Common sense suggests that early treatment is better, but it is still unclear how important it is.

From such studies emerged an interest in treating individuals with schizophrenia as quickly as possible after they developed the disease. This led to a recent NIMH-funded study carried out at 34 mental health centers to try and measure the effects of early treatment. This was the Recovery After an Initial Schizophrenia Episode (RAISE) project that offered some patients with schizophrenia medication management, psychotherapy, family education, case management, and vocational support. These patients were then compared with controls who received treatment as usual. Not surprisingly, the RAISE patients did better in the short term and the program was said to be cost effective. Whether the RAISE program will have any effect on the long-term course of these patients has yet to be determined.

The next logical step in the early treatment of schizophrenia was to move one step back and try to intervene just as the patients were developing the earliest symptoms. Past studies that have tried to predict who will develop schizophrenia have not been promising. One study showed that efforts to detect college students who were schizophrenia-prone by using questionnaires on magical thinking were virtually worthless. In another retrospective study, prediction by high school teachers regarding which of their students would develop schizophrenia was "barely better than chance." A study from Scotland was more promising in terms of identifying individuals who are likely to develop schizophrenia; such individuals scored higher on characteristics such as withdrawal, social anxiety, and odd thinking. However, all of us who have raised adolescent children are aware that they can be quite strange at times, and clinically differentiating such strangeness from early schizophrenia in the absence of a biological marker is a Herculean task.

The most recent attempt to identify those who were in the early stages of developing schizophrenia and intervene was a program set up by Dr. William McFarlane in Maine. Called the Portland Identification and Early Referral (PIER) program, it identified individuals thought to be at high risk for developing the disease and provided them with assertive community treatment, family education, supported education or employment and, if indicated, low dose medication. This group was then compared to a low risk comparison over two years at six study sites. Not surprisingly, those who received the PIER services had fewer symptoms and a better school and work record. Whether this will make a clinical difference over time or is cost effective remains to be determined.

The next logical step is to take another step back and ask whether schizophrenia can be prevented. A group in Australia focused on individuals who were thought to be at high risk for developing the disease and treated them with fish oil (omega-3) for three months. A control group of high-risk patients did not receive the fish oil. In the initial study at the end of one year it appeared that the fish oil had had some effect in preventing the emergence of some cases of schizophrenia. Unfortunately, however, two attempts to replicate these results were negative.

Thus at this point in time there is no evidence that any case of schizophrenia has ever been prevented. It remains an attractive goal to which we should aspire, but true prevention probably depends on having a better understanding of the cause of the disease than we currently have.

Recommended Further Reading

Buchanan, R. W., J. Kreyenbuhl, D. L. Kelly, et al. "The 2009 Schizophrenia PORT Psychopharmacological Treatment Recommendations and Summary Statements." *Schizophrenia Bulletin* 36 (2010): 71–93.

Cohen, C. I., and S. I. Cohen. "Potential Cost Savings from Pill Splitting of Newer Psychotropic Medications." *Psychiatric Services* 51 (2000): 527–29.

Deegan, P. E., and R. E. Drake. "Shared Decision Making and Medication Management in the Recovery Process." *Psychiatric Services* 57 (2006): 1636–39.

Dickerson, F. B., and A. F. Lehman. "Evidence-Based Psychotherapy for Schizophrenia." *Journal of Nervous and Mental Disease* 194 (2006): 3–9.

Dixon, L. B., F. Dickerson, A. S. Bellack, et al. "The 2009 Schizophrenia PORT Psychosocial Treatment Recommendations and Summary Statements." *Schizophrenia Bulletin* 36 (2010): 48–70.

Fenton, W. S. "Prevalence of Spontaneous Dyskinesia in Schizophrenia." *Journal of Clinical Psychiatry* 61 (Suppl. 4) (2000): 10–14.

Francell, E. G., Jr. "Medication: The Foundation of Recovery." *Innovations and Research* 3 (1994): 31–40.

Goren J. L., A. J. Rose, E. G. Smith, et al. "The Business Case for Expanded Clozapine Utilization." *Psychiatric Services* 67 (2016): 1197–1205.

Kelly, D. L., J. Kreyenbuhl, R. W. Buchanan, et al. "Why Not Clozapine?" *Clinical Schizophrenia & Related Psychoses* 1 (2007): 92–95.

Leucht, S., K. Komossa, C. Rummel-Kluge, et al. "A Meta-Analysis of Head-to-Head Comparisons of Second-Generation Antipsychotics in the Treatment of Schizophrenia." *American Journal of Psychiatry* 166 (2009): 152–63.

Leucht, S., M. Tardy, K. Korhossa, et al. "Antipsychotic Drugs Versus Placebo for Relapse Prevention in Schizophrenia: A Systematic Review and Meta-Analysis." *Lancet* 379 (2012): 2067–71.

Opler, L. A., R. S. Laitman, A. M. Laitman, et al. Clozapine: Meaningful Recovery From Schizophrenia, order from website of teamdanielrunningfor receeovery.org.

The Medical Letter on Drugs and Therapeutics (The Medical Letter, Inc.), http://secure.medicalletter.org/medicalletter.

Tandon, R., and M. D. Jibson, "Efficacy of Newer Generation Antipsychotics in the Treatment of Schizophrenia," *Psychoneuroendocrinology* 28 (2003): 9–26.

Torrey, E. F., M. Knable, C. Quanbeck and J. Davis. Clozapine for Treating Schizophrenia: A Comparison of the States. Treatment Advocacy Center (Arlington, VA) 2015. http://www.treatmentadvocacycenter.org/storage /documents/clozapine-for-treating-schizophrenia.pdf

Torrey, E. F., and John Davis. "Adjunct Treatments for Schizophrenia and Bipolar Disorder: What to Try When You Are Out of Ideas." *Clinical Schizophrenia & Related Psychoses* 5 (2012): 208–16.

Worst Pills, Best Pills (Public Citizen's Health Research Group), http://worst pills.org/.

8

The Rehabilitation of Schizophrenia

Expecting the chronically ill patient to use the current mental health system is like expecting a paraplegic to use stairs.

> J. Halpern, et al.,
> The Illness of Deinstitutionalization, *1978*

In recent years, the "recovery model" of schizophrenia has become fashionable in the United States. Although the model is disingenuous in implying that most individuals with schizophrenia can recover most of their function, the model does contain one important truth: the better the opportunities for rehabilitation, the better the individual with schizophrenia is likely to do.

The basic concept that underlies the rehabilitation of schizophrenia was clearly articulated by Dr. Werner M. Mendel, a psychiatrist who spent more than forty years treating patients with this disease in both the private and the public sector. In his book *Treating Schizophre-*

nia, Mendel likens an individual with schizophrenia to an individual with a physical disability:

> If, for example, someone has a paralyzed right arm that cannot be fixed, we then provide her with a brace to help with function. We may modify her car so that she can drive and work the controls with only one hand. We may retrain her to use her left hand for all the things she used to do with her paralyzed right hand. We may also give her psychological support for accepting herself with the defect and help her focus on what she can do rather than what she cannot do.

Treating individuals who have schizophrenia with medication alone, then, is not sufficient. A complete treatment program includes rehabilitation as well. Although patients vary widely in their rehabilitation needs depending on the severity of their symptoms, all of them have to address the basic problems of money, food, housing, employment, friendship, and medical care.

Before addressing these specific problems, it should be noted that one concept underlies all rehabilitation efforts—hope. If the individual with schizophrenia has hope, then rehabilitation efforts are likely to succeed. If the person has no hope, these efforts are likely to fail. This was shown in a recent Swiss study of forty-six individuals with schizophrenia in which poor rehabilitation outcomes were predicted by "pessimistic outcome expectancies . . . and depressive-resigned coping strategies," in short, "whether the patient has already given up or not." Treatment and rehabilitation programs will succeed, therefore, only insofar as they also engender hope.

Money and Food

For over a century, most individuals with schizophrenia were locked away in state psychiatric hospitals, usually for many years at a time. If they got out at all it was to live with their families. It was not until the advent of antipsychotic medication and deinstitutionalization that money, food, and housing became major problems for the hundreds of thousands of individuals who were subsequently released from the hospitals.

Some persons with schizophrenia can work part-time or full-time and are self-supporting. The vast majority, however, must rely on their families or on two government programs, Supplemental Security Income (SSI) and Social Security Disability Insurance (SSDI), for the money to pay for their food and housing.

SSI, a program to provide income for needy aged, blind, and disabled persons, is administered by the Social Security Administration. It defines disability as "an inability to engage in any substantial gainful activity by reason of any medically determined physical or mental impairment which . . . has lasted, or can be expected to last, for a continuous period of not less than twelve months." SSDI is a similar program, except that to be eligible the person must have worked prior to becoming ill and accumulated sufficient credit under Social Security. Benefits from the two programs vary; SSDI varies according to how long the person had worked before becoming ill, while SSI varies from state to state depending upon how much that state supplements the federal SSI payment; approximately half of the states provide some supplement. SSDI and SSI are the most important sources of financial support for individuals with schizophrenia in the United States.

Applications to establish disability and receive SSI and SSDI funds should be made at the local Social Security office. The person's assets and other income are taken into consideration in computing eligibility. If the person has savings worth more than $2,000, he/she may not be eligible; in computing assets, a home, car, and basic household goods do not count toward the $2,000. The application for SSI or SSDI is evaluated by a team consisting of a disability examiner and a physician; they may request additional medical information or request an examination of the applicant in selected cases. In evaluating the application, they pay special attention to evidence of a restriction of daily activities and interests, deterioration in personal habits, marked impairment in relating to other people, and the inability to concentrate and carry out instructions necessary to hold a job. Thus, you should submit whatever medical records are pertinent to establishing this at the time you submit your application. Assessing eligibility for SSI and SSDI is necessarily a subjective task, and studies have reported disagreement among reviewers as much as 50 percent of the time. A decision on an initial application usually takes three to six months; approximately half of all initial applications are denied.

If the applicant is denied SSI or SSDI, he/she has the right to appeal. This must be done within sixty days of the denial, and additional evidence of disability can be included at that time. The initial reconsideration of the appeal occurs in the local Social Security office and results in approval only 15 percent of the time. However, the applicant may appeal again, and this time the hearing is before an administrative law judge of the Bureau of Hearings and Appeals of the U.S. Department of Health and Human Services. At this level a higher percentage of appeals are approved. Further appeals are possible to the Appeals Council Review Board and then to a U.S. district court. It is clear that persistence in pressing a legitimate claim for SSI or SSDI benefits will often result in success.

For applicants who are approved for SSI and SSDI benefits, payments are made retrospectively from the date of the initial application. Since the appeals process can take a year or longer, it is not unusual for SSI and SSDI recipients to receive, as their initial payment, a check for thousands of dollars. For individuals who are not capable of managing their own funds, especially those with concurrent substance abuse, it is customary for the Social Security Administration to appoint a representative payee who may be a family member, case manager, or other person (see chapter 10, "Assisted Treatment").

People with schizophrenia usually require assistance with SSI and SSDI applications and, when necessary, with the appeals processes. Social workers who are submitting these applications on a regular basis are often very helpful, especially in ensuring that the correct clinical information is included so that the person's degree of disability can be assessed fairly. Persons applying for SSI or SSDI for psychiatric disability for the first time would be wise to utilize the services of a knowledgeable social worker. Application forms and appeals processes are confusing even for persons whose brains are working perfectly; to a person with schizophrenia they must appear completely Kafkaesque.

SSI payments, but not SSDI payments, are reduced when the disabled recipient lives with his/her family. In theory this takes account of the room and board the person receives, but in fact it penalizes people with schizophrenia for living at home. Many families resent this discriminatory living aspect of the SSI program and claim that they have expenses for the person just as surely as a boardinghouse operator does. SSI payments are also stopped if a person is hospitalized for more than ninety days. A portion of the SSI monthly payment is intended for the disabled person to use as spending money for clothes, transportation, laundry, and entertainment. The amount of spending money varies by state.

It is important for persons with schizophrenia to establish eligibility for SSI or SSDI benefits if they can. Even if they have other income, thereby reducing the monthly SSI or SSDI check to a very small amount, it is still worthwhile. The reason is that eligibility for SSI or SSDI also establishes eligibility for other assistance programs that can be worth much more than the SSI or SSDI benefits by themselves. Such programs include Medicaid, Medicare, vocational rehabilitation services, food stamps, and some housing and rental assistance programs of the Department of Housing and Urban Development. In some states, eligibility for SSI or SSDI automatically confers eligibility for the other programs, while in other states a separate application must be submitted.

In January 2018 the federal monthly payment for SSI was increased to $750 for an individual and $1,125 for a married couple; approximately half of all states provide a state supplement to this. Individuals on SSI can earn up to $65 per month without losing any SSI income. For persons earning more than $65 per month, their SSI benefits are reduced by $1 for each additional $2 earned. Also in 2000, Congress passed legislation making it possible for SSI and SSDI recipients who are trying to return to full-time employment to retain their Medicaid and Medicare benefits; previously these benefits were automatically lost, thereby presenting a major disincentive for SSI and SSDI recipients to return to work.

Individuals with schizophrenia who do not receive support from their families or from the SSI and SSDI programs must rely on other income. Many of them, especially those living in public shelters, utilize public assistance or welfare checks. Individuals who were in the military at the time they first became ill often qualify for disability payments from the Veterans Administration; these are often very generous and may total over $2,000 a month when all benefits are included.

Food stamps are another supplementary source of support for persons with schizophrenia and are underutilized. To be eligible, a person must have an income below the poverty level; this level includes most persons with schizophrenia. The amount of food stamps a person can receive varies by state and with income. It also varies with the cost of food and so has been rising as food prices have been rising. Food stamps can be obtained through local welfare or social services offices.

Housing

Housing for individuals with schizophrenia includes facilities with varying degrees of supervision, independent living, and living at home.

Professional Supervision: This type of housing has professionally trained persons who provide supervision for most or all of the twenty-four-hour day. It includes crisis houses, halfway houses, quarter-way houses, and similar facilities. An excellent description of one such home can be found in Michael Winerip's 1994 book, *9 Highland Road.*

Nonprofessional Supervision: These facilities have a supervisor in residence part or all of the time, but the supervisor has no training. These include foster homes, board-and-care homes, boardinghouses, group homes, congregate care homes, and similar facilities that go by different names in different locales.

Intermittent Supervision: These residences include apartments and group homes set up for persons with schizophrenia to live basically on their own. Usually a case manager or other mental health professional stops by periodically (e.g., once a week) to make certain that there are no major problems.

The quality of supervised housing for persons with schizophrenia varies widely. On one end of the spectrum are small foster homes where each patient has a room, the food is adequate, and the foster home sponsors watch over and worry about their charges as if they were their own children. A larger version of this may be a renovated hotel where the manager hires staff that organizes social activities for the residents, checks to be sure they are taking their medicine, reminds them of dentist appointments, and helps them fill out applications for food stamps.

But at the other extreme are foster homes with sponsors who provide insufficient heat, blankets, and food; steal the patients' meager funds; use them as cheap labor; and sometimes even rape them or pimp them. The larger versions of these homes are old hotels that provide no services other than a rundown room and carry out similar kinds of exploitation.

Supervision in many homes for released psychiatric patients often exists on paper only. In a group home in Baltimore, which was licensed as a "graduated independent living program" with twenty-four-hour supervision, the staff failed to discover a young man with diabetes until three days after he had died in his room. And in New York City "the police found the decaying corpse of a former patient lying undisturbed in one home inhabited by six other residents." The depths to which housing for individuals with schizophrenia can descend—squalor, chaos, exploitation of patients, unnecessary surgery—was shockingly documented in 2002 in a *New York Times* series about New York group homes.

Because the living facilities are so poor in many places, the professionals in charge of discharging patients from state hospitals are frequently caught in an ethical dilemma. Is the patient really better off in the community than in the hospital? Are the living conditions and exposure to potential victimization really an improvement? I am always surprised to find how many patients with schizophrenia express satisfaction with their living conditions in the community when I know how shoddy the living conditions are. In one study of patients living in board-and-care homes in Los Angeles, 40 percent claimed to be content or reasonably content. I suspect the contentment is in comparison to being back in the hospital or having to live in public shelters or on the streets.

What are the common denominators of good supervised housing for patients living in the community? There are four characteristics that can be identified. First, the people living there are treated with dignity and warmth, not simply as sources of income. Second, the best housing appears to set a maximum of fifteen to twenty persons living in a single facility. Boarding homes or congregate care homes for fifty, one hundred, or even more released patients almost invariably become mental hospital wards called by another name; this is transinstitutionalization rather than deinstitutionalization.

Third, good community housing for psychiatric patients should exist in a coordinated continuum whereby a person can be moved to a residence with more or less supervision depending on the needs of the person. Because schizophrenia is a disease of remissions and relapses, it is unrealistic to expect a patient to remain in the same kind of facility indefinitely.

Finally, community housing for patients with schizophrenia is most useful where it is integrated with other activities of the patients. An excellent example of this principle is the Fairweather Lodges, in which patients live together and contract for jobs as a group. Such facilities have been deemed to be very successful where they have been tried and are well described in John Trepp's *Lodge Magic*, listed at the end of the chapter.

Studies have also been done on patient characteristics that predict greater degrees of independent living. Those characteristics that were most important were patients having frequent contact with their families (who presumably help them maintain their living situation), having good hygiene skills, having relatively few negative symptoms, and being able to participate in social activities.

There are a handful of excellent housing programs for individuals with schizophrenia and other severe psychiatric disorders. Many of them are affiliated with clubhouses, such as Fountain House in New York and Thresholds in Chicago. The last, for example, has units for more than one thousand individuals; furthermore, the housing units exist with many levels of supervision so that individuals can move to a more appropriate level as their clinical condition improves or deteriorates. For families who are fortunate enough to have the financial means, there are a few excellent living facilities for individuals with schizophrenia. They include homes such as Gould Farm in Monterey, Massachusetts; Spring Lake Ranch in Cuttingsville, Vermont; Clearview Communities in Frederick, Maryland; CooperRiis in Mill Spring, North Carolina; Skyland Trail in Atlanta; Hopewell in Mesopotamia, Ohio; Rose Hill in Holly, Michigan; Hanbleceya San Diego in La Mesa, California, and the John Herman House in Rochester, Minnesota. Many of these are expensive, with costs of $100,000 a year or more, but for some families they may be just what is needed. At a more modest level, I will admit to being partial to a model halfway house in Haverford, Pennsylvania (Torrey House), and an excellent independent living complex in Bartlesville, Oklahoma (Torrey Place).

A practical problem that frequently arises with community housing for psychiatric patients is the issue of zoning and community resistance to such housing. Everybody applauds the placement of patients in the community, it is said, as long as the placement is not in their neighborhood. In some towns and cities in the United States, local fights over this issue have been very bitter. There have now been forty studies done on the effect of residential group homes for the mentally ill and mentally retarded on the surrounding neighborhood. A review of these studies found that "the presence of group homes in all the areas studied has *not* lowered property values or increased turnover, *not* increased crime, *not* changed the character of the neighborhood." Persons with schizophrenia in fact make very good neighbors. This assumes, of course, that they are being followed for their illness and supervised for medication by responsible mental illness professionals.

Independent Living: A large and growing number of individuals with schizophrenia live independently, either by themselves or with other people. In recent years this has been referred to as supported housing, implying that the mental illness professionals will support the choice of housing made by the patients. Independent living may run a wide range in quality from rundown SROs (single-room-occupancy hotels) to nicely furnished apartments or homes. A major problem for individuals with schizophrenia living independently is social isolation; in one recent study, 59 percent of individuals and 71 percent of their families indicated that this was a problem. Some individuals with schizophrenia, especially those with limited awareness of their illness, cannot live independently.

Living at Home: A large number of individuals with schizophrenia live at home or with relatives. For some patients and their families this may be a perfectly satisfactory arrangement and cause minimal problems. For many others, however, living at home is quite unsatisfactory and this is especially true for men. This is not surprising since most grown individuals who do not have schizophrenia also encounter problems living at home. For those who do live at home, some suggested strategies are discussed in chapter 11.

Employment

People with schizophrenia extend over the same broad range as persons without schizophrenia regarding their interest in working. At one end of the spectrum are individuals who will do anything to work and will often continue working even when they are not being paid; individuals at the other end will do anything to avoid work. The only difference in work attitudes between persons with and without schizophrenia is that those with the disorder often have problems working closely with other people, thereby making work more difficult for them. Passage of the Americans with Disabilities Act in 1990 was intended to protect mentally ill workers from discriminatory practices and theoretically should result in increased job opportunities for those who want to work.

The majority of persons with schizophrenia have residual disabilities, such as thinking disorders and auditory hallucinations, that are sufficiently severe that full-time employment is impossible. Many can do part-time jobs, however. Estimates of the number of persons with schizophrenia capable of full-time work range as low as 6 percent; from my own experience, I would estimate that approximately 10 to 15 percent of people with schizophrenia can work full-time and an additional 30 to 40 percent can work part-time *if* proper medication maintenance and rehabilitation programs are available and disincentives to losing medical benefits are removed. Past employment is the best single predictor of future employment for a person with schizophrenia; a person who becomes sick after having had a job is more likely to find work than a person who becomes sick without ever having worked.

Work provides several potential benefits for people, not the least of which is additional income. Improved self-esteem is equally important, for to hold a job is evidence that one is like other people. England's Douglas Bennett, one of the few mental illness professionals who has fought for vocational opportunities for persons with schizophrenia, says that a job magically transforms a patient into a person. Patients will often work very hard to control their psychiatric symptoms in work situations because work is so important to them. It has been observed, for example, that "in the morning at the day center, the same person is fulfilling the role of patient and acts like a patient, exhibiting symptoms and bizarre behavior never seen in the workshop the same afternoon." Work also provides people with a daily structure, a reason to get out of bed in the morning, an identity, and an extended social network.

It is ironic that the civil rights efforts that led to the release of so many patients from psychiatric hospitals also led to sharply decreased availability of jobs for them. In the past, many of these patients had worked on the hospital farms, on the grounds, and on housekeeping and kitchen details. Undoubtedly there was some abuse of this captive work force, and civil rights lawyers went to court with claims of "peonage." The result was a pendulum that swung too far in efforts to correct the situation; hospitals became reluctant to employ patients at all because they could not afford to pay them the minimum wage and other employee benefits. The consequence is that there are thousands of patients in hospitals and in the community who are capable of and enjoy working for brief periods but who are not capable of full-time employment. The part-time jobs of the past that were often tailored to their needs are now gone.

The largest impediment to vocational opportunities for persons with schizophrenia is stigma, as will be discussed in chapters 13 and 15. Employers, like most people in our society, do not understand what schizophrenia is and so react negatively when asked if they would consider employing persons with this disease. "I can't have any psychos working in my place" is a common visceral reaction. Another major impediment is that government rehabilitation programs and sheltered workshops have traditionally shunned the mentally handicapped in favor of the physically handicapped. Vocational rehabilitation in the United States is still stuck in the polio era, and if you don't have a visible physical disability, you need not apply. The failure of traditional vocational rehabilitation to serve individuals with schizophrenia was documented in a scathing 1997 report, *A Legacy of Failure*, by John Noble et al. (see "Recommended Further Reading" at the end of this chapter). Some other countries do a much better job of providing job opportunities for psychiatric patients; Sweden, England, and the Netherlands all have a greater availability of workshops for long-term partial employment.

There are several kinds of vocational rehabilitation programs for individuals with serious mental illnesses. There is an ongoing debate among mental illness professionals regarding which approach is the best, but in reality all approaches should ideally be available, since individuals vary widely in their needs.

Sheltered Employment: These are sheltered workshops in which the person is not necessarily expected to graduate to competitive employment. In the United States, Goodwill Industries operates many of them.

Transitional Employment: This model of vocational rehabilitation was developed by Fountain House, a clubhouse in New York City, and is used in many other clubhouses. Participants are assigned to real jobs in commercial establishments and accompanied by a rehabilitation specialist. Two individuals will often divide a single job (e.g., each working half-time) as they learn the job. The graduation rate from transitional employment to competitive employment is impressive, and a 1991 study of transitional employment showed it to be highly cost-effective.

Supported Employment: In this model the individual is encouraged to select the employment of his/her choice, then is trained intensively in job and related social skills before starting the job. An example of supported employment is the Access program affiliated with the Boston University Center for Psychiatric Rehabilitation. The person attends pre-employment classes for fifteen hours a week for seven weeks, then is given a job coach and extensive support in the initial months on the job.

Job Skills Training: This model utilizes commercial establishments that are specifically set up to train individuals with serious mental illnesses in job skills. An impressive example was a restaurant in

Hayward, California, called the Eden Express, in which patients did all jobs, including food preparation, catering, aide to cook, busing, waiting on tables, hostessing, cashiering, dishwashing, and janitorial work. Between 1980 and 1985 a total of 315 persons, or 80 percent of those who enrolled, completed the fifteen-week training program. Approximately twenty-five trainees were enrolled at any given time, and several job counselors made up the training staff. The staff also taught trainees how to interview for jobs at the completion of their training, and 94 percent of the graduates were able to obtain jobs. The Eden Express was largely self-supporting and served more than four thousand customers each month. Salaries for the job counselors were derived primarily from training funds from the California State Departments of Rehabilitation and Education. Other job skills programs have developed modules specifically designed to teach mentally ill workers how to keep their jobs once employed.

Competitive Employment: Some people with schizophrenia can return to competitive employment but not necessarily at the level they would have achieved if they had not become ill. An especially interesting example of competitive employment is the use of people with schizophrenia to be case managers for others with this illness, as described in chapter 11.

Friendship and Social Skills Training

Friendship is needed by persons with schizophrenia, just as it is by everyone without schizophrenia. For the person with schizophrenia, however, there are often barriers to friendship, including the symptoms and brain dysfunction associated with the disorder.

One young man I provided care for recovered from most of his symptoms and was living at home. He attempted to return to his social group of peers, going to taverns and drinking with them as he had done prior to his illness. He found this very difficult, however, complaining that "I can't make out their words, I don't know what to say. It's just not like it used to be." Another patient complained that in social situations "I get lost in the spaces between words in sentences. I can't concentrate, or I get off into thinking about something else." In view of such difficulties, it is not surprising that many people with schizophrenia often respond inappropriately in social situations and eventually withdraw. Studies of patients living in the community report that approximately 25 percent are very isolated, 50 percent are moderately isolated, and only 25 percent lead active social lives. Almost half have no recreational activity whatsoever, other than watching television.

In addition to their brain dysfunction, which may interfere with social relationships, individuals with schizophrenia must also contend with the stigma that accrues to their illness, as discussed in chapters 13 and 15. One older man, who returned to the hospital because the stigma encountered was so pervasive, expressed it well:

> I just can't make it out there. I know who I am and they know who I am—most of the people out there won't come near me or they spit at me in the eye. I'm just like a leper in their eyes. They treat most of us like that. They're prejudiced, you know. They are either afraid or hate us. I've seen it a thousand times. I don't feel good on the outside. I don't belong. They know it and I know it.

There are several possible solutions to the need for friendship among individuals with schizophrenia. One is patient self-help groups, which are discussed below. Another solution is joining clubhouse programs patterned after Fountain House in New York, as discussed in Chapter 9. Another is the Compeer Program that was begun in Rochester, New York, in 1981 and that has spread to many other cities. Compeer volunteers who are not mentally ill are matched with individuals who have schizophrenia or other serious mental illnesses on a one-to-one basis. The two people then get together once a week to shop, go to a movie, go to dinner, play checkers, or share some common interest. (The Compeer website is www.compeer.org.)

Still another solution to the friendship problem is offered by the Friendship Network in New York, which is run by the Queens Nassau NAMI chapter and is a dating service set up specifically for persons who have schizophrenia or bipolar disorder (www.friendshipnetwork.org). I have personally been very impressed by how much support two individuals with severe mental illnesses can give each other and the strength of the bond that comes from sharing these disorders. Some of the relationships are, of course, disasters, but others are the most important thing that has happened to the people involved; as such, they essentially mirror the range of relationships found among people who do not have severe mental illnesses.

Another approach to friendship is by improving the person's social skills through didactic instruction and supervised group interaction. Social skills training is built into many of the vocational rehabilitation programs mentioned in the previous section, but such training may also be done on its own. Some social skills training programs for individuals with schizophrenia are highly structured programs to make the person more aware of social cues, facial expressions, and the subtleties of normal social interactions (e.g., the person is taught to make eye contact when speaking to others). One of the most widely used such programs is the UCLA Skills Training Modules, created by Dr. Robert Liberman and his colleagues, which provided skills training for more than three thousand mentally ill individuals at the West Los Angeles Veterans Administration Medical Center as well as at many other facilities. It consists of ten training modules, each of which has a trainer's manual, patient's workbook, user's guide, and videocassette. Such educational methods can be extremely useful in helping individuals function better socially and thereby better survive schizophrenia. (Contact Psychiatric Rehabilitation Consultants, www.psychrehab.com.) A variant of social skills training is cognitive remediation, in which attempts are made to improve the person's cognitive deficits. Computer-based programs have been developed and various claims made for their effectiveness, but this has yet to be demonstrated.

Another aspect of friendship for a person with schizophrenia is the nonhuman variety. Pets often make excellent companions, just as they do for some persons without schizophrenia. Dogs are especially good, for they love indiscriminately, are not at all bothered by a person's thought disorders or auditory hallucinations, and are usually understanding when things are not going well. Providing pets for persons with schizophrenia can often bring them much pleasure; this has been discovered by families as well as by some psychiatric hospitals that have allowed the patients to keep pets or to utilize visiting "pets on wheels" programs.

Medical and Dental Care

Like everyone else, individuals with schizophrenia get sick with other illnesses and require medical care. Obtaining medical care may be difficult, however, for many reasons. Perhaps the most important one is that most people with schizophrenia do not have medical insurance and so must utilize Medicaid and Medicare. Medicaid benefits vary widely from state to state, and many physicians will not accept Medicaid patients.

Other impediments to obtaining medical care include the inability of some people with schizophrenia to give a coherent account of their symptoms to a physician or other health care practitioner, the higher pain threshold found in some individuals with schizophrenia leading to a delay in diagnosis (see chapter 1), and the difficulty that some people with schizophrenia have in understanding or following instructions for treatment. In addition, side effects of the person's antipsychotic medications may confuse the clinical picture, and the antipsychotic medication may interact with medication prescribed for the medical problems.

For all these reasons there is known to be a comparatively high incidence of untreated medical problems among persons with schizophrenia, with studies reporting such problems in 26 to 53 percent of patients. A study by Adler and Griffith concluded that "the treatment of the medically ill schizophrenic patient can be one of the most challenging tasks a physician will face." The failure to provide such treatment, however, is one reason why individuals with schizophrenia have a higher mortality rate, as discussed in chapter 4.

Because of concern among mental illness professionals that the physical health of individuals with schizophrenia was being neglected, a two-day conference on this problem was held at Mount Sinai School of Medicine in 2002. The participants agreed on consensus recommendations, targeting especially the known side effects of second-generation antipsychotics. Such patients should receive special attention for weight gain (measurements of body mass), blood glucose and lipid levels, and EKG and other cardiac measures.

Like medical care, dental care is also neglected in many individuals with schizophrenia. A study in Scotland reported that such individuals, compared to the general population, were less likely to brush their teeth each day, had had more dental problems, and had fewer remaining teeth.

Exercise

Regular physical exercise is an important component of rehabilitation for individuals with schizophrenia. In recent years, there has been an outpouring of studies showing that exercise improves many brain diseases, such as Parkinson's disease, as well as psychiatric disorders, especially depression. For individuals with schizophrenia, exercise can help with weight control and also ameliorate symptoms.

In 2016, Dauwan et al. reviewed 29 studies of the effects of exercise on individuals with schizophrenia (see Recommended Further Reading). Fifteen studies with a total of 641 patients reported that exercise significantly reduced positive symptoms. In addition, 18 studies with a total of 765 patients found that exercise improved the negative symptoms of schizophrenia even more impressively than the positive symptoms. This is important because the negative symptoms of schizophrenia respond to our existing medications much less robustly. Depression, which is often associated with the negative symptoms of schizophrenia, improved impressively.

Regarding the type of exercise that was effective, any exercise that increased the heart rate (aerobic exercise), as well as physical yoga, was effective. Thus, brisk walking, biking, vigorous dancing, and walking up 3 flights of stairs can all be helpful. Regarding duration, to be effective for reducing symptoms, individuals should try to exercise for a minimum of 90 to 120 minutes each week.

Peer Support Groups but Not the Hearing Voices Network

As part of the rehabilitation for individuals with schizophrenia, peer support can be very important. Being able to openly discuss your symptoms, medication side effects, and problems associated with having this disorder with others who are similarly afflicted can be a source of great support. This may occur informally, as it does in clubhouse programs (see chapter 9), and in fact such informal peer support is one of the reasons why clubhouse programs have been so successful.

Peer support for individuals with schizophrenia may also take place through the organization of formal peer groups which meet regularly. Leadership of such groups is usually provided by one of the people with schizophrenia; a mental health professional may also be involved in the early stages to help get it started. The group may have a formal agenda or not; many such groups sometimes invite speakers. Some groups also plan joint trips or other social events. Such groups have various names such as "On Our Own."

The main problem with peer support groups is that in many places the leadership of such groups has been taken over by "consumer survivors" who are overtly anti-psychiatry and anti-medication. Such groups can be very harmful to individuals with schizophrenia who are trying to adjust to the fact that they have a brain disease and are working toward recovery. Being told by your peers that there is really nothing wrong with you and that it is a mistake to take antipsychotic medication is distinctly unhelpful. Prior to the change in leadership in 2017 at the Substance Abuse and Mental Health Services Administration (SAMHSA) (see chapter 15), that organization was funding anti-psychiatry leaders for peer support groups. Thus, our federal tax dollars were actually being used to make it more difficult for individuals with schizophrenia to recover.

In recent years, peer support groups under a social movement called Hearing Voices Network (HVN) have become popular. This movement started in the Netherlands, spread to England, and is now becoming widespread in Canada and the U.S. According to a 2017 paper by three American HVN advocates, the HVN groups are based upon "core principles" centered on a belief that "hearing voices is not indicative of pathology, but instead reflects underlying difficulties that are a consequence of traumatic experiences and emotional neglect." The promoters of HVN claim that hearing voices is not pathological since it is part of a continuum. Many people hear voices, and in some cultures it is expected that you will hear the voices of your dead ancestors. HVN advocates even claim that hearing voices can even be helpful at times. As one of the leaders of the HVN proclaimed: "I am proud to be a voice hearer. It is an incredibly special and unique experience."

As noted in Chapter 2, it is of course true that hearing voices is not unusual, especially in some cultures, but that does not mean that hearing voices cannot also be a symptom of brain pathology. Consider coughing, for example. Everyone coughs from time to time, but if a person is coughing up blood we recognize the person's symptom as pathological. Nobody who is coughing up blood would say: "I am a proud blood cougher."

A major problem with the HVN support groups, moreover, is that they are founded on the belief that hearing voices is caused by "traumatic experiences and emotional neglect." Thus the HVN is an extension of the childhood trauma and stress theories of the cause of schizophrenia (see chapter 5), and many of the leaders of the HVN movement have also promoted trauma theories. Participants in HVN support groups are encouraged to try and identify the traumatic experiences that caused them to be hearing voices. This of course leads directly to blaming their family for such experiences as "emotional neglect." It is a return to blaming the family theories of the last century.

Another major problem with HVN support groups is that they encourage participants to stop taking their medication. If your voices are not indicative of illness but merely part of a normal continuum of experience, why should you need medication? Thus it is not surprising to find that 29 percent of participants in a HVN group in England said that the group had led them to consider discontinuing their medication.

In summary, peer support groups can be very helpful for individuals with schizophrenia but not if such groups are sponsored by the Hearing Voices Network.

Recommended Further Reading

Anthony, W., M. Cohen, and M. Farkas. *Psychiatric Rehabilitation*. Boston: Center for Psychiatric Rehabilitation, 1990.

Campbell, K., G. R. Bond, and R. E. Drake. "Who Benefits from Supported Employment: A Meta-Analytic Study." *Schizophrenia Bulletin* 37 (2011): 370–80.

Dauwan, M., M.J.H. Begemann, S.M. Heringa, et al. "Exercise Improves

Clinical Symptoms, Quality of Life, Global Functioning, and Depression in Schizophrenia: Systematic Review and Meta-Analysis. *Schizophrenia Bulletin* 42 (2016): 588-99.

Dincin, J., ed. *A Pragmatic Approach to Psychiatric Rehabilitation: Lessons from Chicago's Thresholds Program.* San Francisco: Jossey-Bass, 1995. No. 68 in the *New Directions for Mental Health Services* series.

Dixon, L. B., F. B. Dickerson, A. S. Bellack, et al. "The 2009 Schizophrenia PORT Psychosocial Treatment Recommendations and Summary Statements." *Schizophrenia Bulletin* 36 (2010): 48–70.

Friedlander, A. H., and S. R. Marder. "The Psychopathology, Medical Management, and Dental Implications of Schizophrenia." *Journal of the American Dental Association* 133 (2002): 603–10.

Gioia, D., and J. S. Brekke. "Use of the Americans with Disabilities Act by Young Adults with Schizophrenia." *Psychiatric Services* 54 (2003): 302–4.

Goff, D. C., C. Cather, A. E. Evins, et al. "Medical Morbidity and Mortality in Schizophrenia: Guidelines for Psychiatrists," *Journal of Clinical Psychiatry* 66 (2005): 183–94.

Lehman, A. F., R. Goldberg, L. B. Dixon, et al. "Improving Employment Outcomes for Persons with Severe Mental Illnesses." *Archives of General Psychiatry* 59 (2002): 165–72.

Liberman, R. P. *Recovery from Disability: Manual of Psychiatric Rehabilitation.* Washington, D.C.: American Psychiatric Press, 2008.

McCreadie, R. G., H. Stevens, J. Henderson, et al. "The Dental Health of People with Schizophrenia." *Acta Psychiatrica Scandinavica* 110 (2004): 306–10.

Marder, S. R., S. M. Essock, A. L. Miller, et al. "Physical Health Monitoring of Patients with Schizophrenia." *American Journal of Psychiatry* 161 (2004): 1334–49.

Marder, S. R., W. C. Wirshing, J. Mintz, et al. "Two-Year Outcome of Social Skills Training and Group Psychotherapy for Outpatients with Schizophrenia." *American Journal of Psychiatry* 153 (1996): 1585–92.

Noble, J. H. "Policy Reform Dilemmas in Promoting Employment of Persons with Severe Mental Illnesses." *Psychiatric Services* 49 (1998): 775–81.

Noble, J. H., R. S. Honberg, L. L. Hall, et al. *A Legacy of Failure: The Inability of the Federal-State Vocational Rehabilitation System to Serve People with Severe Mental Illnesses.* Arlington, Va.: National Alliance for the Mentally Ill, 1997.

Persson, K., B. Axtelius, B. Söderfeldt, et al. "Association of Perceived Quality of Life and Oral Health among Psychiatric Outpatients." *Psychiatric Services* 60 (2009): 1552–54.

Trepp, J. K. *Lodge Magic: Real Life Adventures in Mental Health Recovery.* Minneapolis: Tasks Unlimited, 2000.

Winerip, M. *9 Highland Road.* New York: Pantheon Books, 1994.

9

What Good Services Should Look Like

Madness is, contrary to the opinion of some unthinking persons, as manageable as many other distempers, which are equally dreadful and obstinate.
William Battie, 1758

In general, services in the United States for individuals with schizophrenia and other forms of serious mental illness vary from inadequate to abysmal. There are an inadequate number of competent professionals and psychiatric inpatient beds; outpatient follow-up is very uneven; housing is completely inadequate; and rehabilitation services vary from minimal to non-existent. Most depressing is the fact that these services are worse in 2019 than they were two decades earlier. Although some states do better than others, there is not a single state that can be said to have good, or even minimally adequate services. Individuals with schizophrenia receive better services for their illness in virtually every western European nation, especially the Netherlands and Scandinavian countries.

It does not have to be this way. We know what to do and how to deliver good services. We don't do it, however, for a variety of reasons, many of which are associated with the thought-disordered way we fund public psychiatric services. Despite such problems, there are a few individual programs scattered across the country that do a good job of delivering services. This chapter will briefly outline what model mental illness services for individuals with schizophrenia could—indeed *should*—look like and will cite occasional examples of good services.

Psychiatric Inpatient Beds

It is imperative to have an adequate number of psychiatric inpatient beds so that individuals with acute symptoms of schizophrenia can be properly diagnosed and stabilized on medication. The consequences of not having an adequate number of such beds are that individuals who need treatment are not admitted to hospitals and, even if they are admitted, they are then discharged prematurely. The outcome is a revolving door of readmissions and crowded emergency rooms with patients waiting days, even weeks, for a bed to become available.

In 1955 there were 558,000 public (state and county) psychiatric beds in the United States. Based on the population at that time, there were 340 beds per 100,000 population. Following deinstitutionalization (see chapter 14), in 2018 there were only 35,000 public psychiatric beds available. Based on the population at that time, there were therefore only 11 beds per 100,000 population. Ninety seven percent of the public beds used for hospitalizing individuals with schizophrenia and other serious mental illness had been closed. A 2008 survey by the Treatment Advocacy Center suggested that 50 beds per 100,000 population is the minimum number needed to deliver adequate psychiatric services, meaning the United States currently has less than one-quarter of the necessary beds. Based on 2016 data, the states with the fewest beds per population were Arizona, Iowa, Minnesota, and Vermont.

Once an individual has been initially diagnosed and stabilized on medication, it is sometimes possible to use alternatives to inpatient hospitalization for relapses. In the 1960s, for example, the Louisville Homecare Project demonstrated that, in the majority of cases, individuals with schizophrenia who had an exacerbation of their illness could be stabilized at home by using daily visits from a public health nurse and guaranteed medication compliance. Similarly, in the 1970s, Southwest Denver Mental Health Services contracted with six private homes to each take one or two acutely mentally ill persons for up to three weeks at a time. The homeowners met regularly with the mental health team and a psychiatric nurse was available on call at all times. Both the Louisville and Denver experiments were regarded as successful alternatives to inpatient hospitalization but both died because they did not meet criteria for federal funding with Medicaid.

Although most states have closed their state psychiatric hospitals without regard to future psychiatric inpatient needs, a few states have done better. For example, in 2012 Massachusetts opened the Worcester Recovery Center and Hospital, a new 320-bed, state-of-the-art facility to replace two other state hospitals that were being closed. Although the number of public psychiatric beds is still woefully deficient in the state, at least the new hospital is an acknowledgement that some beds are needed.

The Need for Asylum

When the deinstitutionalization of seriously ill psychiatric patients began in the early 1960s, most people assumed that some patients could be placed in the community but that many others would continue to need long-term hospitalization. By the early 1980s, that assumption had been steadily eroded, and in some states (e.g., California, Vermont) there was serious talk of closing state hospitals altogether. Two decades later, we have come back, full circle, to where we began, and most mental illness professionals who work with seriously ill patients believe that there is, and will continue to be, a need for state hospitals or their equivalents for some patients.

The kinds of patients who will continue to need state hospitals are those whose symptoms are the most severe and/or whose behavior makes placement in the community very difficult. They include the 10 to 20 percent of seriously mentally ill who respond minimally or not at all to antipsychotic drugs, those with a propensity toward aggression or violence, those with inappropriate behaviors such as setting fires or disrobing in public, and those who are so helpless and/or dependent that they need the protection of the institution. It would be nice if there were no such patients, but there are and—until we learn the causes of brain diseases like schizophrenia—there will continue to be. Because of the push to close down hospitals, and because of legal decisions mandating the placement of patients in the community as "the least restrictive setting," many patients are currently being returned to the community who should not be.

How big a group of patients is this? The answer will depend in large measure on the quality of outpatient psychiatric and rehabilitation services available. A county or state with good programs may be able to successfully maintain in the community all except 5 to 10 percent of the individuals with schizophrenia. In every system there comes a point where you have to ask hard questions. Is this patient really better off living in the community than remaining in a long-term, sheltered environment? Is the quality of his/her life really going to be better? Is the community truly the "least restrictive setting" for this person? In our rush to return everybody to the community, we have avoided asking such questions, and many patients with schizophrenia have ended up in nursing homes, boarding homes, and public shelters worse than the hospital ward they left. In my eight years of placing patients in the Washington, D.C. community from St. Elizabeths Hospital, I would estimate that at least one-quarter of them were *worse* off, in terms of the quality of their lives, than they had been in the hospital. And such patients often told me that they would gladly return to the hospital if they had the opportunity.

We need to acknowledge, then, the need for some long-term psychiatric beds for the severely disabled. It is reviving the concept of asylum in the benevolent sense that the term was originally used—as protection for those who cannot protect themselves. We do not expect everyone who gets paralytic polio to necessarily be able to walk again, and we do not place them in boarding homes in the community if they are clearly unable to look after themselves. We maintain long-term hospital beds for patients with other severe brain diseases, such as multiple sclerosis and Alzheimer's disease, who are unable to care for themselves. Why shouldn't we do the same for schizophrenia?

Outpatient Services

The gold standard for psychiatric outpatient services for individuals with schizophrenia and other serious mental illnesses is the Assertive Community Treatment (ACT) model, based on a program developed in 1972 in Madison, Wisconsin. ACT programs consist of teams of approximately 8 to 10 mental illness professionals and paraprofessionals who take full responsibility for approximately 100 to 150 patients with severe mental illness. Full responsibility means 24-hour, 7 days a week on-call coverage by a team member with attention to clinical, housing, and rehabilitation needs. Many of the contacts between treatment team members and those who are mentally ill take place in the patients' homes, workplaces, or elsewhere in the community, not in the professionals' offices. Medication is often delivered rather than requiring the person to come to the clinic to obtain it. Care is assertive insofar as ACT team members actively seek out these patients for follow-up care.

ACT programs have proven to be both clinically effective and cost effective. Randomized trials of the ACT model have been carried out in England and Australia, as well as in the United States, and have shown that persons treated using this model have much lower rates of hospitalization and both the mentally ill and their families are highly satisfied with it. A major reason for its success is the continuity of care with the same team members seeing the same patients, no matter where they are, over many years. Thus, if the person is hospitalized or goes to jail, an ACT team member visits the person there and consults with whoever is in charge of their treatment. The ACT team members also get to know the patients' families. Importantly, if one member of the ACT team retires or otherwise leaves, other members of the team who know that patient are still available. Thus, ACT teams offer not only continuity of care, they also offer *continuity of caregiver*, which is the key to their effectiveness.

ACT teams may also become specialized for particular kinds of problems. A few ACT teams in large urban areas, for example, have responsibility exclusively for individuals with serious mental illness who also have major substance abuse problems. Another type of ACT team that has proven to be very useful focuses exclusively on individuals with serious mental illness who have incurred criminal charges. These are referred to as forensic ACT or FACT teams and include corrections personnel as additional team members. One of the first FACT teams was in Monroe County (Rochester), New York. It resulted in a significant reduction in re-arrests, jail days, and hospitalizations among the participants and received the 1989 Gold Award for innovation from the American Psychiatric Association. Another successful FACT program operates in King County (Seattle), Washington. A 2012 report on the programs' first year results indicated that participants had a 45 percent reduction in jail or prison bookings, a 38 percent reduction in days incarcerated, and a 38 percent reduction in psychiatric hospitalizations. Such forensic outpatient programs are clearly cost-effective.

Another effective psychiatric outpatient program for individuals with serious mental illness and criminal charges is the use of a Psychiatric Security Review Board (PSRB). Such boards have the legal authority to determine when mentally ill individuals with criminal charges can be released, the conditions for living in the community, and whether they need to be returned to the hospital. Oregon set up the first PSRB in 1977 and it has been regarded as being very successful. Connecticut created a similar PSRB in 1985 and studies up to 2015 reported a very low re-arrest rate for seriously mentally ill individuals followed in this same manner.

Critical to all psychiatric outpatient programs for individuals with schizophrenia is the ability to ensure that the individuals are continuing to take the medication needed to control their symptoms. As noted in Chapter 1, approximately half of people with schizophrenia have anosognosia and are thus not aware that they are sick. There are a variety of options for ensuring that people take their medications, as described in chapter 7. For individuals with anosognosia, it is often necessary to legally mandate that they continue to take their medication as a condition for living in the community. As described in chapter 10 under Assisted Treatment, the use of outpatient commitment, usually called Assisted Outpatient Treatment (AOT), is becoming increasingly widespread and is legally available in all states except Massachusetts, Connecticut, Maryland, and Tennessee. Examples of especially good AOT programs include those in Essex County, New Jersey; Butler and

Summit Counties in Ohio; Seminole County in Florida; Bexar County in Texas, and Nevada County in California. Such well-regarded AOT programs offer quality services, stress the importance of medication compliance, and use judges who take the time to establish rapport with participants, congratulate them on their successes, and involve the patient as much as possible in treatment decisions.

In addition to ACT teams, good outpatient services for individuals with schizophrenia should also include specialized teams to deal with two major problems—individuals who are being charged with crimes and those who are homeless. Crisis Intervention Teams (CIT) of specially trained police officers, as originally developed in Memphis, have become widespread with the goal being to prevent arrests and obtain treatment for the mentally ill person. Once they have been arrested, mental health courts, initially introduced in Broward County, Florida, in 1997, have proven to be effective in getting patients into mental health treatment instead of incarceration. There are now over 400 mental health courts in the United States. Of course, the existence of CIT-type programs and mental health courts can also be viewed as a failure of the inpatient and outpatient mental health system; if all individuals with serious mental illness were receiving proactive proper care, there should be little need for these programs for this group of patients.

Scattered across the United States are a handful of especially interesting outpatient treatment programs for schizophrenia that include elements of model programs. One such example is in northeast Ohio, centered on Summit County (Akron) and the Department of Psychiatry at the Northeast Ohio Medical University (NEOMED). Summit County has a model Assisted Outpatient Treatment (AOT) program for individuals with psychotic disorders that has evolved into what is called the New Day Court. Using a model common to mental health courts, the New Day Court judge actively engages with individuals under a civil court order in regular status meetings in order to help individuals with serious mental illness engage in treatment and live successfully in the community. The Department of Psychiatry at NEOMED functions as an educational and consultative resource for mental health professionals in the community. Specifically, NEOMED established a Best Practices in Schizophrenia Treatment

(BeST) Center that promotes such interventions as the use of clozapine, long-acting injectable antipsychotics, family education, cognitive remediation, and cognitive behavioral therapy for psychosis. In 2018, NEOMED also opened the nation's first ECHO (Extension for Community Healthcare Outcomes) tele-mentoring program specifically focused on improving the treatment of schizophrenia. Community providers can tune into the weekly NEOMED video conference program to obtain treatment information and consultation on specific case histories. This unusual combination of schizophrenia treatment services is a product of exceptional leadership by local mental health professionals, combined with support by local judges and fiscal support by a local foundation, Peg's Foundation.

Another noteworthy outpatient approach for individuals with serious mental illness, including schizophrenia, is in southern Arizona's Pima county and covers approximately one million people. A variety of innovative programs have been developed to minimize the number of mentally ill individuals who end up in the criminal justice system via strong collaborations between the County, local law enforcement, the Regional Behavioral Health Authority (Cenpatico Integrated Care), and multiple mental health provider organizations. The community mental health system incorporates the liberal use of Assisted Outpatient Treatment, an active mental health court, and extensive CIT training for police officers. In addition, both the Pima County Sheriff's Office and the Tucson Police Department have developed specialized Mental Health Support Teams. Their work is supported by a robust crisis system that includes a 24/7 crisis hotline, over a dozen mobile crisis teams, and the Crisis Response Center.

The Mental Health Support Team consists of 10–12 specially selected officers and detectives, many of whom have relatives with a serious mental illness, whose only job is to respond to mental illness-related police calls. Team members wear civilian clothing and drive unmarked cars to minimize the stigma associated with their calls. The use of the team has markedly reduced the use of force in serving orders for civil commitment and transporting the patients. Since the same team members are responding to all of the major mental illness-related calls, the team becomes familiar with the serial users of police services and high-risk patients, and investigates options for improving the access of such patients to mental health services. More recently, new co-responder teams were created that pair a detective and mobile crisis clinician together.

The Crisis Response Center was built with county bond funds in order to reduce the numbers of people with mental illness in jails and emergency departments. Located on the Banner-University Medical Center South Campus and managed by Connections Health Solutions, the CRC serves 12,000 adults and 2,400 youth annually. CRC clinicians provide psychiatric consultation and backup to the Mental Health Support Team 24/7. It also provides psychiatric triage, urgent care, and observation for up to 23 hours and is located contiguous to the civil commitment court, hospital emergency department, and psychiatric inpatient facility. Police bring most mental illness-related cases directly to the Crisis Response Center with an average turnaround time for police officers of 10 minutes or less. One of the strongest features of the Pima County Program is widespread data collection and sharing across all phases of the program, including both clinical and cost data. The success of the program is a product of unusual leadership in both the mental health and criminal justice sectors and has also received support from the MacArthur Foundation.

Special outpatient outreach programs to homeless individuals with schizophrenia and other serious psychiatric disorders have been developed in many cities since the 1980s. For example, the Los Angeles LAMP (originally the Los Angeles Men's Place) program has been providing psychiatric, medical, housing, and other services to the city's mentally ill homeless population since 1985. New York City has tried a variety of programs over the years, the most recent being the Mental Health Services Corps that utilizes early career mental health professionals and trainees through Hunter College. Another example is the I.M. Sulzbacher Center for the homeless in Jacksonville that has been providing outreach to homeless mentally ill individuals for almost two decades. Such efforts are meritorious and especially useful to train students on the nature of the problem. In terms of reducing the numbers of seriously mentally ill homeless individuals, such programs have had little effect. Most seriously mentally ill homeless people have anosognosia regarding their own illness and will never agree to voluntarily take medication for an illness that they do not think they have. Most outreach programs, in turn, are reluctant to use existing commitment laws to involuntarily force treatment.

Rehabilitation

Just as ACT programs are the gold standard for outpatient services for individuals with schizophrenia, so clubhouses are the gold standard for rehabilitation services. The first clubhouse was Fountain House, founded in 1948 in New York City by patients who had been discharged from a state hospital. A clubhouse is a community facility that is open 7 days a week, in which members, as they are called, congregate for social and educational activities. Medications are usually not given out, but members are strongly encouraged to take them as prescribed. Since all members have been mentally ill, no stigma accrues to that status. Vocational rehabilitation is an integral component, with all members being expected to participate on work teams that maintain the clubhouse by preparing lunch, cleaning, or answering telephones. Many members also participate in formal vocational training programs, and clubhouses have proven to be one of the most successful models for job rehabilitation. Most clubhouses are also associated with housing programs in which members share apartments or homes. As mentioned in chapter 8, the Thresholds Clubhouse Program in Chicago has a housing program for over one thousand members.

Clubhouses have also been shown to be cost effective because they decrease the rehospitalization of its members. A study done at Thresholds, for example, reported a nine-month rehospitalization rate of 14 percent for members compared with 44 percent among a matched control group who were not members. Despite the many advantages of clubhouses, there are only about 160 of them in the United States, mostly because of restrictions on funding them using Medicaid or other public funds. Among the best clubhouses currently operating are Genesis Club in Worcester, Massachusetts; Gateway House in Greenville, SC; Magnolia House in Cleveland; Grand Avenue Club in Milwaukee; and Independence House in St. Louis.

Quality of Life Measures

In the 1990s, interest increased in assessing the outcome of treatment and rehabilitation for individuals with schizophrenia. One outcome measure is the quality of the person's life. Scales to measure this quality have been developed by Dr. Douglas A. Bigelow and colleagues at the University of Oregon Health Sciences Center, and Dr. Anthony F. Lehman and colleagues at the University of Maryland Center for Mental Health Services Research, as well as others. They include such issues as the person's living situation, family relations, social relations, employment, health, finances, safety, and legal problems. Some quality of life surveys also include questions regarding the person's inner experiences, such as pleasure, self-reliance, and self-fulfillment.

To date, these quality of life measures are little-used by mental illness professionals. However, they may well be the wave of the future. Imagine how different services for mentally ill individuals would be if measures of the quality of their lives were included as a routine part of rehabilitation. Imagine, moreover, how different the service system would be if rehabilitation outcome measures were used to determine the compensation of the mental illness professionals.

Quality of life can be assessed either subjectively (by asking the person) or objectively (by having another person rate the quality of life). Both of these measures should be integral parts of all outcome measurements of treatment and rehabilitation for schizophrenia. Measurements can be done at any one of three levels: the person, the program, or the outcome from the family and community's point of view. This is schematically summarized in the table on the following page.

When measures such as these start being widely used, and when the compensation of the providers is tied to the outcomes, then mental illness services for individuals with schizophrenia and other severe psychiatric disorders will improve rapidly.

METHODS OF MEASURING THE OUTCOMES OF TREATMENT AND
REHABILITATION FOR INDIVIDUALS WITH SCHIZOPHRENIA

	SUBJECTIVE MEASURES	OBJECTIVE MEASURES
Person	Self ratings of quality of life	Interviewer ratings of the person's quality of life and severity of symptoms
Program	Patient ratings of inpatient, outpatient, rehabilitation, housing, and other services	Patient care indicators; JCAHO and other surveys and site visits, preferably unannounced
Family and community	Family satisfaction surveys; surveys of police and jail personnel, public shelter and soup kitchen managers	Quantitative information from family surveys; number of mentally ill persons using soup kitchens or sleeping in parks; number of police calls for cases related to mental illness

Recommended Further Reading

Allness, D. J., and W. H. Knoedler. *The PACT Model of Community-Based Treatment for Persons with Severe and Persistent Mental Illness: A Manual for PACT Start-up.* Arlington, VA: National Alliance for the Mentally Ill, 1998.

Balfour, M. E. , J. Winsky and J. Isely. "The Tucson Mental Health Support Team (MHST) Model: A Prevention Focused Approach to Crisis and Public Safety." *Psychiatric Services* 68 (2017): 211–212.

Doyle, A., J. Laneil, K. Dudek. *Fountain House: Creating Community in Mental Health Practice.* New York: Columbia University Press, 2013.

Flannery, M. and M. Glickman. *Fountain House: Portraits of Lives Reclaimed from Mental Illness.* Center City, MN. Hazelden, 1996.

Fuller, D.A., E. Sinclair, J. Geller, et al. "Going, Going, Gone: Trends and Consequences of Eliminating State Psychiatric Beds, 2016." Treatment Advocacy Center (Arlington, VA), 2016. TACReports.org/going-going-gone.

Lamb, H. R. "The Need for Continuing Asylum and Sanctuary." *Hospital and Community Psychiatry* 35 (1984): 798–800.

Lehman, A. F. "Measures of Quality of Life among Persons with Severe and Persistent Mental Disorders." *Social Psychiatry and Psychiatric Epidemiology* 31 (1996): 78–88.

Torrey, E. F. "Continuous Treatment Teams in the Care of the Chronic Mentally Ill." *Hospital and Community Psychiatry* 37 (1986): 1243–47.

Torrey, E. F. "Economic Barriers to Widespread Implementation of Model Programs for the Seriously Mentally Ill." *Hospital and Community Psychiatry* 41 (1990): 526–31.

Torrey, E. F. *American Psychosis: How the Federal Government Destroyed the Mental Illness Treatment System*. New York: Oxford University Press, 2013.

Torrey, E. F. *The Insanity Offense: How America's Failure to Treat the Seriously Mentally Ill Endangers its Citizens*. New York: W.W. Norton, revised paperback edition, 2012.

Torrey, E. F., K. Entsminger, J. Geller, et al. "The Shortage of Public Hospital Beds for Mentally Ill Persons," Treatment Advocacy Center (2008). Arlington, VA.

Wasow, M. "The Need for Asylum for the Chronically Mentally Ill." *Schizophrenia Bulletin* 12 (1986): 162–67.

Wing, J. K. "The Functions of Asylum." *British Journal of Psychiatry* 157 (1990): 822–27.

10

Ten Major Problems

Although insanity is a disease to which every man is liable, a feeling prevails regarding it obviously different from any that prevails regarding most diseases. It is so incapacitating, and involves such complete dependence; its effects upon the civil and social condition of a man are so distinctive; and it is the subject of so much popular apprehension and horror, that it demands a consideration, especially if a cure is expected, that is peculiar to itself.

American Journal of Insanity, *1868*

Having the misfortune to be afflicted with schizophrenia brings with it many problems, both for those affected and for their families. Of all those problems, ten stand out as among the most common, the most persistent, and the most perplexing.

TEN MAJOR PROBLEMS	
• cigarettes and coffee	• medication noncompliance
• alcohol and street drugs	• assisted treatment
• sex, pregnancy, and AIDS	• assaultive and violent behavior
• victimization	• arrest and jail
• confidentiality	• suicide

Cigarettes and Coffee

One cannot overstate the importance of cigarettes and coffee in the daily lives of many people with schizophrenia. They are a major focus of social interaction, expenditure of funds, accumulation of debt, and trading of favors. Some individuals with schizophrenia are so obsessed with obtaining cigarettes and coffee that it appears to dominate their daily activities.

Studies have shown that between 65 and 85% of individuals with schizophrenia smoke cigarettes, in contrast to about 18% of the general population. Although the smoking rate in the general population has decreased significantly in recent years in response to anti-smoking campaigns, a recent study reported that between 1999 and 2016 the prevalence of smoking among individuals with schizophrenia did not similarly decline. What did decrease was the number of cigarettes smoked each day, probably in response to the rising price of cigarettes. When they smoke, individuals with schizophrenia tend to buy cigarettes with more nicotine and to extract more nicotine and carbon monoxide from each cigarette.

The consequences of smoking for individuals with schizophrenia are severe. As noted in chapter 4, the life expectancy for individuals with schizophrenia is approximately 25 years less than the general population, and smoking-related deaths are major contributors to this disparity. Deaths from heart and lung diseases are especially common, not including lung cancer which, for unknown reasons, is not elevated in schizophrenia. The importance of smoking on life expectancy can be illustrated by the fact that people who quit smoking between 25 and 34 years of age add on average 10 years to their life expectancy;

35 and 44 add 9 years; 45 and 54 add 6 years; and 55 and 64 add 4 years. Smoking by people who are psychotic or mentally confused can also be dangerous, and fires in group homes where large numbers of such patients are living are not uncommon.

Another consequence of smoking by individuals with schizophrenia is that it may lower their blood level, and thus the efficacy, of their antipsychotic medication. This is because smoking activates a specific cytochrome enzyme that causes the liver to get rid of the antipsychotic more rapidly. This is especially true for particular antipsychotics, especially haloperidol, fluphenazine, asenapine, olanzapine, and clozapine. Thus when individuals who are taking these drugs stop smoking, the blood level of the drug will rise and they might experience side effects. Conversely, if the person later resumes smoking the blood level will decrease making the drug seem less effective. Clinicians should adjust the drug dose accordingly when people are trying to quit smoking.

It is not known why individuals with schizophrenia become so heavily addicted to nicotine. For many years it was thought that they were self-medicating since nicotine is known to transiently improve some cognitive functions such as attention. Recent studies have cast doubt on this self-medication hypothesis, and in fact it has been shown that chronic smoking actually decreases cognitive function. Since nicotine is known to affect many brain neurotransmitters and since there are known to be nicotine receptors in the brain, it seems likely that the strong addiction to nicotine experienced by individuals with schizophrenia has a biological, though not yet understood, explanation.

Given the problems associated with smoking, all individuals with schizophrenia should be given the opportunity to quit smoking through smoking cessation programs. It has been shown that behavioral and psychotherapeutic treatments alone are not effective. However, the use of smoking cessation drugs, especially in conjunction with nicotine replacement therapy such as nicotine patch, are quite effective. In 2016 the results of a large study of smoking cessation drugs was published. Varenicline (Chantix, Champix) was reported to be superior to bupropion (Wellbutrin, Zyban), which in turn was superior to placebo in helping psychiatric patients to stop smoking. It is important to continue the drugs since the relapse rate is high when they are discontinued. Another approach to smoking cessation for individuals with schizophrenia is to switch their antipsychotic to clozapine; it is the only psychotic which decreases nicotine craving in some, but not all, patients.

Caffeine intake among individuals with schizophrenia is also very heavy but has not been quantified as precisely as has smoking. Patients have been documented as drinking thirty or more cups of coffee each day as well as drinking many colas, which also contain caffeine; each cup of coffee contains approximately 80 mg. of caffeine, and each cola, approximately 35 mg. There are also some individuals with schizophrenia who buy instant coffee and eat it directly from the jar with a spoon. Like nicotine, it is not understood why individuals with schizophrenia are so strongly addicted to caffeine, although caffeine is known to affect adenosine receptors in the brain and, through them, the metabolism of dopamine, serotonin, GABA, glutamate, and norepinephrine. One study also suggests that caffeine may decrease Parkinsonian symptoms such as stiffness and tremor.

It is known that high caffeine intake in anyone can produce the symptoms of caffeine intoxication, including nervousness, restlessness, insomnia, excitement, flushing of the face, rapid heartbeat, and muscle twitching. Studies of individuals with schizophrenia who ingest large amounts of caffeine have demonstrated that some patients have a worsening of their symptoms. It was previously thought that coffee, and especially tea, may interfere with the absorption of antipsychotic drugs, but this is now uncertain.

Just as some antipsychotics interact with nicotine to decrease blood level, and thus effectiveness of the antipsychotic, so these same antipsychotics interact with caffeine to increase the blood level. In one study, patients taking clozapine had their serum levels measured while using caffeine and again after they had abstained from caffeine for five days. The clozapine levels while using caffeine were approximately twice as high as while not using caffeine. Thus, alterations in caffeine intake could markedly affect both the effectiveness of these medications and their side effects. These effects of caffeine are not true for the other second-generation antipsychotics, because they are metabolized by different liver enzymes.

One thing that is clear about both smoking and caffeine intake among individuals with schizophrenia is that more studies are needed to clarify the consequences of the behavior. Until they are done, I would suggest the following:

1. Recognize the strength of these addictions in many individuals with schizophrenia. Obviously some reasonable maximum limits must be set, such as one pack of cigarettes and four cups of coffee or colas per day, but setting limits is different from trying to prohibit the behavior altogether.

2. Everyone with schizophrenia who expresses the desire to quit smoking should be given the opportunity to do so with smoking cessation drugs and replacement therapy.

3. Demand that individuals with schizophrenia who smoke do so in a safe manner (e.g., not in bed) and only in specified places. Nonsmokers have the right to not be exposed to the known dangerous effects of secondhand smoke. Establish clear penalties for not adhering to such rules, and enforce them.

Alcohol and Street Drugs

Alcohol and street drug abuse among individuals with schizophrenia is a large and apparently growing problem. A community study reported that 34 percent of individuals with schizophrenia abused alcohol, 26 percent abused street drugs, and altogether 47 percent abused one or both of these. A 2002 national survey reported that individuals with severe psychiatric disorders are twice as likely to abuse drugs and alcohol compared to individuals who are not affected. The severity of the problem may vary considerably, from an occasional episode of abuse to almost continual abuse.

There are many reasons why individuals with schizophrenia abuse alcohol and drugs. Probably the most important one is the same reason why individuals who do *not* have schizophrenia abuse alcohol and drugs—it makes them feel good. Substance abuse is endemic in the general population, and there is no reason why individuals with schizophrenia should be exempt. It is important to realize, therefore, that many individuals with schizophrenia who are abusing alcohol and street drugs would also be doing so if they had never become sick.

There are other reasons for alcohol and drug abuse that are specific to schizophrenia. Substance abuse provides a social network and something to do for individuals who are often socially isolated and bored. There is also evidence that some individuals with schizophrenia are self-medicating with the alcohol or street drugs, resulting in decreased anxiety, decreased depression, and increased energy. One study reported that alcohol decreased depression and improved sleep in individuals with schizophrenia, but it also increased auditory hallucinations and paranoid delusions. It is also probable that there is a genetic connection between having a predisposition to schizophrenia and a predisposition to alcoholism since recent genetic studies show some overlap in predisposing genes.

Many of the consequences of alcohol and street drug abuse for individuals with schizophrenia are identical to the general population and include impaired family and interpersonal relations, job loss, loss of housing, financial debt, medical problems, and arrests and jailings. In addition, it has been shown that individuals with schizophrenia who are substance abusers have many more symptoms, more frequent violent episodes, a higher use of emergency psychiatric services, lower compliance with antipsychotic medication, and a much higher relapse rate compared to non–substance abusers (see chapter 11). A large number of them end up among the homeless population.

The treatment of individuals with schizophrenia who also are severe substance abusers is quite unsatisfactory. Many are ping-ponged back and forth between the mental illness treatment system and the substance abuse treatment system, rejected on both sides. They are the patients nobody wants. Clozapine may be worth trying in individuals who are alcohol dependent, since preliminary studies suggested that it may decrease the person's drinking.

The most effective treatment programs for individuals who are dually diagnosed with schizophrenia and substance abuse are integrated treatment programs in which both conditions are treated by a single team of mental health professionals. The efficacy of such integrated treatment has been well demonstrated by Dr. Robert Drake and his associates at the Dartmouth Psychiatric Research Center in New Hampshire. In 2015 they published data showing comparatively good outcomes on the majority of both rural and inner city patients (see Recommended Further Reading). However, they also emphasize that a minority of patients do not respond and continue their substance abuse.

A variety of treatment approaches have been tried. The Twelve-Step self-help methods of Alcoholics Anonymous (AA) and Narcotics Anonymous (NA) are effective for a minority of individuals with schizophrenia, although some do better with a lower-key modified Six-Step program. A disadvantage of some such groups is that they encourage total abstinence from all drugs, sometimes interpreted as including antipsychotic medications as well. Individuals with schizophrenia also do not do well in the confrontational groups promoted by some AA and NA chapters. Individual psychotherapy is of limited effectiveness with the dually diagnosed patients, and a large trial using cognitive behavioral therapy in England also was not effective. By contrast, treatment programs in which housing and/or jobs are part of the integrated program have shown more success.

In some cases it is necessary to utilize compulsory monitoring techniques to decrease alcohol and drug abuse in individuals with schizophrenia. This is especially true for those patients who become violent or otherwise get in trouble when abusing alcohol or street drugs. Urine testing can be used to ascertain street drug use, and skin patches are being developed that change color if alcohol is ingested. Hair analysis can also be useful because it detects the use of amphetamines, barbiturates, cocaine, and heroin (but not marijuana) for up to three months after use. Alcohol abuse can sometimes be controlled by the use of disulfiram (Antabuse), which, if taken each day, makes the person physically ill if they then drink alcohol during the ensuing twenty-four hours. Disulfiram can be used in individuals with schizophrenia, but it tends to decrease blood levels of antipsychotics, so the person may need to take a higher dose of the antipsychotic while on disulfiram.

Families of individuals with schizophrenia who are abusing alcohol or street drugs need to be aware of how common this problem is and learn to recognize it. A useful clue is the disappearance of large amounts of the person's money that cannot be accounted for. Making the substance abuser aware of the effects and consequences of their substance abuse, setting and adhering to clearly defined limits, and utilizing compulsory treatment modalities (often mandated by the regular courts, drug courts, or mental health courts for individuals who have pending legal charges) are all important parts of a comprehensive treatment plan.

Should an individual with schizophrenia be allowed to drink at all? Many clinicians say no. I would agree with this if the person has a history of violent behavior or if alcohol appears to exacerbate the symptoms of his/her illness. However, if these are not factors and the person has had no tendency to abuse alcohol, I know of no reason why someone with schizophrenia should not have an occasional social drink if that is something he/she enjoys doing and is part of his/her culture. Having a beer at the end of the day with friends or having a glass of wine with dinner is for many people a pleasurable part of life. People who have had the misfortune to have been afflicted with schizophrenia should not be further penalized or deprived of small pleasures that are available to other people unless there is a clear reason to do so. At the same time I personally tell patients and their families to set clear limits on any alcohol intake (e.g., two cans of beer or two glasses of wine or one ounce of alcohol per day) and to be constantly alert for any signs of alcohol abuse.

Street drug use by persons with schizophrenia can be summed up in one word: NO. For many patients, even marijuana may set off psychotic symptoms in an unpredictable way, and it may take days to recover from them fully. One young man I treated remained almost symptom-free on medication except when he smoked marijuana; he then became floridly psychotic for several days. Not every person with schizophrenia reacts so dramatically, of course, but there is no way to predict who will do so. Some researchers have even claimed that there is a small group of individuals with schizophrenia for whom marijuana *improves* their symptoms. Stronger drugs, especially PCP and amphetamines ("speed"), are like poison for anyone with schizophrenia. Families should discourage their use in every way possible, and should not allow a family member with schizophrenia in the home if street drug use is suspected. This rule is absolutely mandatory if the person has a history of assaultive or violent behavior; many of the homicides committed by those afflicted with schizophrenia appear to occur following use of street drugs. Draconian measures to discourage street drug use are perfectly legitimate, including requiring the person with schizophrenia to periodically submit to urine testing or hair analysis for street drug use as a condition of living at home, receiving support from the family, or remaining out of the hospital.

Sex, Pregnancy, and AIDS

Sex is an important issue for most men and women, and there is no reason to think that it should be any different for individuals with schizophrenia. Mentally ill individuals are commonly consigned to an asexual status in our imaginations, but that is a mistake. Individuals with schizophrenia run a wide range, from having practically no interest in sex to being preoccupied with it, the same range found in individuals who do not have schizophrenia.

Studies suggest that approximately two-thirds of individuals with schizophrenia are sexually active in any given year. One study of women outpatients reported that 73 percent of them were sexually active; another study of men and women outpatients reported that 62 percent were sexually active, including 42 percent of the men and 19 percent of the women who had had multiple sexual partners within the past year. A study of individuals in a psychiatric admissions unit similarly found that 66 percent had been sexually active within six months, whereas a survey of long-term patients in a state psychiatric hospital noted that "sexual activity was extensive and far-ranging at the hospital." The reverse side of the picture is the group who is not sexually active; a study in England reported that more than one-third of adults with schizophrenia "had never had a sexual relationship."

Sexual activity for individuals with schizophrenia, however, is more difficult than for individuals who do not have schizophrenia. Imagine how complex sex would seem if you had delusions that the person was trying to harm you or you were hearing constant auditory hallucinations. Dr. M. B. Rosenbaum, in a sensitive article on the sexual problems of persons with schizophrenia, described one patient who "vividly described all the angels and devils in his bedroom telling him what and what not to do" while having intercourse. Dr. Rosenbaum concluded: "It is hard for most of us to 'get it together' sexually—how much harder for the schizophrenic with his or her many very real limitations!"

Antipsychotic medications may also interfere with the sex lives of individuals with schizophrenia; this appears to be as true for second-generation antipsychotics as it is for first-generation antipsychotics. One study reported antipsychotic medication side effects affecting sexual function in 30 to 60 percent of individuals taking the medications. These effects included decreased libido, male impotence, orgasmic dysfunction, and female menstrual irregularities. Such side effects are a major reason why some patients discontinue taking their medications, although they usually do not verbalize this. In evaluating sexual side effects of antipsychotic medications, however, it must be remembered that some of the individuals reporting side effects had sexual dysfunction before they became sick or started taking medication, since sexual dysfunction is not uncommon in the general population. One recent study, for example, reported sexual side effects in 45 percent of individuals with schizophrenia taking antipsychotic medication but also in 17 percent of normal controls; thus, the true rate of sexual side effects due to the medication was 28 percent. A few individuals have had their sexual lives improved by antipsychotic medications; for example, one report described two heterosexual men who "would routinely engage in continuous sexual activity for two to six hours while taking the medication at a properly adjusted dose."

Another problem is how to assess whether the patient is a consenting adult or is being taken advantage of in the sexual situation. This usually applies to women, although occasionally men will be taken advantage of by other men. Questions the family should ask include: Is she able to say no to men in nonsexual situations? Is her judgment reasonably good in other areas of her day-to-day functioning? Is she discreet, which suggests good judgment, in her sexual encounters? Is she trying to avoid men or is she seeking them out? Is she agreeing to sex primarily to obtain specific payment, most often cigarettes or food?

Consultation with the patient's psychiatrist and/or nursing staff at the group home or the psychiatric ward where the patient is known will often clarify the consent issue for the family. The family of one woman, for example, became upset when they found that she was having intercourse regularly at the halfway house, and she told her parents she was being taken advantage of. Discussion with halfway house staff established that the woman was seeking out the sexual encounters, and her claim of being taken advantage of was designed to assuage the disapproval of her parents. If a woman really is being taken advantage of, however, increased supervision and restrictions in her activity may be indicated. Women who consent to intercourse merely to acquire cigarettes or food need a plan formulated by the families and psychiatric staff to provide these items reliably, so the woman with schizophrenia will be less tempted to prostitute herself.

Protection against pregnancy is another problematic area for individuals with schizophrenia, since many such individuals have difficulties in planning ahead. According to one authority "the rate of children born to psychotic women is estimated to have tripled since deinstitutionalization first began in the United States." Unplanned pregnancies are relatively common among women with schizophrenia; in one study 31 percent of the women had had induced abortions. As noted in chapter 7, it is also known that women being switched from a first-generation antipsychotic to a second-generation antipsychotic have an increased risk of becoming pregnant unless they use contraceptives. The first-generation antipsychotics elevate prolactin and thus make ovulation less likely, whereas the second-generation antipsychotics, except risperidone and paliperidone, do not elevate prolactin.

Condoms are the first choice for contraception because they provide protection against AIDS and other sexually transmitted diseases as well as against pregnancy; however, many men will not use them. Four methods of long-term contraception have been approved by the Food and Drug Administration and are now available for use by women. One is a skin patch (Ortho Evra) that lasts for one week and then must be replaced. Another is injections of medroxyprogesterone acetate (Depo-Provera), which need to be given only every three months. The third is progestin implants beneath the skin (Norplant), which last for five years. The fourth is the intrauterine device. All these methods can produce some menstrual irregularities but are highly effective and satisfactory contraceptives for many women.

Ethical aspects of contraception in women with schizophrenia can also pose major problems. Some women may not wish to use contraception for religious reasons. Others may not wish to do so because they want to become pregnant. It is easy to empathize with a thirty-six-year-old single woman with schizophrenia who wants to have a baby before it is too late; it is also easy to empathize with the infant who is born into such a situation and who is totally dependent for care on its mother. The genetic facts on a baby born to two persons with schizophrenia are harsh—an estimated 36 percent of these children will eventually develop schizophrenia (see chapter 12). It is also true that most people with schizophrenia have enough difficulties looking after their own needs without the burden of a dependent infant. One study reported that "schizophrenia was associated with a markedly increased risk of poor parenting. . . ." Another study of eighty female "chronic psychiatric outpatients" reported that only one-third of the seventy-five children they had borne were being reared by the mothers. Indeed, the loss of child custody by mothers with schizophrenia is very common because many of them are unable to care for the child. One study of mothering among women with major psychiatric disorders reported that, not surprisingly, women who had better insight into their own illness were better mothers than those who did not have such insight. To assist in thinking through ethical issues regarding contraception in women with schizophrenia, some guidelines have been proposed by McCullough et al. at the Center for Ethics, Medicine and Public Issues at Baylor College of Medicine (see "Recommended Further Reading" at the end of this chapter).

Once a baby has been conceived, the couple and their families are often caught between a rock and a hard place. Abortion and adoption should both be considered; responsible decisions frequently involve consultation with the psychiatrist, family physician, lawyer, religious adviser, and social worker; Coverdale et al. have proposed guidelines for such decision making (see "Recommended Further Reading"). Often from such consultations a consensus will emerge on the best course of action, and this sharing of decision making will alleviate the burden on both the patient and the patient's family. In the past, putting such children up for adoption was commonly done, and many families adopted children without being told that one or both parents had schizophrenia.

It is known that women with schizophrenia are less likely to seek prenatal care or to follow instructions for it. Some studies have claimed that women with schizophrenia have an excess number of complications of pregnancy and birth, whereas other studies have concluded that this is not so. A study from Denmark reported that women with schizophrenia had a higher than expected rate of preterm deliveries and low birth-weight babies. Especially disturbing was a preliminary report from Australia indicating that women with schizophrenia give birth to an increased number of children with mental retardation and an increased number who die before age one.

The major dilemma of pregnancy in women with schizophrenia is whether to take antipsychotic medications during the pregnancy. The safest advice regarding medications to give any pregnant woman is to not take anything, but that may be impossible for women with schizophrenia. Antipsychotic drugs have been used by thousands of women while pregnant and appear to be safe compared to many other drugs used in medicine. Recent studies, however, have shown that these drugs occasionally cause malformations or congenital anomalies to the growing fetus, so they should not be considered completely safe and should be taken only when absolutely necessary. The most critical time for such damage appears to be the first three months of pregnancy.

Regarding the taking of antipsychotic drugs while breastfeeding, this should not be done. Antipsychotic drugs are transmitted in the breast milk in small amounts, but because the baby's liver and kidneys are not mature the drugs may accumulate in the baby's body. Since a woman who needs medication has the option of bottle feeding, it seems an unnecessary risk to take.

AIDS is an important threat to the health of individuals with schizophrenia. Surveys of the HIV positivity rate among admissions to state psychiatric hospitals have ranged from 1.6 percent in Texas to 5.5 percent in New York, but these surveys include patients with all diagnoses. The only survey done to date of HIV positivity of psychiatric admissions specifically with schizophrenia reported that 3.4 percent were positive in a university hospital in New York City. As expected in all such studies, it has been emphasized that concurrent substance abuse markedly increased the chance of becoming HIV positive; a study of seriously mentally ill homeless individuals who

MEDICATIONS AND PREGNANCY

Given what is currently known, a reasonable plan for pregnant women with schizophrenia is the following:

1. Stop antipsychotic medication for the first three months of pregnancy if she can do so without a serious relapse.

2. Remain off medication for as much of the pregnancy as possible beyond three months unless symptoms start to recur.

3. If it is necessary to restart the medication, use whichever antipsychotic medication she has responded to in the past. There are insufficient data yet to say that one type of antipsychotic medication is more dangerous than another during pregnancy.

4. There are data, however, to suggest that lithium, carbamazepine (Tegretol), valproic acid (Depakane), and divalproex sodium (Depakote), which are sometimes used as ancillary medications in schizophrenia, should be avoided during pregnancy.

5. Do not be heroic by avoiding medications at all costs. If the woman needs medication, use it. Having a pregnant woman who is acutely psychotic has risks of its own for both the woman and the fetus.

6. Discuss the issue of medication in detail before the pregnancy or as early in the pregnancy as possible. Be certain that the woman's family and all concerned understand the options. If the decision is made to stop medication, draw up a contract that specifies that the woman will resume medication if the doctor deems it advisable. The contract must be binding on the woman—even if she changes her mind because of her psychosis—so that she can be medicated involuntarily if necessary.

were also abusing drugs and alcohol reported that 6.2 percent of them were HIV positive.

Studies on individuals with schizophrenia regarding their knowledge about AIDS and its risk factors have reported a remarkably poor understanding. In one study of women with schizophrenia, 36 percent said that you can get AIDS by shaking hands, 58 percent said you can get it from a toilet seat, and 53 percent did not know that condoms help prevent AIDS. A 1993 study of condom use in the previous six months among individuals with schizophrenia found that condoms had been consistently used by only two of eight individuals who had had a single sexual partner and one of fifteen individuals who had had multiple sexual partners. In another study, one-third of seriously mentally ill individuals had been treated for a sexually transmitted disease, a major risk factor for HIV transmission.

What can patients and families do about the problems connected with AIDS? Open discussion, education, and the use of condoms are obvious needs and should be given high priority. AIDS education programs for patients with serious mental illnesses have been developed by Dr. Robert M. Goisman and his colleagues at the Massachusetts Mental Health Center and by Dr. Jeffrey A. Kelly and his colleagues at the Medical College of Wisconsin.

Victimization

Individuals with schizophrenia are commonly victimized, although such events are only rarely reported. Many individuals with schizophrenia have impaired thought processes and mental confusion, making it difficult for them to keep track of money or personal belongings. It also results in their putting themselves into dangerous situations because they cannot assess the situation correctly. This is especially true for individuals with both schizophrenia and substance abuse; as a Connecticut study concluded, "social isolation and cognitive deficits leading to poor judgment about whom to trust may leave people with serious mental illness vulnerable to drug dealers." Criminals thus view individuals with schizophrenia as "easy marks"; this situation is exacerbated by the common practice of locating group homes in rundown neighborhoods in which criminals congregate. It is rather like placing unlocked rabbit hutches in the middle of a forest filled with foxes.

Theft and assault are the most common crimes perpetrated against individuals with schizophrenia. In a study of 278 residents living in a Los Angeles board-and-care home, of whom two-thirds had schizophrenia, one-third reported having been robbed or assaulted within the previous year. A study of 185 individuals with schizophrenia admitted to a psychiatric hospital in North Carolina found that 20 percent of them had been the victim of a nonviolent crime, and an additional 7 percent had been a victim of a violent crime, in the preceding four months. The danger is especially great for individuals with schizophrenia living in public shelters. In a New York shelter, for example: "The mentally ill are often preyed upon by criminals who come to the shelter straight from prison. Those who receive Social Security disability checks become targets for muggers."

For women with schizophrenia, rape is a constant danger. A study of twenty women with schizophrenia in New York reported that ten of them had been raped, and half of those had been raped more than once. In Washington, D.C., among forty-four women who had a serious psychiatric disorder and who were intermittently homeless, 30 percent had been physically assaulted and 34 percent had been sexually assaulted. In France fourteen out of sixty-four women with schizophrenia had been raped, and nine of these had been raped multiple times. The director of a public women's shelter in San Francisco described the brutality of the streets: "I know one woman who has been raped seventeen times. . . . She doesn't report it because it's just what happens out there."

Fewer than half of all individuals with schizophrenia bother to report to the police crimes such as assault, robbery, and rape. A study of the reporting of such crimes by individuals with severe psychiatric disorders found that approximately half the time the police responded with disbelief, rudeness, anger, or offered no help. It is also difficult for many individuals with schizophrenia who have a thinking disorder to construct a coherent narrative regarding the crime. The police, therefore, view them as poor potential witnesses if the perpetrator of the crime should be brought to trial.

Several steps can be taken to improve the safety of individuals with schizophrenia. Most important is not placing group homes or other living facilities in high-crime neighborhoods. For individuals with schizophrenia who are living on their own, partially subsidized housing is needed because in many cities the only housing units that are affordable on SSI or SSDI are in high-crime areas. This is also a major reason why many people with schizophrenia have a better quality of life living in a small town rather than in a large city.

Another step that will improve the safety of individuals with schizophrenia is organized training sessions on self-defense, how to avoid being victimized, and how to report a crime to the police. Bringing members of the local police force to the group home, day program, clubhouse, or other gathering place would make such training sessions more effective as well as making both the police and the patients more comfortable with one another.

Confidentiality

Issues of confidentiality are one of the most common and most irritatingly irrational problems faced by relatives of individuals with schizophrenia. This situation has become even worse since passage of a privacy rule under the Health Insurance Portability and Accountability Act, widely known as HIPAA, in 2002. Confidentiality between physicians and patients are governed by state laws, which differ somewhat from state to state. They are designed to protect the physician–patient relationship and have been extended to other mental illness professionals. However, these laws are not absolute and can be changed. They can also be justifiably breached when the interests of the patients or the public clearly take precedence. For example, when a person with schizophrenia (or any other mental disorder) confides to a mental illness professional a wish or plan to harm another person; at one time such communications were considered to be confidential and legally exempted from disclosure under physician–patient confidentiality. In 1976, however, courts in California ruled that mental illness professionals have a duty to warn the potential victim in such situations. This ruling, generally referred to as the Tarasoff decision, has been extended to many other states.

Abuse of confidentiality statutes is currently causing many problems not only for families but also for the public mental illness system generally. In many cases, the problem is that mental illness professionals themselves are unsure about what information can be released. A study reported that 54 percent of the professionals "were confused about the types of information that are confidential," and 95 percent "interpreted confidentiality policies conservatively." Relatives thus cannot get the information they need to provide appropriate care for their family member. And mental illness professionals in one sector of the mental illness care system (e.g., the psychiatric unit of the county jail) often cannot access the person's psychiatric records from another sector of the system (e.g., the Community Mental Health Center).

There are of course legitimate instances when confidentiality must be maintained. Such cases usually involve an individual with schizophrenia who has good awareness of his/her illness and who has expressly instructed the mental health professional to not share information with his/her relatives. The reasons may vary, and include anger at the relatives, a belief that they are overcontrolling, a wish to prevent disclosure of a recent abortion, etc.

Far more often, however, confidentiality is invoked in instances when the patient has little or no awareness of his/her illness and is clearly not competent to make an informed judgment regarding whether disclosure of information would be helpful to him/her. There is a Catch-22 quality to such situations, with the patient essentially saying: "I'm not sick, so you can't tell my relatives about my sickness because it doesn't exist."

In such situations the mental health professional will often return the relative's call with words such as: "I'm sorry, but I cannot answer your question because of confidentiality issues." If you then point out the logical absurdity of the situation, the mental health professional may become defensive. One of the most difficult aspects of solving the confidentiality problem is translating this phrase: "I'm sorry, but I cannot answer that because of confidentiality issues." Although the same words are used, the phrase may be translated into one of several different meanings, depending on the speaker. If you can make the proper translation, you will be on your way to solving the problem. The most common translations are the following (I have used male gender for convenience; such individuals are found equally among females):

Dr. Freud: "I personally think that you are part of the cause of your relative's schizophrenia, and the less you have to do with him/her, the better. So don't bother me again."

Mr. Milquetoast: "I would need permission from my supervisor to tell you anything, and besides, as an employee of this organization, I've learned that the less I say to anybody, the better."

Mr. Incharge: "I have information that you want and need, but I'm not going to share it, at least for now, until you have groveled a little and acknowledged my superiority."

Mr. Lawyer: "The less I tell you the better, because then you are less likely to sue me/my hospital, and besides, if I tell you too much, you will realize how badly we have botched the treatment of your relative."

The heights of absurdity to which the confidentiality problem may ascend was well illustrated by the mother of a young man with schizophrenia. She described how she attempted to get information about his condition during the six months he was committed to a psychiatric hospital in Boston:

> I was never told how he was doing. I was in complete darkness about his prognosis, whether positive or negative. Each time I questioned the social worker assigned to his case, which was almost daily, the answer would be, "Danny would not give us permission today to tell you how he was doing."
>
> This was the reply I received for the first month or so. Then one day, moved by pity because of the state of anxiety I was in, she replied to my inquiry, "Danny would not give us permission today to tell you how he was doing but the patients on the ward are doing well today."
>
> I grasped at her coded message with much relief. But after hearing that same coded message and only that for the remainder of his commitment, it became quite evident to me that the system was as ill as my son and needed much help.

The key to resolving the confidentiality problem is to recognize that, for many individuals with schizophrenia, the relatives are not *merely* relatives but are also essential members of the treatment team. Individuals with schizophrenia are no longer hospitalized for long periods of time; rather, they are treated in the community, often in the family's home. Relatives have become increasingly sophisticated about schizophrenia and its treatment and not infrequently now know at least as much as the mental illness professional. When the relatives are accepted as legitimate care providers, the issue of confidentiality becomes easier to resolve.

Pioneering work on the development of release-of-information forms, a protocol to guide confidentiality problems, and confidentiality staff training programs have been developed by the Department of Mental Health in Riverside County, California, and adopted elsewhere. The protocol emphasizes the benefits of family involvement and the fact that mental illness professionals can (and should) accept information *from* the families at any time. If the individual with schizophrenia refuses to consent to any release of information, mental illness professionals can still provide much information to the family by speaking of hypothetical cases rather than the specific individual.

Families should also familiarize themselves with the confidentiality statutes governing the release of information in their states. If faced with uncooperative professionals such as Dr. Freud, Mr. Milquetoast, Mr. Incharge, or Mr. Lawyer, appeal first to the person's supervisor and, if necessary, to the supervisor's supervisor. Put your request in writing and send it by registered mail. Indicate your familiarity with your state's statute, and state that it does not apply in this case.

If that fails, have a lawyer friend send a letter on law firm stationery reiterating your request for information needed to provide adequate care for your relative. State clearly that you will hold the mental illness professionals and/or psychiatric care center legally responsible for any consequences of failed psychiatric care attributable to their failure to provide you with the necessary information. Most important, do not accept any less information than you would expect to be forthcoming from professionals if your family member had another brain disease, such as multiple sclerosis or Alzheimer's disease.

In recent years it has become increasingly clear to everyone that the HIPAA law, as currently written, is impeding the treatment of individuals with schizophrenia and other serious mental illnesses. In 2016, members of Congress introduced legislation to amend the HIPAA law and, although such legislation has not yet been passed, it is likely to do so in the near future. It has also become clear that HIPAA is protecting public officials more than it is protecting patients. Whenever a high-profile homicide occurs in which a mentally ill person is thought to have been the perpetrator, public officials invoke the HIPAA law to justify not giving out any information, including information on how they had failed to provide treatment for that individual. Indeed, the greatest utility of the HIPAA law to date is in protecting the backsides of public officials.

Medication Noncompliance

Medication noncompliance by individuals with schizophrenia is a major source of frustration for families and the single biggest cause of relapse and rehospitalization. It is extremely common, with studies showing that approximately 70 percent of patients are noncompliant with medication by the end of the second year following hospitalization. It is also extremely costly; one research group estimated that medication noncompliance for schizophrenia costs approximately $136 million per year. Medication noncompliance is also found in other medical conditions, such as hypertension, heart disease, rheumatoid arthritis, and tuberculosis, but it appears to be of greater magnitude in schizophrenia.

There are eight principal reasons for medication noncompliance in schizophrenia. The most important reason is anosognosia, the lack of awareness that one is sick. As described in chapter 1, such lack of insight is biological in origin, caused by damage to the frontal lobe, cingulate, and areas in the right cerebral hemisphere. One of the con-

---

REASONS FOR MEDICATION NONCOMPLIANCE

1. Anosognosia: person unaware of illness (biological)
2. Denial: person aware of illness but wishes not to be ill (psychological)
3. Medication side effects
4. Poor doctor–patient relationship
5. Delusional beliefs regarding medication (e.g., that it is poison)
6. Cognitive deficits, confusion, disorganization
7. Fears of becoming medication dependent or addicted, or threats to masculinity
8. Loss of feeling of importance

sequences of lack of awareness of illness is completely predictable—if a person does not believe he/she is sick, why take medication? In one study of schizophrenia, for example, the number of patients who were compliant with medication was twice as high among those with awareness of their illness as compared to those without such awareness. It is therefore not surprising that several studies have also reported an inverse correlation between awareness of illness and rehospitalization rates. Lack of awareness produces medication noncompliance, which leads to relapse and rehospitalization.

Anosognosia, or lack of awareness of illness, should be distinguished from denial. In denial, the person is aware that he/she is sick but wishes not to be. Taking medication is a daily reminder of one's illness; not taking medication is therefore an attempt to deny that the illness exists. Denial is often temporarily effective until the symptoms of the illness recur. Whereas anosognosia is biological in origin, denial is psychological in origin. A seriously mentally ill woman illustrated such denial:

> I did not want to believe I was sick, falling to the false logic of medication. Instead of thinking, "I am sick; therefore I need medication," I thought, "I am taking medication; therefore I am sick, and if I stop taking medicine, I will be well."

Another excellent description of denial was written by Mike Earley, the seriously mentally ill son of blogger Pete Earley, originally published on March 12, 2010 and reposted on August 24, 2016.

> Denial was a strong factor in my understanding and even when evidence of my own madness would be presented, my mind would find a way to weave out of the circumstance and an obtuse reasoning would somehow form that would keep my own pride intact. Always two steps ahead of the truth, my brain would tap dance its way into a room where I was not at fault, where it was everybody else versus me, where I was some sort of prophet or special medium who was undergoing visions, not hallucinations, and I was important, not a victim.
>
> It is very hard to understand that one's own credibility is broken. There is a lot of personal shame one undergoes when they

realize that they are no longer in line with society's understanding of sane. It makes one doubt one's own instincts and second guess the movements and decisions that one makes. Suddenly, the veil of confidence and ability has been lifted and one is a wreck, struggling to piece together the remnants of what are left of one's self image.

A third major reason for medication noncompliance among individuals with schizophrenia is the side effects of the medication. As expressed by Esso Leete, who has schizophrenia:

"Unfortunately the side effects of antipsychotic medications can often be more disabling than the illnesses themselves, and I have even experienced side effects from the pills I took to control the side effects of the antipsychotic medications." With the introduction of the second-generation antipsychotics, which have fewer EPS side effects, it was hoped that medication compliance would improve; recent studies, unfortunately, have found that medication compliance for patients on the second-generation drugs is no better than for those on first-generation drugs.

Studies have shown that many psychiatrists are not clinically astute in their ability to diagnose side effects. In one study of psychiatrists, for example, "the major finding was a high rate of clinical underrecognition of all major extrapyramidal syndromes." Another study reported that "psychiatrists misjudged the bothersomeness to patients of 24 percent of side effects and 20 percent of symptoms." Among the most troubling side effects of antipsychotic medication are akathisia (feelings of restlessness), akinesia (decreased spontaneity), and sexual dysfunction. An early study of drug refusal by patients with schizophrenia found that "the reluctance to take antipsychotic medication was significantly associated with extrapyramidal symptoms—most notably a subtle akathisia." The author noted that the akathisia could change over time "so that a patient could be optimally medicated on one visit, and experience an akathisia or other EPI [extrapyramidal involvement] on the same dosage of phenothiazines two weeks later." Giving the patient an extra supply of anti-Parkinson drugs to take on an as-needed basis is a suggested solution. Akinesia is also especially difficult for clinicians to appreciate because it is primarily a subjective experience and may be confused with depression.

Another major cause of medication noncompliance in individuals with schizophrenia is a poor doctor–patient relationship. Arriving at the best antipsychotic medication and the right dose of that medication for any given individual should be a shared undertaking between the doctor and patient. Dr. Ronald Diamond, in a lucid paper on the subject, says that "it is still important to listen to what patients say and to take seriously their experience with their medication." Betty Blaska, writing from a patient's point of view, makes the same point: "Many of the mistakes [of the psychiatrists] previously described come down to one thing: a refusal to see the consumer as an expert on his or her illness. The person with schizophrenia is *the* authority on *his* schizophrenia."

Instead, the norm for doctor–patient relationships in American psychiatry is complaints such as, "I have this side effect, but my doctor won't listen or take it seriously." One reason for this problem with doctor–patient relationships is that many of the psychiatrists in American public sector jobs were trained in other countries, where the doctor is considered to be *the* authority and patients are not supposed to question his/her advice or judgment. Another reason is that the norm in many community mental health programs is for the psychiatrist to see the patient for fifteen minutes every two or three months to check the medications; such a time frame precludes discussion of any except the most severe side effects.

Still other patients refuse to take medication because of their delusions, which may be either grandiose (e.g., a belief that you are all-powerful and therefore do not need the medication) or paranoid (e.g., a belief that people are using the medication to poison you). Other patients do not take their medication because of confusion, disorganization, or other cognitive deficits. A few individuals do not comply with medication because of fears that they will become dependent on or addicted to it; such fears are found more frequently in men for whom taking medication may also impugn their masculinity.

Finally, a few individuals with schizophrenia stop taking their medication because it takes away their delusional system and makes them feel less important. This is especially true for individuals with paranoid schizophrenia who, while delusional, often believe themselves to be the object of attention from government officials, etc. Richard McLean, in *Recovered, Not Cured,* described this:

> A few months after I began medication many of my symptoms had disappeared. I no longer chased cars to look at numberplates, or tuned into the radio for messages. I began to enjoy radio again. The drawback was that life was less interesting. Instead of feeling that I was always at the centre of something, albeit unpleasant, I found reality enveloped me in greyness and boredom. . . . It's not that I missed being psychotic; the difference was that I went from being waves on a beach to a particle of sand.

What are the answers to medication noncompliance? It is important for families and mental illness professionals to recognize how common noncompliance is, including the high frequency of surreptitious noncompliance when others think the patient is taking his/her medicine. It is also important to ascertain the reasons for the noncompliance, because solutions to the problems of lack of awareness of illness, denial, medication side effects, a poor doctor–patient relationship, and other reasons such as delusional thinking are somewhat different.

Better education of the patient should be helpful in most cases. One recent study of psychiatric patients' knowledge of their medication at the time of hospital discharge found that 37 percent of the patients did not know why they were supposed to take their medication and 47 percent did not know when to take it. Part of this is undoubtedly owing to the cognitive impairment of the person secondary to the illness. Using pill containers that have separate compartments for each day and using once-daily dosing also simplifies medication taking. A variety of automated systems (e.g., the Medi-Monitor System) are also being developed that remind you which pill to take when; when attached to a computer or a telephone line, they also beep or send a message to your computer to allow feedback to the treating physician or clinic. Using injectable depot medications such as the antipsychotics listed in chapter 7, which only have to be given every two to four weeks, can also be very helpful for individuals who respond to these medications.

POSSIBLE SOLUTIONS TO IMPROVE MEDICATION COMPLIANCE

1. Educate the patient regarding the benefits of medication and the risks of non-compliance.

2. Improve the doctor–patient relationship or find a better doctor.

3. Change medications, reduce dose, and/or treat side effects.

4. Simplify the medication regimen (e.g., single daily dosing, use of compartmentalized pill containers, or automated pill-notification systems).

5. Use injectable, long-acting medications.

6. Use positive reinforcement (e.g., cigarettes, coffee, money, travel).

7. Make the treatment provider the payee for the person's SSI or other benefits check, then tie medication compliance to receiving the money.

8. Use assisted treatment (e.g., assertive case management, conditional release, outpatient commitment, conservatorship).

The doctor–patient relationship can be improved if the psychiatrist is willing to accept the patient as a partner, not as an underling to carry out orders. Changes in medication or dose and attention to side effects are essential. Having the patient keep a daily diary of side effects and giving the patients some autonomy to increase or decrease medication dosage as needed can both be helpful. Medication should be approached as a joint venture with risks and benefits weighed against each other. The risks of medication noncompliance include rehospitalization, violence, jail, homelessness, and suicide, whereas the benefits include no medication side effects. The risks of medication compliance include side effects, whereas the benefits include living a more normal life and achieving a modified form of some of the person's original life goals.

For individuals who lack awareness of their illness, none of the above may be effective in persuading them to take medication. One strategy worth trying is taking videos of the person during periods of psychosis, then replaying it for him/her; one family found this to be effective (see Anonymous under Recommended Further Reading). Positive reinforcement is always worth trying, and coffee and cigarettes are sometimes sufficient. A higher stakes positive reinforcement is to have the clinic or case manager become the representative payee for the person's Supplemental Security Income (SSI) or other benefits, which will be discussed in the next section as one form of assisted treatment.

Additional information on medication noncompliance can be found in the briefing papers on the website of the Treatment Advocacy Center, www.treatmentadvocacycenter.org.

Assisted Treatment

Assisted treatment is necessary for many individuals with schizophrenia who lack awareness of their illness and, when unmedicated, are unable to provide for their needs or become a danger to themselves or others. Assisted treatment is used for conditions such as tuberculosis when patients refuse to take medication and, because of their untreated illness, are a danger to themselves or others. For schizophrenia, however, assisted treatment has become a lightning rod and has ignited opposition from civil libertarians, antipsychiatry groups such as the Scientologists, and others who are dissatisfied with the psychiatric care system for other reasons.

Assisted treatment has become increasingly necessary in the era of deinstitutionalization. In the past, when most individuals with schizophrenia were hospitalized, compliance with medication was not an issue. Now, however, most individuals with schizophrenia who previously would have been hospitalized are living in the community, and approximately half of them have anosognosia, as described in chapter 1, and thus lack awareness of their illness. For many of these, assisted treatment, or the *threat* of assisted treatment, is necessary. This difference is, in fact, important because experience with assisted treatment programs has clearly demonstrated that the majority of individuals with schizophrenia will comply with medication based on the *threat* of assisted treatment alone and that assisted treatment programs such as outpatient commitment have to be actually implemented in only a very small number of cases. Possible options for assisted treatment are the following:

1. *Advance directives:* Increasingly used in all areas of medicine, individuals formulate directives at a time they are well regarding what they want to happen when they become sick. In a few states, individuals with severe psychiatric disorders, during a period of remission, can sign an advance directive instructing that they be treated (in which case it would be a form of assisted treatment) or that they may not be treated if they become sick again. Advance directives are also known as "Ulysses contracts" after the Greek hero who, while sailing past the island of the deadly seductive Sirens, instructed his crew to bind him to the mast and "be strictly enjoined, whatever he might say or do, by no means to release him till they should have passed the Sirens' island."

The efficacy of advance directives as assisted treatment has not been studied. One possible problem is that advance directives could be signed by individuals who had no awareness of their illness at the time they signed. In states where advance directives must be certified by a psychiatrist, the certification could be done by psychiatrists who are unalterably opposed to assisted treatment under any circumstances. In such cases, advance directives would become an impediment to necessary treatment rather than being a form of assisted treatment. This has actually occurred in some cases in Ontario, Canada.

2. *Assertive case management:* Under assertive case management, case managers actively seek out patients at their homes or elsewhere in the community who do not follow up with appointments. The Program of Assertive Community Treatment (PACT or ACT teams) is the best-known example of this. Multiple studies have demonstrated that PACT teams decrease rehospitalization days. In a Baltimore study of homeless individuals with severe psychiatric disorders, 77 were assigned to a PACT team and compared with 75 others assigned to traditional outpatient treatment. During the following year, those treated by the PACT team had fewer hospital days (35 versus 67), fewer days living on the streets (10 versus 24), and fewer days in jail (9 versus 19). Those treated by the PACT team also had increased medication compliance (either intermittently or fully compliant) from 29 percent at the start to 55 percent after one year; however, "approximately one-third of the subjects were noncompliant at any given time point." As-

sertive case management would therefore appear to be an effective method of assisted treatment for some patients but not others.

3. *Representative payee:* To assist with money management, a patient's SSI, SSDI, or VA disability check can be assigned to the patient's family, case manager, or psychiatric clinic as the representative payee. Studies have shown that using a representative payee reduces hospitalization days, substance abuse, and days spent homeless. No study has been done on the effect of using representative payees to improve medication compliance. Anecdotal information, however, suggests that this arrangement is not unusual (e.g., the patient must accept a depot antipsychotic injection as a condition for being given his/her monthly check). In a U.S. Third Circuit Court of Appeals ruling, the court ruled that a man with epilepsy and borderline mental retardation was not entitled to SSDI benefits unless he demonstrated compliance with his anti-epileptic medication.

4. *Conditional release:* Patients who have been legally committed to a hospital can be released on the condition that they are compliant with medication. Violation of the condition can result in rehospitalization. In most states the hospital director has the authority to do this without asking permission of the courts. Forty states have laws permitting conditional release. In the past, this form of assisted treatment was widely used for both civil and forensic (criminal) cases, but now it is used mostly for the latter.

New Hampshire was previously the leading state using conditional release for civilly committed patients; in 1998, 27 percent of patients released from the New Hampshire State Hospital were put on conditional release. In the only study of the effectiveness of conditional release on medication compliance reported to date, twenty-six severely psychiatrically ill patients were conditionally released from the New Hampshire State Hospital with assessment of various measures for the year prior to hospitalization and the two years following conditional release. The results are shown in the following table.

The patients on conditional release thus had markedly improved medication compliance and decreased episodes of violence.

Among forensic (criminally committed) psychiatric patients, conditional release is much more widely used. The best-known example is Oregon's Psychiatric Security Review Board, which has been stud-

EFFECTIVENESS OF CONDITIONAL RELEASE		
	YEAR PRIOR TO HOSPITALIZATION	*FIRST YEAR ON CONDITIONAL RELEASE*	*SECOND YEAR ON CONDITIONAL RELEASE*
Months of medication compliance	2.9	10.4	10.7
Episodes of violence (rated on a 7-pt. scale)	5.6	2.4	1.1

ied and reported to be highly effective in reducing future criminal behavior. Additional studies on the effectiveness of conditional release for insanity defense acquittees have been carried out in Maryland, Illinois, California, New York, and Washington, D.C. The states that use conditional release most widely per population for their forensic population are Arkansas, Maryland, and Missouri. By contrast, seven states do not even have laws allowing for the use of conditional release for forensic patients (Idaho, Indiana, Massachusetts, New Mexico, North Carolina, Pennsylvania, and Texas). For more information on this issue see the 2017 report on the Treatment Advocacy Center Website, "Treat or Repeat: A State Survey of Serious Mental Illness, Major Crimes and Community Treatment."

5. *Outpatient commitment:* Outpatient commitment involves a court order for the patient to comply with treatment (usually including medication) as a condition for remaining in the community. Violation of the condition can result in rehospitalization. Some form of outpatient commitment is available in all state except Connecticut, Maryland, Massachusetts, and Tennessee but is used in very few of them.

The effectiveness of outpatient commitment in decreasing hospital admissions has been clearly established. In Washington, D.C., admissions decreased from 1.81 per year to 0.95 per year before and after outpatient commitment. Similarly, in Ohio the decrease was from 1.5 to 0.4, and in Iowa from 1.3 to 0.3. In one study in North Carolina, admissions for patients on outpatient commitment decreased from 3.7 to 0.7 per one thousand days. In another study in North Carolina, "subjects who underwent sustained periods of outpatient commitment beyond that of the initial court order had approximately 57 percent fewer readmissions and 20 fewer hospital days than control subjects."

Outpatient commitment has also been shown to be effective as a form of assisted treatment in increasing treatment compliance. In North Carolina only 30 percent of patients on outpatient commitment refused medication during a six-month period compared to 66 percent of patients not on outpatient commitment. In Ohio, outpatient commitment increased patients' compliance with outpatient psychiatric appointments from 5.7 to 13.0 per year and with attendance at day treatment sessions from 23 to 60 per year. In Arizona, among patients who had been outpatient committed "71 percent of the patients voluntarily maintained treatment contacts six months after their orders expired" compared to "almost no patients" who had not been put on outpatient commitment. And in Iowa "it appears as though outpatient commitment promotes treatment compliance in about 80 percent of patients while they are on outpatient commitment. After commitment is terminated about three-quarters of that group remain in treatment on a voluntary basis."

Most important, outpatient commitment has been shown to decrease violent behavior by individuals with schizophrenia and other severe mental illnesses. In a randomized trial in North Carolina of 262 individuals who were on court-ordered outpatient commitment for longer than six months, the authors reported that "the results were striking." Specifically, "the predicted probability of any violent behavior was cut in half from 48 percent to 24 percent, attributable to extended OPC [outpatient commitment] and regular outpatient services provision." Similarly, in New York, assisted outpatient commitment resulted in a 66 percent reduction in "serious violent behavior" during the first year.

The most impressive study of outpatient commitment came from New York State. In 1999 the state implemented an outpatient commitment law, Kendra's Law, named after a young woman who was killed by a man with schizophrenia who was not being treated. A 2003 study of the effects of Kendra's Law reported that individuals subjected to the law had dramatic reductions in hospitalization (87 percent to 20 percent) and medication noncompliance (67 percent to 22 percent) and even more dramatic reductions in homelessness (21 percent to 3 percent), arrest (30 percent to 5 percent), and jailings (21 percent to 3 percent). Similarly, the outpatient commitment statute in California, named Laura's Law after a young woman who was killed by a man with untreated schizophrenia, has been shown in studies of one county to decrease hospitalizations, homelessness, arrests, and incarceration of mentally ill individuals and to ultimately save the county money.

6. *Conservatorship:* Conservatorships and guardianships occur when a court appoints an individual to make treatment decisions for another individual who is believed to be mentally incompetent. They are used most frequently for individuals with mental retardation and with severe neurological diseases such as Alzheimer's disease; they are used much less often for individuals with severe psychiatric illnesses. In one study done in California, "of the 35 patients who were placed on conservatorship, 29 (83 percent) remained stable as long as the conservatorship lasted, but for the 21 patients whose conservatorship was terminated, only 9 (43 percent) remained stable after termination."

7. *Substituted judgment:* This is closely related to outpatient commitment and conservatorship. In Massachusetts, which does not have an outpatient commitment statute, patients with severe psychiatric illnesses have the right to refuse medication. A mental health professional can take such an individual to court; if the court finds that the patient is incompetent, it may use a substituted judgment standard, appoint a guardian, and order the patient to take medication. In a six-month study of patients subjected to such a procedure, their admissions decreased from 1.6 to 0.6, and hospital days decreased from 113 to 44. Reflecting on substituted judgment, Dr. Jeffrey Geller noted: "In one of the more ironic outcomes of mental health law over the last two decades, the right to refuse treatment court decisions have become the basis in Massachusetts for involuntary community treatment orders."

8. *"Benevolent coercion":* This is Dr. Geller's term for threatening to institute legal proceedings to compel treatment for patients who do not comply with treatment. Geller reported that he informed his patients that "if the lithium level fell below 0.5 meq./liter, the patient would be involuntarily admitted to a state hospital." According to Geller, such "benevolent coercion" is an effective method of assisted treatment.

Anecdotal evidence suggests that it is used widely but rarely discussed publicly.

9. *Mental health courts:* In the last two decades, mental health courts have become a popular means of enforcing treatment for individuals with schizophrenia and other severe psychiatric disorders. A court in Broward County, Florida, in 1997 is often credited with being the first such court, but similar courts had existed previously in places such as Marion County, Indiana, and a county in upstate New York where a knowledgeable judge for many years sentenced mentally ill people who had committed misdemeanors to comply with their mental health center treatment plan or go to jail. There are now more than four hundred mental health courts nationwide, and they are growing in number.

Mental health courts are in essence psychiatric outpatient clinics with a judge in place of a psychiatrist—a black robe is substituted for a white coat. Since all the mentally ill individuals who are brought to such courts have misdemeanor or felony charges against them, the judge gives them the choice of either complying with a treatment plan or going to jail. Not surprisingly, most patients opt for the former, with good effects. Recent studies have shown that mental health courts reduce the rearrests of mentally ill individuals by one-third and the days incarcerated by half. Even after the person has been discharged by the court, studies have shown that the positive effects of the courts is sustained for at least two years—a lingering "black robe effect." As one observer summarized it: "Mental health courts can be a powerful force to reduce violence and recidivism. By applying the principles of therapeutic jurisprudence, these courts can protect society and improve the lives of mentally ill offenders who have been violent."

At the same time that we praise mental health courts, we should recognize them for what they are. Just as jails and prisons have become the nation's psychiatric inpatient units (see chapter 14), so too are mental health courts becoming the nation's psychiatric outpatient system. The care of the mentally ill in the United States is effectively being transferred from the medical sector to the corrections sector. If medical officials were doing their job and using outpatient commitment, conditional release, guardianship, and other appropriate means of assisted treatment, the mental health courts would not be necessary.

Assisted treatment for individuals with schizophrenia can there-fore be achieved using several different options. In published accounts of these procedures, it is usually implied that only one such method is being used, but in fact more than one are often being used at the same time. For example, the PACT program of assertive case management is sometimes combined with the use of guardianship in Wisconsin. And many of the patients in the Baltimore PACT study of homeless individuals were given representative payees as well as assertive case managers.

Although all forms of assisted treatment appear to be effective for some patients with schizophrenia, efficacy for treatment compliance has been clearly established only for outpatient commitment. The paucity of research on the various forms of assisted treatment is sur-prising, given its importance.

A common problem for those supervising individuals with schizo-phrenia on assisted treatment is how to know whether the person is taking the medication. Using long-acting, injectable medications such as the antipsychotics listed in chapter 7 is effective for individuals who respond to those medications. Research is also in progress to develop a slow-release antipsychotic capsule that could be implanted beneath the skin that would gradually release the medication over several months; it could be removed at any time by a physician. Many anti-psychotics also come in liquid form that can be mixed with juice, and the person can be observed swallowing it. Patients taking lithium pills can be monitored by taking blood samples and checking their lithium level. For individuals taking other kinds of pills or capsules, it is possi-ble to mix substances such as riboflavin or isoniazid with the medica-tion and then take urine samples to see whether the person is taking the medication. These measures have been used to assess medication compliance in other diseases, such as tuberculosis, but to date they have not been used to routinely monitor medication compliance in in-dividuals with schizophrenia.

What is the effect on individuals with schizophrenia who lack awareness of their illness of being forced to take medication? Oppo-nents of assisted treatment have alleged that the effects are devastat-ing and drive those so treated permanently away. In fact, studies done on assisted treatment have found it to be remarkably benign in most cases. In one study, 27 outpatients who "had felt pressured or forced to take medications within the past year" were asked to express their feelings about the forced treatment. Among the 27, 9 were positive, 9 expressed mixed views, 6 said they had no feelings about it, and only 3 reported a negative effect. In another study, 30 patients who had been forcibly medicated during their psychiatric hospitalization were asked about it after being discharged. Retrospectively, 18 of them said that being forced to take medication was a good idea, 9 disagreed, and 3 were unsure.

For some mental illness professionals and other people, however, coercive treatment for individuals with schizophrenia is anathema. It contravenes our beliefs about civil liberties, the rights of individuals to privacy, and the freedom of speech and thought. The American Civil Liberties Union and the Bazelon Center for Mental Health Law in Washington, D.C., have staunchly opposed laws allowing forced treatment and have obtained court rulings in some states that have made such treatment practically impossible.

What these well-meaning but misguided advocates have failed to understand is that approximately half of all individuals with schizophrenia have little awareness of their illness. When such individuals refuse medication they are doing so as part of illogical or irrational thought processes. The right to be free of the symptoms of a brain disease must be weighed against the individual's right to privacy. Safeguards to prevent abuse of forced treatment must, of course, be built into the system, and this can be done using public defenders and individuals who have been mentally ill themselves to monitor the system. As articulated by one observer, the "freedom to be sick, helpless and isolated is not freedom." The rights of the individual must also be weighed against the needs of the person's family and society as a whole, especially in those individuals who become assaultive or violent when not taking medications.

In an effort to focus attention on the consequences of failing to treat large numbers of individuals with schizophrenia and other severe mental disorders, the national nonprofit Treatment Advocacy Center (TAC) in Arlington, Virginia, was founded in 1998. Funded by individual donors and foundations, TAC promotes the use of assisted treatment when needed and is working with many states to revise their outdated statutes and educate officials on better use of the existing laws. The Treatment Advocacy Center is the only national organization that focuses on the issue of assisted treatment. It can be accessed on the Internet at www.treatmentadvocacycenter.org and is also listed in appendix B.

Assaultive and Violent Behavior

Assaultive and violent behaviors are major problems for individuals with schizophrenia. It is true that most individuals with schizophrenia are not dangerous. It is also true that people with schizophrenia contribute only a small fraction of the total amount of violent acts in society. Nevertheless, a small number of people with schizophrenia are dangerous and commit violent acts, often high profile, disproportionate to their number.

Evidence to support this goes back half a century. Two studies of families who belong to NAMI demonstrated a high incidence of assaultive and violent behavior. In a 1986 survey 38 percent of the families "reported that their ill relative was assaultive and destructive in the home either sometimes or frequently." A 1990 NAMI survey of 1,401 families reported that within the preceding year 10.6 percent of the seriously mentally ill individuals had physically harmed another person and an additional 12.2 percent had threatened harm.

These findings are consistent with other studies of assaultive and violent behavior among individuals with serious mental illnesses. Rabkin reviewed studies done in the 1960s and 1970s and reported that for patients discharged from public mental hospitals "arrest and conviction rates for the subcategory of violent crimes were found to exceed general population rates in every study in which they were measured." In another study, it was found that fifteen of twenty individuals who were arrested for attempting to push people in front of subway trains in New York City had a diagnosis of schizophrenia. Steadman et al. also followed up patients discharged from mental hospitals and reported "that 27 percent of released male and female patients report at least one violent act within a mean of four months after discharge."

Other surveys of mentally ill individuals living in the community have reported similar findings. A methodologically excellent study by Link et al. in New York City found that former psychiatric patients were two to three times more likely than other community residents to have used a weapon or hurt someone badly and that most of the excess violence was committed by those individuals who were psychiatrically sickest and presumably not taking medication. Similarly, in the five-site Epidemiologic Catchment Area (ECA) study carried out by the National Institute of Mental Health, individuals with schizophrenia reported having used a weapon in a fight more than twenty times as often as individuals with no psychiatric disorder. There was also found to be a high correlation between violent behavior in schizophrenia and concurrent alcohol or drug abuse.

In reviewing many of these studies in 1992, Professor John Monahan concluded: "The data that have recently become available, fairly read, suggest the one conclusion I did not want to reach: Whether the measure is the prevalence of violence among the disordered or the prevalence of disorder among the violent, whether the sample is people who are selected for treatment as inmates or patients in institutions or people randomly chosen from the open community, and no matter how many social and demographic factors are statistically taken into account, there appears to be a relationship between mental disorder and violent behavior." In a 1996 editorial reviewing such studies, Dr. Peter Marzuk added: "In the last decade, however, the evidence showing a link between violence, crime, and mental illness has mounted. It cannot be dismissed; it should not be ignored."

In recent years additional studies have examined the relationship between schizophrenia and violent behavior. A 2015 summary of 20 such studies concluded as follows: "At least 20 studies have examined violence in patients with schizophrenia spectrum disorders in various clinical and community settings. A meta-analysis of this literature reported that the risk of violence was on average three to five times higher for men with schizophrenia, and four to 13 times higher for women with schizophrenia, compared with their counterparts without schizophrenia in the general population. Odds are substantially higher when homicide is considered as the violence outcome, and for any violence in studies comparing first-episode psychosis patients to population controls."

It is true that individuals with schizophrenia and other serious mental illnesses are responsible for a disproportionate percentage of certain kinds of homicides. Whereas they are responsible for approximately 10 percent of all homicides in the United States, they are responsible for approximately one-third of all mass killings, such as Jared Loughner in Tucson, Jiverly Wong in Binghampton, Issac Zamora in Seattle, James Holmes in Aurora, Aaron Alexis at the Washington Navy Yard, and Elliot Rodgers in Santa Barbara. Another type of homicide in which individuals with serious mental illnesses are heavily involved are intrafamily homicides. In 2016 the Treatment Advocacy Center published a study, "Raising Cain: The Role of Serious Mental Illness in Family Homicides," reporting that 50 percent of parents who kill their children and 67 percent of children who kill their parents have a serious mental illness, mostly schizophrenia. This study is available on the Treatment Advocacy Center website.

It should be emphasized that America is a violent society and, within this broad context, the contribution of individuals with schizophrenia to total violence is very small. It should also be reiterated that most individuals with schizophrenia are not assaultive or violent. However, a minority of individuals with schizophrenia are assaultive or violent and the problem will not go away simply by repeating outdated mantras to the contrary.

The three best predictors of assaultive and violent behavior in individuals with schizophrenia are concurrent alcohol or drug abuse, noncompliance with medication, and a past history of being assaultive or violent. Families that are faced with this problem must learn to recognize cues of impending violence and pay attention to them. If an individual with schizophrenia becomes assaultive or violent, it is best to stay calm (listen mostly, but respond in a calm and sympathetic manner), keep physically distant from the person, and call for help and/or the police as necessary.

Most assaultive and violent behavior can be prevented with planning. If there have been one or more episodes in the past, the family should have safe-proofed the house (e.g., sharp knives are kept locked up), asked for a review of the person's medication, explored options for improving medication compliance (e.g., outpatient commitment), made an effort to reduce alcohol or drug abuse by controlling the per-

---

HOW TO RESPOND TO AN INDIVIDUAL WITH SCHIZOPHRENIA
WHO IS POTENTIALLY VIOLENT

- Be aware that the three most important predictors of violence are a past history of violence, concurrent alcohol or drug abuse, and the failure to take antipsychotic medications.

- Make the person's treatment team aware of your concerns and of the person's past history of violence. This is more effective if done in writing.

- If the person has been violent, suggest to the treatment team that they consider using clozapine, carbamazepine, valproate, beta blockers, or other medications thought to decrease violent behavior.

- Safe-proof your house by removing all potential weapons. Put a good lock on the door of one room that you can use as a refuge if needed; this room should have a telephone.

- If threatened, stay calm, remain physically distant (give the person lots of space), do not look directly into his/her eyes, sympathize, try to find something on which you can both agree.

- Remain physically between the person and an open door; do not allow yourself to become trapped.

- Have the emergency response number posted next to the telephone and do not hesitate to call the police. If in doubt, call.

- Have a Crisis Information Form, already filled out for such emergencies, ready to hand to the police when they arrive. It should include the person's name, age, diagnosis, treating psychiatrist or clinic with telephone number, current medications, and summarized past history of violent behavior.

---

son's funds, and conveyed very clearly to the person the precise consequences (e.g., the person will no longer be allowed to live at home) if assaultive or violent behavior recurs. If it does, then it is mandatory to carry out those consequences.

A family within which the patient has been assaultive or violent is particularly poignant and lives in a special circle of hell. Its members are often afraid of the patient, yet at the same time they feel sorry for him/her and recognize that the behavior is a product of abnormal brain function. The ambivalence inevitably felt by the family members is formidable; fear and love, avoidance and attraction, rest uneasily side by side. Afterward, no matter how well the patient gets, no matter how much time elapses, the memory of the past assault or violence never fully recedes.

Arrest and Jail

Being arrested and jailed has become a common, yet rarely discussed, experience for many individuals with schizophrenia. It is yet another sad measure of the failed mental illness treatment system. In the 1990 study of 1,401 randomly selected members of NAMI, the families reported that 20 percent of their severely mentally ill family members had been arrested within the previous five years and 40 percent had been arrested at some time in their lives. A 1985 Los Angeles study of homeless individuals who had been previously psychiatrically hospitalized found that 76 percent of them had been arrested. Going to jail for individuals with schizophrenia appears to be almost as much a part of their lives as is going to a psychiatric hospital.

Over the past three decades, the number of individuals with schizophrenia who experience arrest has continued to increase. A 2014 study by the Treatment Advocacy Center reported that approximately 20 percent of inmates in jails and 15 percent of inmates in state prisons have a serious mental illness. Based on the total number of inmates in jails and state prisons, this means that there are approximately 356,000 seriously mentally ill individuals in America's jails and state prisons. This is ten times the number of seriously mentally ill individuals remaining in state psychiatric hospitals.

The present situation is an inevitable consequence of deinstitutionalizing hundreds of thousands of individuals with severe psychiatric disorders without ensuring that they received the medication and aftercare necessary to remain well. As early as 1972 in California, psychiatrist Marc Abramson published data showing that the number of mentally ill persons in jails was increasing as deinstitutionalization got under way. Abramson coined the term "criminalization of mentally disordered behavior" and predicated accurately that the situation was going to get much worse.

By the 1980s it had become possible to track mentally ill individuals directly from psychiatric hospitals to jails. In Belcher's study of 132 patients discharged from Columbus State Hospital in Ohio, for example, within six months of discharge 32 percent of those with schizophrenia, manic-depressive illness, or severe depression had been arrested. The reason for arrest in most cases was behavior associated with a recurrence of their illness because of their failure to take medication (e.g., "walking in the community without clothes").

The vast majority of individuals with schizophrenia who are arrested are arrested on misdemeanor charges, usually associated with untreated illness. In the NAMI survey referred to above, only 2.6 percent of the 20 percent arrested had been arrested for "serious acts of violence or other felonies." Most were arrested on such charges as trespassing, disturbing the peace, destroying property, shoplifting, and being drunk and disorderly.

For most individuals with schizophrenia, the experience of being jailed varies from "unpleasant" to "a living hell." Being ridiculed by guards or other prisoners is the least problem; in some jails "mental cases" wear uniforms of a different color and so are readily identifiable. More serious are problems of assault, rape, suicide, and even homicide, all of which have been well documented. Jails require prisoners to follow rules, but following rules assumes that your brain is thinking logically. For many individuals with schizophrenia who are not on medication, logical thinking is impossible. Such individuals commit bizarre acts that cause problems for everyone. In California, a newspaper reported that mentally ill inmates in one jail "try to escape by smearing themselves with their own feces and flushing themselves down the toilet."

For families it is also painful to watch helplessly as a mentally ill family member is arrested and jailed. There is, of course, the stigma attached to it, but much worse is knowing that the person may be abused or assaulted.

For a small number of individuals with schizophrenia, however, the opposite is the case. Because it is so difficult to get psychiatric care for individuals with schizophrenia who are unaware of their illness and who refuse voluntary treatment, and because mentally ill individuals with legal charges pending often can be treated involuntarily, it has become increasingly common for public officials and families to have mentally ill persons arrested *solely as a means for getting them into treatment*. In Massachusetts, for example, one mother noted: "Rather than wait for the patient to become so psychotic that disaster occurs, many families bring charges against a patient for making threats or damaging property." The fact that families have to have their family member arrested in order to get treatment for the person's schizophrenia is indeed a pitiful commentary on our mental illness treatment system.

Suicide

Suicide is a major cause of death in the United States and has been increasing in recent years. According to the National Center for Health Statistics, in 2016 a total of 44,965 people killed themselves, 123 each day. An estimated 5 percent of individuals with schizophrenia commit suicide, a major contributor to their excess mortality as discussed in chapter 4. This is five times the rate of the general population.

Depression represents the single most important cause of suicide among persons with schizophrenia, just as it does among persons without schizophrenia. The majority of patients will experience significant depression at some point during the course of their illness; this realization should lead psychiatrists to remain alert for depression and to treat it more aggressively with antidepressant medication. Depression may arise from the disease process itself (i.e., the schizophrenia affects the brain chemistry so as to cause depression), from the patients' realization of the severity of their illness (i.e., as a reaction to the disease), or occasionally as a side effect of medications used to treat schizophrenia. Depression must also be differentiated in schizophrenia from the slowed movements (akinesia) and slowed thought processes that may be symptoms of the disease.

Most persons with schizophrenia who commit suicide do so within the first ten years of their illness. As might be expected, approximately three-quarters of them are men. Those at highest risk have a remitting and relapsing course, good insight (i.e., they know they are sick), a poor response to medication, are socially isolated, hopeless about the future, and have a gross discrepancy between their earlier achievements in life and their current level of function. Any patient with these characteristics *and* associated depression should be considered at high risk for suicide. The most common time for suicide is during a remission of the illness immediately following a relapse.

Data also suggest that the failure to adequately treat individuals with schizophrenia increases the risk of suicide. In a Finnish study of ninety-two individuals with schizophrenia who killed themselves, it was found that "the majority of victims (78 percent) were in the active illness phase, but among them over half (57 percent) were either not prescribed adequate neuroleptic [antipsychotic] treatment or were not using it." Similarly, a Belgian study of sixty-three individuals with schizophrenia who committed suicide reported that "there were seven times as many patients who did not comply with treatment in the suicide group as there were in the control group."

Occasionally persons with schizophrenia will commit suicide accidentally in a stage of acute psychosis (e.g., they may jump off a building because they think they can fly or because voices tell them to do so). Most suicides in schizophrenia are intended, however, and are often carefully planned by the person. Like all clinicians who have taken care of large numbers of patients with schizophrenia, I have known several who eventually committed suicide, and such deaths evoke great sadness.

There are other suicides, however, that evoke not only sadness but also anger. These are the preventable ones—the patient who is treated inadequately with medications and then told that nothing more can be done, or the patient who is doing nicely on medication until another doctor reduces it and begins insight-oriented psychotherapy. I wish I could say that these suicides were rare occurrences, but they are not. The high suicide rate in schizophrenia is in part due to our inadequate care system (or, more accurately, nonsystem) on which these patients are forced to rely.

What can families and friends of individuals with schizophrenia do to minimize the risk of suicide? The most important thing is to be alert for it, especially in an individual who is depressed and who has recently recovered from a relapse. Past suicide gestures or attempts are an important predictor of future attempts. Expressions of guilt and worthlessness, hopelessness about the future, an unwillingness to make plans for the future, and putting one's affairs in order (e.g., giving away prized possessions or making a will) are all red flags that may indicate serious suicidal intent.

Families and friends should then *ask* and *act*. Ask the person if he/she is planning to commit suicide (e.g., "I know you have been depressed recently and I am very worried about you. Are you planning to harm yourself?"). Some people are afraid to ask about suicide because they fear it will put the idea into the person's head. This is not true, and often the person is relieved to be able to talk about suicidal thoughts and plans. Most people who are planning to commit suicide have mixed feelings about it. Do not directly argue with the person about committing suicide but rather point out the reasons for not doing so. One excellent reason at this time is the promise of more effective medications with fewer side effects that are likely to become available in the next few years.

Act by taking away the person's planned modalities for committing suicide (e.g., a gun or pills) and similar weapons in the immediate environment. Act also by ensuring that the person's treating psychiatrist is aware of the person's suicidal intentions and urge him or her to aggressively treat the person's depression. Specifically, ask the psychiatrist if he/she has considered a trial of clozapine; there are strong suggestions that it may be effective in decreasing suicidal ideation. If the psychiatrist is reluctant to act, put your advice and admonitions in a registered letter to the psychiatrist, if necessary, adding that you have consulted your lawyer about the case. The psychiatrist will get the message. In some cases involuntary commitment to a psychiatric unit may be necessary to ensure the person's safety until antidepressant medication can take effect.

Despite the best efforts of family and friends, however, some individuals with schizophrenia will commit suicide. If family and friends have done what they could do to help, they should not feel guilty or blame themselves. Suicide in schizophrenia is the final and ultimate measure of the tragedy of this disease.

Recommended Further Reading

Anonymous. "Video and Poor Insight in Persons with Schizophrenia." *Schizophrenia Bulletin* 42 (2016): 262–63.

Amador, X. *I Am Not Sick, I Don't Need Help!* Peconic, N.Y.: Vida Press, 2000.

Bogart, T., and P. Solomon. "Procedures to Share Treatment Information among Mental Health Providers, Consumers, and Families." *Psychiatric Services* 50 (1999): 1321–25.

Caldwell, C. B., and I. I. Gottesman. "Schizophrenics Kill Themselves Too: A Review of Risk Factors for Suicide." *Schizophrenia Bulletin* 16 (1990): 571–89.

Cather, C., R. S. Barr, and A. E. Evins. "Smoking and Schizophrenia: Prevalence, Mechanisms and Implications for Treatment." *Clinical Schizophrenia & Related Psychoses* 2 (2008): 70–78.

Choe, J. Y., L. A. Teplin, K. M. Abram. "Perpetration of Violence, Violent Victimization, and Severe Mental Illness: Balancing Public Health Concerns." *Psychiatric Services* 59 (2008): 153–64.

Citrome, L., and J. Volavka. "Management of Violence in Schizophrenia." *Psychiatric Annals* 30 (2000): 41–52.

Coverdale, J. H., L. B. McCullough, and F. A. Chervenak. "Assisted and Surrogate Decision Making for Pregnant Patients Who Have Schizophrenia." *Schizophrenia Bulletin* 30 (2004): 659–64.

De Boer, M. K., S. Castlelein, D. Wiersma. "The Facts about Sexual (Dys)function in Schizophrenia: An Overview of Clinically Relevant Findings." *Schizophrenia Bulletin* 41 (2015): 674–86.

Diamond, R. "Drugs and the Quality of Life: The Patient's Point of View." *Journal of Clinical Psychiatry* 46 (1985): 29–35.

Dickerson, F., J. Schroeder, E. Katsafanas, et al. "Cigarette Smoking by Patients With Serious Mental Illness, 1999-2016: An Increasing Disparity." *Psychiatric Services* 69 (2018): 147–53.

Drake, R. E., C. Mercer-McFadden, K. T. Mueser, et al. "Review of Integrated Mental Health and Substance Abuse Treatment for Patients with Dual Disorders." *Schizophrenia Bulletin* 24 (1998): 589–608.

Drake, R.E., A.E. Luciano, K.T. Muesser, et al. "Longitudinal Course of Clients With Co-Occurring Schizophrenia-Spectrum and Substance Use Disorders in Urban Mental Health Centers: a 7-Year Prospective Study." *Schizophrenia Bulletin* 42 (2016): 202-211.

Empfield, M. D. "Pregnancy and Schizophrenia." *Psychiatric Annals* 30 (2000): 61–66.

Hyde, A. P. "Coping with the Threatening, Intimidating, Violent Behaviors of People with Psychiatric Disabilities Living at Home: Guidelines for Family Caregivers." *Psychiatric Rehabilitation Journal* 21 (1997): 144–49.

Jamison, K. R. *Night Falls Fast: Understanding Suicide.* New York: Alfred A. Knopf, 1999.

Lamb, H. R., and L. E. Weinberger. "Mental Health Courts as a Way to Provide Treatment to Violent Persons with Severe Mental Illness." *Journal of the American Medical Association* 300 (2008): 722–24.

Malik, P., G. Kemmler, M. Hummer, et al. "Sexual Dysfunction in First-Episode Schizophrenia Patients: Results from European First Episode Schizophrenia Trial." *Journal of Clinical Psychopharmacology* 31 (2011): 274–80.

Marshall, T., and P. Solomon. "Professionals' Responsibilities in Releasing Information to Families of Adults with Mental Illness." *Psychiatric Services* 54 (2003): 1622–28.

McCullough, L. B., J. Coverdale, T. Bayer, et al. "Ethically Justified Guidelines for Family Planning Interventions to Prevent Pregnancy in Female Patients with Chronic Mental Illness." *American Journal of Obstetrics and Gynecology* 167 (1992): 19–25.

Minkoff, K., and R. E. Drake, eds. *Dual Diagnosis of Major Mental Illness and Substance Abuse.* San Francisco: Jossey-Bass, 1991.

Monahan, J., A. D. Redlich, J. Swanson, et al. "Use of Leverage to Improve Adherence to Psychiatric Treatment in the Community." *Psychiatric Services* 56 (2005): 37–44.

Petrakis, I. L., C. Nich, and E. Ralevski. "Psychotic Spectrum Disorders and Alcohol Abuse: A Review of Pharmacotherapeutic Strategies and a Report on the Effectiveness of Naltrexone and Disulfiram." *Schizophrenia Bulletin* 32 (2006): 644–54.

Roy, L., A.G. Crocker, T.L. Nicholls, et al. "Criminal Behavior and Victimization Among Homeless Individuals With Severe Mental Illness: A Systematic Review." *Psychiatric Services* 65 (2014): 739–50.

Swanson, J. W., M. S. Swartz, R. Borum, et al. "Involuntary Out-Patient Commitment and Reduction of Violent Behaviour in Persons with Severe Mental Illness." *British Journal of Psychiatry* 176 (2000): 224–31.

Torrey, E. F. *Out of the Shadows: Confronting America's Mental Illness Crisis.* New York: John Wiley and Sons, 1997.

Torrey, E. F., and M. Zdanowicz. "Outpatient Commitment: What, Why, and for Whom?" *Psychiatric Services* 53 (2001): 337–41.

Torrey, E. F., J. Stieber, J. Ezekiel, et al. *Criminalizing the Seriously Mentally Ill: The Abuse of Jails as Mental Hospitals.* Washington, D. C.: Health Research Group and National Alliance for the Mentally Ill, 1992.

Torrey, E. F., M. T. Zdanowicz, A. D. Kennard, et al. "The Treatment of Persons with Mental Illness in Prisons and Jails: A State Survey." Treatment Advocacy Center (2014). http://www.treatmentadvocacycenter.org/storage/documents/treatment-behind-bars/treatment-behind-bars.pdf

Velligan, D.I., M. Sajatovic, A. Hatch, A. et al. "Why do Psychiatric Patients Stop Antipsychotic Medication? A Systematic Review of Reasons for Nonadherence to Medication in Patients with Serious Mental Illness." *Patient Preference and Adherence* 11 (2017): 449–68.

11

How Can Patients and Families Survive Schizophrenia?

The wretchedness of those families upon whom devolve the care and maintenance of the insane can be estimated only by those who, from personal observation, have become acquainted with its extent. Their peace is interrupted,
their cares are multiplied, their time is engrossed, and their fortunes reduced
or entirely dissipated in attempting to restore to reason one unfortunate
member. . . . The misery which they suffer is communicated to a large circle
of friends and the whole neighborhood is indirectly disturbed by the malady
of one.

Samuel B. Woodward, 1821

Schizophrenia brings with it myriad practical problems. Other chronic
diseases, such as polio, kidney failure, and cancer, may drain patients
and families emotionally, physically, and sometimes financially. When
the disease affects the person's brain, however, the management of the
disease assumes Herculean dimensions. Whatever one does and however hard one tries, there is always the lingering feeling that it is not
quite enough.

One of the main reasons why having schizophrenia is so problematic is that most people do not understand the disease. A mother of two sons illustrated this point poignantly. Her elder son, affected with muscular dystrophy, "gets emotional support everywhere he turns. His handicap is visible and obvious and the community, family, and friends open their hearts to him and go out of their way to make his life better." By contrast, her younger son, affected with schizophrenia, "is misunderstood by all. He is also terribly disabled, but his disability is not visible. He looks like a healthy, strong young man, . . . but the neighbors ignore him. . . . They don't understand him. All in all, they wish he'd go away."

The Right Attitude

Developing the right attitude is the single most important thing an individual or family can do to survive schizophrenia. The right attitude evolves naturally once there is resolution of the twin monsters of schizophrenia—blame and shame. These lie just beneath the surface of many families, impeding the family from moving forward, souring relations among family members, and threatening to explode in a frenzy of finger pointing, accusations, and recriminations. Blame and shame are the Scylla and Charybdis of schizophrenia.

As should be clear from chapter 5, feelings of blame and shame are completely irrational. There is no evidence whatsoever that schizophrenia is caused by how people have been treated either as children or as adults; it is a biological disease of the brain, unrelated to interpersonal events of childhood or adulthood. But many people believe otherwise, and their feelings have often been based on what a mental health professional has said (or at least implied) to them. An excellent description of this process is recounted by Louise Wilson in *This Stranger, My Son:*

Mother: "And so it is we who have made Tony what he is?"
Psychiatrist: "Let me put it this way. Every child born, every mind, is a tabula rasa, an empty slate. What is written on it"—a stubby finger shot out, pointed at me—"you wrote there."

The consequences are predictable, with the mother lying awake at night remembering all the things she did that might have caused the schizophrenia.

There is, of course, not a mother, father, brother, or sister in the world who has not done things he or she regrets in past relationships with other family members. We are, after all, rather imperfect human beings, and it is not surprising that at times we all speak or act impulsively out of jealousy, anger, narcissism, or fatigue. But fortunately we have resilient psyches, capable of absorbing random blows without crumbling or being permanently damaged. People do not cause schizophrenia; they merely blame each other for doing so.

Moreover, not only do the well family members blame one another for causing the schizophrenia in the family, but the person with schizophrenia may also do so. James Wechsler's son, in *In a Darkness*, once turned to him and angrily exclaimed, "You know, Dad, I wasn't *born* this way." And in *This Stranger, My Son*, Louise Wilson recounts the following comment from her son:

> "I read a book the other day," Tony said. "It was in the drugstore. I stood there and read it all the way through."
>
> We waited, alarmed by the severity of his expression.
>
> "It told what good parents ought to be. It said that people get ... the way I am ... because their parents weren't qualified to be parents."

The blaming of one another for the illness magnifies the tragedy of schizophrenia manyfold. By itself it is a chronic disease of the brain and a personal and family disaster of usually manageable proportions. But when family members add blame to its burden, the disease spreads its roots beneath the whole family structure and becomes a calamity of boundless dimensions. The pain that blame causes in such circumstances must be seen to be believed.

Few members of the mental health profession have focused on the amount of harm that has been done by the idea that parents and families cause schizophrenia. Psychiatrists especially, as members of the medical profession, see themselves as unlikely to cause harm. We now know that this is not so, and it is likely that in the twentieth century psychiatrists as a group did more harm than good to persons with schizophrenia. The harm was not done maliciously; indeed I know of few psychiatrists who could be characterized as mean-spirited. Rather the harm was done inadvertently because of prevailing psychodynamic and family interaction theories of the disease (see chapter 5). But it was harm nonetheless. William S. Appleton is one of the few professionals who have written about this and analyzed the undesirable consequences that follow when professionals blame the families for causing the disease:

> Badly treated families retaliate in ways that are detrimental to the patient. They become less willing to tolerate the problems he causes, are less agreeable to changing their behavior toward him, do not give much information when interviewed, and pay few visits to the hospital.

Occasionally, families are reluctant to give up the blame and guilt they feel. This may occur, for example, in a family where there are still young children; if the parents believe themselves to be responsible for the schizophrenia in their older child, then by changing their behavior they can theoretically prevent it in the younger children. If, on the other hand, they believe that schizophrenia is a random biological happening, as all the evidence suggests, then they are helpless to prevent it. Guilt in such families provides an illusion of control. Another type of family that resists giving up guilt is one in which guilt is the family's way of life. Usually one or more members of such families are in long-term psychotherapy and the family seems to thrive on guilt, wallowing in it and blaming one another as their principal pastime. In such families, as one mother explained to me, "guilt is the gift which keeps on giving." I encourage individuals with schizophrenia who come from such families to minimize time spent within the family setting because it is detrimental to progress and to getting on with life despite a handicap.

The obverse of blame is shame. Inevitably, if families believe that they have somehow caused the schizophrenia, they will try to hide the family member affected, deny the illness to their neighbors, and otherwise dissociate themselves from the victim in a multiplicity of ways.

Persons with schizophrenia sense this and feel more isolated than ever. It is not unusual for the patient then to react angrily toward the family, retaliating by making less effort to control bizarre behavior, and perhaps disrobing in front of elderly Aunt Agatha. Such behavior generates more shame in the family, producing more isolation and anger in the patient, and the downward spiral of shame and anger continues.

Education, as noted below, may resolve the problem of blame and shame. When family members come to understand that they did not cause the disease, the blame and shame felt by them are usually markedly reduced and the living situation for the person with schizophrenia improved. The question of who is responsible for the disease should be asked of all family members, and the person with schizophrenia should participate in the discussion if possible. Once this is opened up, the beliefs and fears that will sometimes emerge in the ensuing discussion are extraordinary. And once the issue of blame and shame is resolved and put to rest, schizophrenia becomes much easier to live with. One parent expressed it this way:

> Once you have unloaded your guilt, laid upon you by well-meaning professionals, the next step is easier. If you have done nothing wrong and have been doing the best you can, then you have nothing to be ashamed of. You can *come out of the closet*. The relief experienced by this act gives you strength to go on, and support starts coming out of the woodwork.

Once blame and shame have been put aside, the right attitude naturally evolves. The right attitude has four elements and can be called a SAFE attitude: Sense of perspective, Acceptance of the illness, Family balance, and Expectations that are realistic.

THE RIGHT ATTITUDE

Sense of perspective
Acceptance of the illness
Family balance
Expectations that are realistic

Sense of Perspective: At first glance, a sense of perspective seems antithetical to schizophrenia. How can the most tragic disease known to mankind elicit perspective of any kind? And yet it is precisely because schizophrenia is such a tragic disease that a sense of perspective is mandatory. Without perspective the family burns out and loses its resiliency to handle the inevitable ups and downs inherent in the disease. The people I have seen that were most successful in coping with schizophrenia were those who had retained a sense of perspective and an appreciation of the absurd.

What do I mean by a sense of perspective? I certainly do not mean laughing *at* a person with this disease. Rather it is laughing *with* them. For example, one family in which the son relapsed each autumn and required rehospitalization had a standing family joke with the son that he always carved his pumpkins in the hospital. In another family, a woman went to a Halloween party dressed as a Cogentin tablet, a medication used for side effects in schizophrenia. In my own family, I once sent my sister with schizophrenia a new suit as a gift, and she replied, "The suit looks ghastly on me, and I gave it away." It is the kind of ingenuous reply that is often heard from individuals with schizophrenia, a reply stripped of the social graces to which we have become accustomed, a reply that we would all like to make on occasion but usually do not. Being able to laugh with a person with schizophrenia on such occasions is good therapy for everyone; becoming indignant is not.

Perhaps the best example of the sense of perspective so necessary in schizophrenia was told by researcher H.B.M. Murphy, while surveying a small Canadian village for individuals with schizophrenia:

> One of our other informants learnt first of another case in a fashion which still less suggests shame or embarrassment. To use his own words, it happened that my wife had been making a social visit to them and she noticed a blanket over the parlour sofa as if some stuff had been covered up there. After a time, while they were having tea, it moved. She must have seemed a little startled, for they said: "Oh, that's just Hector. He always hides himself like that." Then they went on with tea!

Acceptance of the Illness: For both the patient and the family, this is the second important ingredient in the right attitude. Acceptance does not mean giving up, but rather an acknowledgment that the disease is real, that it is not likely to just go away, and that it will impose some limitations on the person's abilities. It is acceptance of things as they are, not things as you wish them to be.

Esso Leete, an articulate woman who has schizophrenia, described the problems she has had in accepting her disease as follows: "I am haunted by an evasive picture of what my life could have been, whom I might have become, what I might have accomplished." Once acceptance has been achieved, however, the person is freed up from a huge burden, as Judith Baum, another mentally ill woman, described it: "There came the morning, sunny and bright and cold, when I accepted the fact that I had a mental illness. It was a stormy, angry and tearful time. But with acceptance came release."

Some parents experience prolonged grief in reaction to their child's schizophrenia and find acceptance very difficult to achieve. Rosalynn Carter, in her book *Helping Someone with Mental Illness*, quoted a letter from such a mother:

> "I cry most every night before I go to sleep," she continued. "I cry when I see street people. I cry when I think that even if a 'miracle' drug is produced, Stephanie will still have lost a part of her life. I cry when I think she's never gone to a dance with a boy; that she'll never marry; never be a mother; never experience life in the way others do.
>
> "I cry when my older daughter gets to travel the world as a representative of her law firm while Stephanie sits on her bed and rocks. I cry when my middle daughter published articles in our local newspapers and Stephanie smokes and listens to her 'voices.'"

Many individuals with schizophrenia and their families never learn to accept the disease. They go on, year after year, denying it and pretending it does not exist. When acceptance can be achieved, it becomes easier for everyone. One mother wrote about her sick daughter's reaction when the daughter fully realized her diagnosis and that she had been the one in one hundred to get the disease: "Well, I guess if it's percentage-wise it might as well be me. I have such a terrific family to hold my hand, and since I've been tagged someone else has escaped." Such an extraordinary attitude is an ideal to be striven for but rarely achieved, because such insight and kindness are so unusual.

More common, unfortunately, is anger in both the patient and the family. The anger may be directed at God for creating a world in which schizophrenia exists, at fate for dealing a bad hand, at the patient for becoming sick, or at one another for causing the illness. It varies from being a mild resentment bubbling to the surface when social activities must be curtailed because of the person with schizophrenia to a more virulent bitterness flowing beneath the surface of their daily activities like a caustic acid. Occasionally the anger does not achieve overt expression but rather turns inward; it is then seen as depression.

Whenever I encounter such families, I wish I could send them to a Buddhist monastery for a month. There they might learn the Oriental acceptance of life as it is, an invaluable attitude in surviving this disease. Such acceptance puts schizophrenia into perspective as one of life's great tragedies but stops it from becoming a festering sore eating away at life's very core. As one mother told me, "You can't stop the bird of sorrow from flying over your head, but you can stop it from making a mess in your hair."

Family Balance: An important aspect of the right attitude in surviving schizophrenia is an ability to weigh the needs of the ill family member against those of others in the family. Families that selflessly sacrifice everything for the person with schizophrenia are usually doing so because they feel irrationally guilty about possibly having caused the disease. To provide care for a seriously disabled person living at home may be a job requiring 168 hours per week; furthermore, it is unpaid and offers few thanks. Who is to care for the caregiver, who more often than not is the mother? How are we to weigh the needs of other children? Or the needs of the parent or parents to get away periodically? It is important to weigh these conflicting needs calmly and rationally, recognizing that the person with schizophrenia does not always come first. It may be necessary, for example, to occasionally rehospitalize a person with schizophrenia for the needs of the family and not the needs of the patient; perceptive mental illness professionals recognize such dilemmas and support the family in such decisions.

Expectations That Are Realistic: Modifying assumptions about a person's future is difficult to accomplish but important to attempt, for it often follows directly from acceptance of the disease. It is especially difficult if the person with schizophrenia had been unusually promising prior to becoming ill. Such families tend to hang on to the hope, year after year, that the person with schizophrenia will someday become normal again and resume his or her career. Grossly unrealistic plans are made, money is saved for college or a big wedding, and family members fool one another with the shared myth of "when he gets well again."

The problem with the myth is that the ill person knows it is a myth, and it puts him/her in a no-win situation. There is nothing the person can do to please the family except to get well, and that is beyond his or her control. Several observers have noted this problem and have urged families to lower their expectations for the person. If this is done, the families themselves become happier. Creer and Wing noted in their interviews with such families:

> Several relatives mentioned that giving up hope had paradoxically been the turning point for them in coming to terms with their unhappiness. "Once you give up hope," one mother said, "you start to perk up." "Once you realise he'll never be cured you start to relax." These relatives had lowered their expectations and aspirations for the patient and had found that doing this had been the first step in cutting the problem down to manageable size.

Another parent said, "You've got to reach bedrock, to become depressed enough, before you are forced to accept the reality and the enormity of the problem. Having done that, you don't allow your hopes to become too high and thus leave yourself open to disappointment when they are not fulfilled."

This does not mean that families should have no expectations at all of the person with schizophrenia. H. Richard Lamb, one of the few psychiatrists who have worked assiduously on the rehabilitation of such patients, has said, "Recognizing that a person has limited capabilities should not mean that we expect nothing of him." Expectations must be realistic, however, and consonant with the capabilities of the person with schizophrenia. Just as the family of a polio victim should not expect the person's legs to return to complete normality, so too the family of a person with schizophrenia should not expect the person's brain to return to complete normality. Psychiatrist John Wing wrote:

> A neutral (not overemotional) expectation to perform up to *attainable* standards is the ideal. This rule, if difficult for the specialist to adopt, is a thousand times more difficult for relatives. Nevertheless, we should be humbled to recognize that a large portion of relatives, by trial and error, do come to adopt it, without any help from professionals.

The effect of lowering one's expectations is often to be able to enjoy and share things with the person for the first time in many years. Thus, if someone who was an accomplished flutist prior to becoming ill takes up the flute again to play simple pieces, both the person and the family can enjoy that accomplishment. It is no longer going to be seen, implicitly or explicitly, in the light of when-you-are-well-you'll-be-able-to-give-concerts-again-dear. Similarly, if the person is able to ride a bus for the first time alone or go to the store by himself or ride a bicycle, these accomplishments can also be celebrated for what they are—often magnificent accomplishments for a person whose brain is not functioning properly. The person with schizophrenia and the family need to be able to find joy in such accomplishments just as a polio victim finds joy in relearning to walk. Oliver Sacks, in his book *The Man Who Mistook His Wife for a Hat*, expresses this attitude well in his story about brain-damaged and deformed Rebecca who could still see beauty in life:

> Superficially she *was* a mass of handicaps and incapacities . . .
> but at some deeper level there was no sense of handicap or in-

capacity, but a feeling of calm and completeness, of being fully
alive, of being a soul, deep and high, and equal to all others. . . .
We paid far too much attention to the defects of our patients,
as Rebecca was the first to tell me, and far too little to what was
intact or preserved.

The Importance of Education

Achieving the right attitude about schizophrenia becomes increasingly possible the more one learns about the disease. As Ed Francell
succinctly put it: "My advice to consumers and families is to get your
hands on anything and everything. . . . The more information you
know, the better you can put the illness in perspective."

Much learning about schizophrenia takes place in local support
groups for patients and families. The monthly or bimonthly meetings
of local groups throughout the United States sponsored by NAMI and
analogous groups in Canada sponsored by the Schizophrenia Society
of Canada have been the single most important contributions of these
organizations. They provide a forum for individuals with schizophrenia and their families to learn about the disease and to learn from one
another how to survive.

At a more formal level, the "Family-to-Family" twelve-week education course developed by Joyce Burland and NAMI Vermont has
been a great success. Under NAMI sponsorship it has been taught in
forty-nine states to more than three hundred thousand family members. The course curriculum has been translated into Spanish, Italian, Mandarin, Vietnamese, and Arabic and consists of 250 pages of
resource material that is updated each year. The Family-to-Family
course has been evaluated and is said to reduce stress and improve
problem solving by family members.

Survival Strategies for Patients

For a person with schizophrenia, surviving the disease is often a major
challenge. In recent years, however, a large number of suggestions

have been put forward by individuals who are affected and by mental illness professionals. Such suggestions can make survival easier.

Most individuals with schizophrenia do better if they have a daily routine and a predictable schedule. This allows them to anticipate stresses and minimize surprises. One patient, Esso Leete, believes that "a controlled environment is probably so important to me because my brain is not always manageable. Making lists organizes my thoughts."

Most individuals who successfully manage their schizophrenia also have specific plans for doing so. Identifying and coping with specific stressors is one aspect of this. For example, Leete describes her four-part approach as "recognizing when I am feeling stressed; identifying the stressor; remembering from past experience what action helped in the same situation or a similar one; and taking that action." Keeping a card in one's wallet or purse listing what to do when under stress may also be useful.

General coping strategies for surviving schizophrenia consist of activities such as exercise, good diet, and pursuing hobbies. A study of exercise in individuals with schizophrenia reported that it improved their sleep pattern, improved self-esteem, and decreased auditory hallucinations. Other approaches for dealing with auditory hallucinations include cognitive behavioral therapy, described in chapter 7, and a variety of self-developed methods summarized in the article "Patients' Strategies for Coping with Auditory Hallucinations" by Dorothy Carter et al., listed under "Recommended Further Reading" at the end of this chapter.

Specific coping strategies for other symptoms are both varied and imaginative. Esso Leete minimizes her paranoia by always choosing "a seat where I can face the door, preferably with my back to the wall instead of to other people" and by "asking the people I am with questions like who they are calling, where they are going, or whatever."

In 2017 a useful article was published on "How Occupationally High-Achieving Individuals with a Diagnosis of Schizophrenia Manage Their Symptoms" (see Recommended Further Reading). It described the coping strategies of 16 such individuals, including the avoidance of stressful situations; having a social support network; taking medications; enacting specific coping strategies; engaging spirituality; and using work or further education to provide meaning.

One of the most important things that individuals with schizophrenia can do to survive is to join self-help groups, but not those associated with the Hearing Voices Network (see chapter 8). These go under a variety of names such as Recovery Inc., GROW, Schizophrenics Anonymous, On Our Own, and Psychosis Free. All such groups provide support and education and a place where, as one patient put it, "I can just be myself." Schizophrenics Anonymous, for example, was established in Michigan in 1985 by Joanne Verbanic, who had schizophrenia, to provide fellowship, to educate, and "to help restore dignity and sense of purpose for persons who are working for recovery from schizophrenia or related disorders." There are now more than one hundred sixty Schizophrenics Anonymous chapters (www.sardaa.org).

One of the most exciting recent developments among individuals with schizophrenia is the increasing role they are playing in providing mental illness services. In many communities they run drop-in centers for mentally ill persons. In San Francisco, they have been trained and hired as "peer counselors" on locked psychiatric inpatient units. And in San Mateo County, California, "peer counselors" have been hired to do AIDS education and to provide support for other patients who are being moved from psychiatric hospitals to apartment living. In Denver, individuals with schizophrenia have been trained in a six-month training program as case management aides and have played an important role in the state's Community Mental Health Centers. The Denver consumer provider program was replicated in Texas, Washington, and Massachusetts, and logically should represent a wave for the future of mental illness services.

The development of self-help groups, "peer counselors," and consumer provider programs has, unfortunately, proceeded much more slowly than should have been the case. The major reason for this is the "consumer survivor" movement, described in chapter 15. The small but highly vocal group of "consumer survivors" has frequently encouraged individuals with schizophrenia to stop taking their medication, and some "consumer survivors" even deny that schizophrenia exists as a brain disorder. This small group has widely discredited the much larger and respectable movement in the eyes of many families and agencies who provide mental illness services.

One of the most important survival strategies for patients is to become medication-savvy. Read up on the medications you are on until you know as much as, or even more than, your treating psychiatrist. Indeed, one of the goals for a medication-savvy patient is to be able to (politely) tell the treating psychiatrist something that he/she didn't know. A second step in being medication-savvy is to keep a list of all medications taken, the length of time they were taken, the dose, and the adverse effects. This continuously updated list should be given to any new treating psychiatrist encountered in the course of the illness. If you see a psychiatrist for only fifteen minutes every three months, it is also helpful to give the psychiatrist a list of your present medications and adverse effects; with limited time, it helps him/her focus on the important issues. Patients who have had a very bad reaction to a medication or who are taking medications with potentially severe drug interactions (e.g., clozapine and benzodiazepines) should also wear a Medical Alert bracelet, so that if they become unconscious or very psychotic, they will not be given the wrong medication.

The final step in being a medication-savvy patient is to keep a list of things you wish you could do but that the illness prevents you from doing. These are essentially the goals you wish to achieve by taking medication and participating in other forms of recovery and rehabilitation. The list reminds you *why* you are taking medication and *why* you are willing to try new medications as they become available to possibly ameliorate your symptoms. The list should, of course, be realistic and consistent with your abilities prior to your illness (e.g., being able to read a book, go into a crowded room without panicking, hold a job at least half-time, have a boyfriend, etc.). It should not include items such as "be a concert pianist" if you have never played the piano!

Survival Strategies for Families

In recent years, there has been an outpouring of studies documenting the burden for families of having a family member with schizophrenia living at home. One review article summarized twenty-eight such studies, of which seventeen were published in the 1990s. These studies described the family members' loss of personal time, decreased social relationships, poorer health, and decreased finances because someone had to stop working in order to be at home. The family is frequently asked to act as the ill person's case manager, psychotherapist, nurse, landlord, cook, janitor, banker, disciplinarian, and best friend. This impossible array of family tasks is relatively new, since, prior to the 1960s, the majority of people with schizophrenia were hospitalized at least intermittently. The frustrations that are inevitable in such situations were described by one mother as follows:

> Sometimes I feel like a social director. It is my job to think of stimulating things for my daughter to do and places for her to visit. I arrange outings and provide transportation and amiable companionship. It is not that I dislike my personal role in Carrie's life, but I admit to some frustration. I have a life of my own that I want to get back to, and I'm ready for Carrie to take more responsibility for hers.

A 2018 online survey of 1,142 caregivers for individuals with schizophrenia and schizoaffective disorder confirmed the high level of distress and caregiver burden experienced by these individuals, especially problems associated with the monitoring of medication and the lack of social support. Such families need support from mental illness professionals for their caregiving activities but often do not receive it. In an effort to improve the support of mental illness professionals for families, a group of families and professionals in Australia created a training program for the professionals. In the United States, the Riverside County Department of Mental Health in California created a position called "family advocate" to support the families and train the professionals; this idea has spread to other counties in California.

Whether the family member with schizophrenia is living at home or not, the family must confront some basic questions. One that frequently comes up is how should the family members behave toward someone with schizophrenia? In general, people who get along best with individuals with schizophrenia are those who treat them most naturally. This can be verified by watching the nursing staff in any psychiatric hospital. The staff who are most respected by both professionals and patients treat the patients with dignity and as human beings, albeit with a brain disease. The staff who are least respected treat the patients in a condescending manner, frequently reminding them of their inferior status. Often this is because the staff member does not understand schizophrenia or is afraid of it. The simple answer, then, to the question "How should I behave toward a person with schizophrenia?" is, Kindly.

Beyond this, however, there are certain aspects of schizophrenia as a disease that do modify to some degree one's behavior toward a person who has it. These modifications arise directly and predictably out of the nature of the brain damage and the symptoms of the disease as described in chapter 1. Persons with schizophrenia have great difficulty in processing sensory input of all kinds, especially two or more simultaneous sensory stimuli. If this is kept in mind, then determining how to behave toward the person becomes much easier.

Make communications, for example, brief, concise, and unambiguous. As explained by one family member: "Look at the person. Talk in short, concise, adult statements . . . be clear and practical . . . give one set of directions at a time with no options."

Another mother described how she communicates with her adult son with schizophrenia:

> My son seemed to have difficulty dealing with all the stimuli around him. He responded slowly and said that he had difficulty with "everything coming at me." At those times it was important for me to speak in simple, slow sentences. Requests were made for one thing at a time. Keeping down complexity was very important. Strong emotion increased his difficulty in processing what I was saying. However much in a hurry I felt, there was no way to hurry him. Patience was absolutely necessary.
>
> Sometimes leaving requests by way of memo or over the telephone seemed to work better than face to face—I am not sure why—sometimes he seemed to be overstimulated by my presence.
>
> Ask the person with schizophrenia one question at a time. "Did you have a nice time, dear? Who went with you?" may seem like a straightforward two-part question for a normal person, but for a person with schizophrenia it may be overwhelming.

It is also counterproductive to try to argue people with schizophrenia out of their delusional beliefs. Attempts to do so often result in misunderstanding and anger, as described by John Wing:

> Patients tended to develop sudden irrational fears. They might, for instance, become fearful of a particular room in the house. Maybe they would tell the family the reason for their fear. "There's a poisonous gas leaking into that room" or "There are snakes under the bed in that room." At first relatives are baffled by this. Some admitted they had grown frustrated with a patient's absolute refusal to abandon some idea, despite all their attempts to reason with him, and had lost their temper. But they found this only resulted in the patient becoming very upset, and in any case the idea continued to be held with as much conviction as ever.

Rather than arguing with the patient, simply make a statement of disagreement; this can be done without challenging or provoking him or her. Thus, a reasonable response to "There are snakes under the bed in that room" is "I know you believe there are snakes there, but I don't see any and I doubt that there are," rather than a peremptory "There are *no* snakes in that room." The patient has some reason for believing that there are snakes there—perhaps he/she heard them or even saw them. It is often useful for the family member to acknowledge the validity of the patient's sensory experiences without accepting the person's interpretation of the experiences. Such a statement might be "I know you have some reason to believe there are snakes there, but I think that the reason has to do with the fact that your brain is playing tricks on you because of your illness."

Family members and friends of patients are often tempted to deal with the patient's delusional beliefs in a sarcastic or humorous manner. The statement about snakes, for example, might be responded to as follows: "Oh yes, I saw them there too. And did you see the rattlesnakes in the kitchen as well?" Such statements are never useful and are often very confusing for the patient. It also reinforces their delusional belief and makes it more difficult for them to separate their personal experiences from reality. One patient, who believed he had a rat in his throat and asked the doctors to look at it, was told sardonically by the doctors that the rat was too far down to see. When the patient recovered, he recalled, "I would have been grateful if they had stated quite plainly that they did not believe that there was a rat in my throat." This is good advice.

Another useful way to handle the delusional thinking of people with schizophrenia is to encourage them to express such thinking only in private. Talking about snakes being under the bed is not harmful within the context of family and friends, but if said in a crowded elevator or announced to the saleslady in a store, it can be embarrassing for everyone concerned. Discuss this frankly and straightforwardly with the person and it will often be appreciated. As Creer and Wing point out: "A more realistic aim is to try to limit the effect of such ideas upon the patient's public behavior. Many patients were well able to understand this and to limit odd behavior, such as talking to themselves, and the expression of odd ideas, to private occasions."

An impediment to communicating with persons with schizophrenia is their frequent inability to participate in normal back-and-forth conversation. "One patient returned home each evening from the day center, ate in complete silence the meal her aunt provided, and then went straight to her room. . . . Her aunt, who was lonely and elderly, would have been very glad for a chat in the evenings. She was puzzled by the patient's almost total lack of communication." Such patients often are aware of conversations around them but are unable to participate. "One young man generally sat in silence, or muttering to himself, while his parents were conversing about family matters. Later, however, they learned that he had quite often spoken to a nurse at the hospital about such topics of conversation at home and had clearly been taking in what was said despite all appearances to the contrary." Many such patients like to have other people around them but do not like to interact with them directly. "One lady said she had been surprised to hear from a friend that her nephew suffering from the disease liked to come and visit her. 'I would never have guessed it because when he comes he just sits in a chair and says absolutely nothing.'"

An analogous problem families have in their efforts to relate to persons with schizophrenia is their impaired ability to express emotions. Frequently the patient will relate to even close family members in what appears to be a cold and distant way. This emotional aloofness is quite normal for many persons with this disease and should be respected. Difficult though this coldness may be, do not take it personally. The patient may find it easier to express emotion or verbal affection toward a family pet, and it is sometimes a good idea to provide the person with a cat or dog for this purpose.

A common problem is how the family should behave toward a person with schizophrenia when he/she is withdrawn. It is important to recognize the need of many persons with this disease to withdraw. One mother wrote me that while chatting with her ill daughter as they were doing the dishes, the daughter turned and said: "Leave me alone now, Mom, so I can enjoy my own world." Sometimes the withdrawal can be pronounced. I once had a patient who remained in her room at home for weeks at a time, coming out only during the night to eat.

It can be puzzling to know what to do in these cases of social withdrawal. Should you insist that the person emerge from the bedroom and interact socially, or should you leave him or her alone? The answer is, as a general rule, to leave the person alone. If the withdrawal seems excessive or too persistent, it is possible it may herald the recurrence of more severe symptoms and will require evaluation by the patient's psychiatrist. But in most cases the withdrawal is being used as a means for coping with the internal chaos in the patient's brain and is an appropriate response. Family members should remind themselves not to take such withdrawal as a personal rejection but should keep themselves available. As described usefully by one mother: "When our son was acutely ill we managed best by not being too intrusive, by not trying too hard to draw him out of his world and into ours, but by always being available at the times when he needed our support and tried to communicate."

In social situations it is important not to expect too much from persons with schizophrenia. Remember that they may be having problems assimilating sensory input or understanding what is being said. Minimize the number and scale of social events in the house in order to relieve pressure on the person. Patients can often handle one visitor at a time, but groups are usually overwhelming to them. Similarly, taking the person to group gatherings or parties outside the home is often a difficult and confusing experience for the person.

Experiment to find leisure time activities that are enjoyable. Those with a single (or dominant) sensory input are usually most successful. Thus, a person with schizophrenia will often enjoy cartoons or a travelogue on TV but will not be able to understand a show with a plot. A boxing match may be preferable to a baseball game. Visual spectacles, such as a circus or ice show, are often very enjoyable, while a play is often a total failure. Individuals are, of course, different in this regard, and it is necessary to explore different possibilities. The fact that people enjoyed something before they became ill does not mean that they necessarily will enjoy it after they become ill.

A common trap that families frequently fall into is to blame *all* the person's undesirable or unwanted behavior on the disease. It should be called "the disease trap." Every little shortcoming, including the person's failure to pick up dirty socks or replace the cap on the tube of toothpaste, is blamed on schizophrenia. Families need to remind themselves that human beings come with peccadilloes built in and that there are few around who have achieved perfection. Resist the temptation to blame everything on schizophrenia and ask how many mistakes *you* made in the last week. Along the same line, allow individuals with schizophrenia to have a bad day now and then, just as we allow those of us without schizophrenia to have a bad day. We all need such days since our neurochemical and neurophysiological machinery does not work perfectly all the time; extending the privilege of a bad day to individuals with schizophrenia is both common sense and common courtesy.

Above all, cultivate the art of being unflappable. Radiate quiet confidence that you can handle any idea, however strange, that your relative may come up with. If the person's auditory hallucinations are worse that morning, simply comment on it matter-of-factly, just as if you noticed that a person's arthritis is worse: "I'm sorry to see that the voices are bothering you more today." One parent said, "The most remarkable lesson I have learned about managing a schizophrenic person at home is to try to stay as calm as possible. The upsets and delusions have not been caused by me, and being calm keeps my son that way also. I might be heaving inside but my behavior on the outside is controlled." The epitome of unflappability was illustrated by Pliny Earle, one of the best-known nineteenth-century American psychiatrists. Earle described the superintendent of an insane asylum who went to the top of the hospital's tower accompanied by one of his patients:

> While admiring the extensive and beautiful prospect spread before them, the patient, with much excitement, suddenly seized the superintendent by the arm, and pressed him toward the edge of the tower, exclaiming, "Let's jump down, and thus immortalize ourselves!" The superintendent very coolly arrested the patient's attention, and replied: "Jump down! Why, any fool can do that. Let's go down and jump up!" The proposition struck the fancy of the patient, and thus the two were saved from their impending peril.

If the family member with schizophrenia lives at home, two things are essential—solitude and structure. A person with schizophrenia needs his or her own room, a quiet place that can be used for withdrawing. Families solve this problem in a variety of ways, including putting a small house trailer in the backyard. Structure is also helpful for most persons with schizophrenia, and they function better with regular meal hours, chores, and a predictable daily and weekly routine. One mother said:

> I found structure was very important during the more difficult days. Things were done similarly each day and at designated times, and every day of the week had its individual character which was kept as consistent as possible. This seemed to give him a sense of order, that life was predictable, and also established a sense of time.

At the same time that routines are established, realize that the person with schizophrenia may deviate from them for no apparent reason. This is especially true of sleeping and eating routines. One father complained about his son, "My wife will cook a meal, and then he doesn't want it. Then two hours later he suddenly decides he does." An admirable solution to this kind of problem was outlined by this mother:

> The second practical suggestion concerns the schizophrenic's need for a sudden intake of food. At least in the case of our son, available

wholesome snacks are very important. I've learned to keep yogurt, cheese, cold meat, etc., in the refrigerator; fruit on the table; and quick canned meals on the shelves. All this has seemed more important than a regular schedule of meals, although three good meals a day helps, too. The strict time doesn't matter. If Jim fixes himself a can of stew at four in the afternoon, I simply leave his dinner ready for him to heat up when he's ready.

Another thing needed for a family member with schizophrenia whether he/she is living at home or just visiting is a set of clearly defined limits regarding which behaviors are not acceptable. A failure to bathe for several weeks has consequences that affect all family members. No family should tolerate assaultive behavior (as discussed in chapter 10) or dangerous behavior (e.g., smoking in bed), and this message must be conveyed clearly and unambiguously. The consequences for such behaviors should also be spelled out in advance and the family must be willing to follow through on the consequences if it becomes necessary to do so.

Another problem that perplexes many families is the amount of independence and autonomy that can be given to a person with schizophrenia. The problem is similar to that faced by parents of adolescent children. As a general rule, persons should be given as much autonomy and independence as they can handle, and this should be done in a graduated series of steps. For example, a person who believes he or she should be able to travel alone to a concert and stay out late should be given the opportunity to demonstrate readiness by successfully going to the store regularly, traveling alone to the halfway house during the day, avoiding street drugs, and not getting into trouble in public because of bizarre behavior. I have known families who discreetly followed their family member on initial forays into the community to ensure that no harm befell the patient. When the patient asks for more autonomy, the family should set up a series of conditions that must be met before the autonomy can be granted; for example, a patient who asks to travel home alone from the halfway house might be told that this can be tried once the patient has demonstrated familiarity with the bus route and has successfully gone for two weeks without forgetting to lock the door of the house.

Chores are another means by which persons with schizophrenia may demonstrate their readiness for more independence. Sweeping, cleaning, doing the dishes, taking out the garbage, feeding the dog, and weeding are all examples of chores that may be appropriate to assign to the ill family member. Families are sometimes reluctant to assign such chores, fearing that any stress will cause a recurrence of the patient's symptoms. Patients who are lazy may encourage such fears, pleading illness whenever there is work to be done. One mother described the resentment that is an inevitable consequence of this situation: "It's so annoying when you've got lots of housework to do, and there he is, a fine healthy-looking young man, and he just *sits* there doing absolutely nothing." Doing chores will not cause a patient to become sicker, and such chores are used extensively in halfway house settings and club-house programs. They are an ideal way for patients to assume more independence and they increase the person's self-esteem at the same time. I have seen some extremely psychotic patients doing chores quite nicely and feeling better for having done so.

The management of the patient's money may cause the most difficulty of all. Most patients know that a portion of their SSI check is earmarked for their personal needs, and they believe they should have the right to spend it however they please. They should be reminded, however, that the personal portion of the check is intended to cover necessities, such as clothes, as well as cigarettes and sodas.

Occasionally persons with schizophrenia can take total responsibility for their money and can manage it with minimal difficulties. I knew one woman severely affected with paranoid schizophrenia, for example, who was very delusional much of the time but was able to take monthly trips to the bank and manage her funds. Predictably, she would not tell the doctors or nurses how much money she had. More common, however, is the person who cannot manage money at all; some patients, for example, will repeatedly give away any money they have to the first person who asks for it. For such persons it may be useful to link autonomy in money management to other behaviors indicating independence. For example, if patients have difficulty with personal hygiene and grooming, it may be appropriate to agree to give them more money to spend as they wish every week that they successfully take a shower without being told. The successful performance of chores is another way that patients can demonstrate that they are ready for greater financial responsibility.

Issues of independence and money management may also cause problems for families because of the family's inability to understand that their family member is getting better. When one has lived with a severely psychotic individual who may have even needed help in dressing himself, it is often difficult to recognize a few weeks later that the person is now able to travel by bus alone and manage a weekly allowance. Families have often been both scared and scarred, and their ability to respond and adapt sometimes becomes constricted.

As discussed previously, education for families is extremely important in helping them to survive schizophrenia. Support groups, such as those organized by state and local NAMI organizations (see appendix B), are also very helpful.

A final survival strategy for families is to become a strong advocate for your ill family member. Aggressively take on the mental health treatment system and make it work for your family member. Since the treatment system is completely dysfunctional in most states, this strategy is not for the faint of heart, but exercising one's chutzpah can be remarkably therapeutic. An example of this strategy was posted on the website of the Treatment Advocacy Center (www.treatmentadvocacycenter.org) in 2012 by Doris Fuller, regarding her efforts to get her daughter properly treated. It is called "It Pays to Be Shameless."

Three months after she was committed to the state hospital, my darling twenty-five-year-old daughter is free of the demons that emerge when she's psychotic and getting ready for discharge from her third involuntary hospitalization in three years.

She says she learned from the relapse that quitting her medications is really dangerous. Like every other parent of a child with a severe mental illness who is moving into recovery, I pray this is true.

What I learned from her latest setback is that it pays to be shameless. All those admonitions my mother gave me about not imposing on others, not asking too much, not being stubborn? "Go over heads"? Always. When she was too ill to tell me anything about her own condition, I shamelessly asked for the top person on duty every time I called the hospital to find out how she was doing. I knew that the charge nurse would have the most complete answers and be in a position to order changes if anything was amiss.

"Know what services are available in your community"? Absolutely. I explored discharge housing within days of her commitment and then shamelessly and regularly called and e-mailed the best facility I found, to keep track of space and begin a relationship with the people who might be taking care of her.

I found that it paid to be shameless outside the system, too. My daughter spent Christmas, New Year's, and Valentine's Day not only in a psychiatric hospital but in isolation. Even with infallibly kind and patient staff nearby, it's lonely in there. So I posted not-very-subtle messages on Facebook about how much she loved getting mail at the holidays. Cards and notes poured in, to her delight. When family members said they never called because they didn't know what to say to her, I told them, "Ignore the part of her you don't recognize and just talk to the part you do. It's still there." Some called. In the dark hours when she was too tortured by inner voices even to make conversation with me, I'd tell her, "Then I'll read to you." I probably looked pathetic reading children's picture books to her over the telephone, but it was comforting to us both.

When I was growing up, my mother always admonished me not to impose on others, not to be demanding, not to be stubborn. If I did, she would scold me that I ought to be ashamed. With my daughter's well-being at stake, I do all the things Mom said I shouldn't do, but I'm never ashamed, because they pay off.

Effects of Schizophrenia on Siblings, Children, and Spouses

Although most family accounts of schizophrenia focus on the effects of the disease on mothers and fathers of ill individuals, schizophrenia is a problem for other family members as well. Brothers, sisters, sons, daughters, husbands, wives, uncles, aunts, grandfathers, and grandmothers may all be profoundly involved in the care of family members with schizophrenia. As such they have all of the same problems as do mothers and fathers. There are certain problems, however, that other family members confront frequently.

Shame and Embarrassment: Family members may be profoundly embarrassed by the psychotic behavior of their ill relative. Roxanne Lanquetot, whose mother had schizophrenia, recalls being "convinced that I would have been better off an orphan, I tried to hide my mother and deny her existence by pretending she didn't exist." Kathleen Gordon's ill mother would take her children "and sit us down on the side of a busy street and count trucks for hours on end. And write down the names of all the trucks that went by." One young woman I know almost literally stumbled over her mother, homeless and psychotic, in an airport as she was returning to college. And Meg Livergood, who stopped for a red light in Miami, saw her homeless sister with schizophrenia shuffle across the street in front of her car but was too embarrassed to call out to her. One common reaction to such shame and embarrassment is to move as far away from the family home as possible.

Anger, Jealousy, and Resentment: Individuals with schizophrenia frequently occupy an inordinate amount of their family's energy and time, leaving little for other family members. Wendy Kelley recalled that when her sister developed schizophrenia "suddenly both my brother and I felt there was no time for us; everyone was consumed by what was going on with my sister." Jody Mozham, whose father had schizophrenia, remembers being "envious watching my friends have regular conversations with their fathers. . . . I had a father, yet I didn't." Anger and resentment may become exacerbated if large amounts of the family's financial resources, such as money set aside for college, must be used to pay for the ill person's treatment.

Depression and Guilt: When a person develops schizophrenia, other family members may lose a valued relationship. Ami Brodoff expressed this loss poignantly:

That day, many days before it, and many days since, I've missed my older brother with the persistent ache and longing usually reserved for a loved one lost through death. Although grieving for someone who has died is painful, some sense of peace and acceptance is ultimately possible. However, mourning for a loved one who is alive—in your very presence and yet in vital ways inaccessible to you—has a lonely, unreal quality that is extraordinarily painful.

One man whose wife developed schizophrenia described the loss of the relationship as follows:

I feel such great sorrow towards my wife of twenty-five years. The person I knew died in 1985. I try to grieve, but it's complicated by the body that keeps reappearing. It looks like her, but it's not.

And a woman whose husband developed schizophrenia noted:

My husband's schizophrenia is like a third member in our marriage. It is always there. Even with medication, we still deal with his paranoia, his isolation, and his need for my full attention on a daily basis.

The family members who did not develop schizophrenia may also develop survivor guilt, a common phenomenon in airplane accidents and other random tragedies. Paul Aronowitz described this when he announced to his brother, who was afflicted with schizophrenia, that he was getting married: "'It's funny,' his brother answered matter-of-factly. 'You're getting married, and I've never even had a girlfriend.'"

Pressure to Succeed: The siblings or children of individuals with schizophrenia often try to compensate for their ill family member by being as perfect as possible. In a study of the children of mentally ill parents, Kauffman et al. labeled the extremely competent offspring as "superkids."

Fear of Becoming Sick: Most siblings and children of individuals with schizophrenia are themselves haunted by a fear that they too will develop the disease. As Roxanne Lanquetot recalls: "Growing up with a mentally ill mother was oppressive and worrisome and it interfered with the development of my sense of self. I was terrified that I was like my mother and therefore had something wrong with me."

Forced to Play Unwanted Roles: Schizophrenia changes family relationships, often profoundly. Margaret Moorman in *My Sister's Keeper* described how difficult it was to change from being a younger sister to being, in essence, a mother for her older sister. Husbands and wives whose spouse becomes ill often must become their spouse's parent. Jody Mozham described the effect of her father's illness on her mother: "She once knew this dream man that turned into an invalid. No longer did she have the role of being a wife, she was his guardian." Kathleen Gordon, both of whose parents had schizophrenia, even at age four "was aware that I could not trust my parents in what they told me to do or in their behavior" and by age nine was the "virtual head of her household."

There are many things that family members can do to alleviate some of the burden of having a relative with schizophrenia. Education is most important, and this should always include even small children in the family whose ability to understand is much greater than most adults assume. Some articles and books targeting the problems of relatives of individuals with schizophrenia are listed at the end of this chapter under "Recommended Further Reading." Support groups can be extremely helpful, including groups specifically set up for other relatives. Julie Johnson, whose brother has schizophrenia, developed an eight-stage healing process for siblings as outlined in her book *Hidden Victims—Hidden Healers.* Acceptance of the inevitable role shifts comes slowly but is necessary because siblings often end up with at least some responsibility for their ill brother or sister once their parents have died.

Finally, many brothers, sisters, husbands, wives, sons, and daughters are learning to cope with schizophrenia by becoming advocates for better services and more research, working with organizations such as NAMI and the Treatment Advocacy Center. Advocacy, in fact, is one of the most useful and therapeutic means for coping by the unaffected family members, and many suggestions are listed in chapter 15. A corollary of this is that many schizophrenia researchers, including myself, began working in this field primarily because we had a family member afflicted with the disease. I also know many clinical psychiatrists, psychologists, psychiatric social workers, and psychiatric nurses whose work is motivated by the fact that someone in their family has schizophrenia; they tend to be among the best professionals. Similarly, many state legislators who have affected family members are leading efforts to improve state treatment laws.

Minimizing Relapses

One of the keys to surviving schizophrenia is to minimize relapses. The threat of relapse is a perpetual shadow hanging over individuals with schizophrenia and their families. Each minor deviation from the person's usual behavior is regarded as suspect. The question hangs in the air, often not expressed in words but rather as a sideways glance: "Is this the beginning of another episode?" "Should I/he/she take additional medicine?" "Should I say anything?" Doris Fuller of the Treatment Advocacy Center once described it as waiting for the return of her daughter's demons: "It's in my mind that they continue to lurk, monstrous sentries that keep me from passing from hope to optimism."

As discussed in chapter 10, medication compliance is the single most important thing a person with schizophrenia can do to minimize relapses. Individuals who take their medication regularly will have far fewer relapses than those who are intermittently compliant or noncompliant. Substance abuse is another powerful predictor of relapse; in one study of thirty-seven individuals with schizophrenia, all of whom were on long-acting injectable antipsychotic medication, those who were abusing alcohol or drugs had four times as many relapses as those who were not substance abusers.

In one of the largest studies of relapse in schizophrenia, 145 patients were questioned regarding the symptoms they experienced in the early stages of their relapses. The symptoms reported most frequently were being tense and nervous, eating and sleeping problems, having trouble concentrating, enjoying things less, and experiencing restlessness. Marvin Herz, one of the study's authors, concluded that "it is extremely important to educate both patients and families" about the symptoms and signs of relapse, and that "family involvement is a crucial component in the treatment of schizophrenia."

In England, Max Birchwood and his colleagues have done studies to ascertain which symptoms are the best predictors of impending relapse. Out of this work has evolved a "Warning Signals Scale," which should be kept by all individuals with schizophrenia and their families. It includes eight questions that, if answered in the affirmative, may indicate an impending relapse.

In many cases the patient and/or family has learned over time which symptoms and signs heralded relapse. One woman who had had multiple episodes of schizophrenia described to me the things she looked for: "My main prodromal symptoms are quick irritability and anger and, when out-of-doors, thinking that everyone I see looks familiar although I do not know *whom* they remind me of." Another woman described her relapse as occurring in four stages:

> In the first stage, I feel just a bit estranged from myself. From my eyes the world seems brighter and more sharply defined, and my voice seems to echo a bit. I start to feel uncomfortable being around people, and also uncomfortable in sharing my changing feelings.
>
> In the second stage, everything appears a bit clouded. This cloudiness increases as does my confusion and fear, especially fear of letting others know what is happening to me. I try to make logical excuses and to get control over the details of my life, and often make frantic efforts to organize everything; cleaning, cataloging, and self-involved activity is high. Songs on the radio begin to have greater meaning, and people seem to be looking at me strangely and laughing, giving me subtle messages I can't understand. I start to misinterpret people's actions toward me, which increases my fear of losing control.
>
> In the third stage, I believe I am beginning to understand why terrible things are happening to me: others are the cause of it. This belief comes with a clearing of sight, an increasing level of sound, and an increasing sensitivity to the looks of others. I carry on an argument with myself as to whether these things are true: "Is the FBI

WARNING SIGNAL SCALE

This questionnaire concerns *new or worsened* problems and complaints you have experienced during the *last 2 weeks*.

		Yes	No
1.	Sleep has been restless or unsettled	☐	☐
2.	Feeling tense, afraid, or unsettled	☐	☐
3.	Having difficulty concentrating	☐	☐
4.	Feeling irritable or quick-tempered	☐	☐
5.	Feeling unable to cope, difficulty in managing everyday tasks and interests	☐	☐
6.	Feeling tired or lacking energy	☐	☐
7.	Feeling depressed or low	☐	☐
8.	Feeling confused or puzzled	☐	☐

or the devil causing this? . . . No, that's crazy thinking. I wonder why people are making me crazy."

In the fourth and last stage, I become chaotic and see, hear, and believe all manner of things. I no longer question my beliefs, but act on them.

Each person with schizophrenia has their own particular symptom pattern when relapsing, and that pattern tends to be similar from relapse to relapse. Personally, I find changes in the person's sleep pattern an especially useful indicator, and I ask about this frequently.

How can relapses be minimized? First, everyone with schizophrenia should keep their own relapse symptom list, and it should be familiar to their family and friends. Individuals with schizophrenia should try to identify those things that tend to exacerbate relapses (e.g., the stress of social situations) and avoid them when necessary. For example, it may be possible to attend the wedding of a friend when things are going well, but it may be best to call and say you cannot come if you think that you might be in the early stages of a relapse. Spending more time alone, reducing work hours, and getting more exercise are all examples of strategies used by some people with schizophrenia to reduce stress.

Always keep in mind that the single most common cause of relapse is not getting enough medication. This may be because the person stopped taking it, or because the doctor reduced the dosage, or simply because the person needs more medication at this point in his/her illness. And extra medication in the early stages of relapse will frequently abort it and get the person back to baseline. For this reason I give many patients an extra supply of medication and allow them to increase it on their own if they feel that they need it. Physicians do this all the time with patients with diabetes who may need more insulin on some days and less on other days, and I find the same principle useful in schizophrenia.

All of this assumes, of course, a best-case scenario in which the person with schizophrenia has awareness of his/her illness and therefore can assess warning signs of relapse. As discussed in chapters 1 and 10, approximately half of individuals with schizophrenia have limited awareness. One possible strategy for minimizing relapses in such cases is to take videotapes of the persons when they are very psychotic, then to show them the videotapes when they are in remission.

Finally, remember that schizophrenia has ups and downs for no apparent reason, just as multiple sclerosis and Parkinson's disease do, and most people have occasional relapses no matter how hard they try to avoid them. This is part of the disease process and must be accepted. For most people with schizophrenia, then, relapses can be reduced, but they cannot be prevented altogether.

Recommended Further Reading

In the past two decades, there has been an outpouring of articles and books written to help patients and families survive schizophrenia. Many of these are listed below without annotation. Appendix A includes my selections of the most useful books, with annotation. Some of the books are out of print but may be available at your local library or on the Internet.

For Families in General

Adamec, C. *How to Live with a Mentally Ill Person.* New York: John Wiley, 1996.
Amador, X., and A.-L. Johanson. *I Am Not Sick: I Don't Need Help.* Peconic, N.Y.: Vida Press, 2000.

Backlar, P. *The Family Face of Schizophrenia*. New York: G. P. Putnam, 1994. Paperback by Tarcher, 1995.

Baronet, A.-M. "Factors Associated with Caregiver Burden in Mental Illness: A Critical Review of the Research Literature." *Clinical Psychological Review* 19 (1999): 819–41.

Beard, J., P. Gillespie, and G. Karser. *Nothing to Hide: Mental Illness in the Family*. New York: New Press, 2002.

Bernheim, K. F., and A. F. Lehman. *Working with Families of the Mentally Ill*. New York: Norton, 1985.

Bernheim, K. F., R. R. J. Lewine, and C. T. Beale. *The Caring Family: Living with Chronic Mental Illness*. New York: Random House, 1982.

Busick, B. S., and M. Gorman. *Ill Not Insane*. Boulder, Colo.: New Idea Press, 1986.

Carter, R. *Helping Someone with a Mental Illness*. New York: Times Books, 1998.

Creer, C., and J. Wing. *Schizophrenia at Home*. London: Institute of Psychiatry, 1974.

Dearth, N. S., B. J. Labenski, E. Mott, et al. *Families Helping Families*. New York: Norton, 1986.

Deveson, A. *Tell Me I'm Here*. New York: Penguin, 1992.

Dixon, L. B., A. Lucksted, D. R. Medoff, et al. "Outcomes of a Randomized Study of a Peer-Taught Family-to-Family Education Program for Mental Illness." *Psychiatric Services* 62 (2011): 591–97.

Esser, A. H., and S. D. Lacey. *Mental Illness: A Homecare Guide*. New York: John Wiley, 1989.

Farhall, J., B. Webster, B. Hocking, et al. "Training to Enhance Partnerships Between Mental Health Professionals and Family Caregivers: A Comparative Study." *Psychiatric Services* 49 (1998): 1488–90.

Flach, F. *Rickie*. New York: Fawcett Columbine, 1990.

Garson, S. *Out of Our Minds*. Buffalo: Prometheus Books, 1986.

Hatfield, A. B. *Family Education in Mental Illness*. New York: Guilford Press, 1990. Paperback edition, 1999.

Hatfield, A. B., ed. *Families of the Mentally Ill: Meeting the Challenge*. San Francisco: Jossey-Bass, 1987.

Hatfield, A. B., and H. P. Lefley, eds. *Families of the Mentally Ill: Coping and Adaptation*. New York, Guilford Press, 1987.

Hatfield, A. B., and H. P. Lefley. *Surviving Mental Illness: Stress, Coping and Adaptation*. New York: Guilford Press, 1993. Paperback edition, 1999.

Hinckley, J., and J. A. Hinckley. *Breaking Points*. Grand Rapids, Mich.: Chosen Books, 1985.

Howe, G. *The Reality of Schizophrenia*. London: Faber and Faber, 1991.

Howells, J. G., and W. R. Guirguis. *The Family and Schizophrenia*. New York: International Universities Press, 1985.

Jeffries, J. J., E. Plummer, M. V. Seeman, and J. F. Thornton. *Living and Working with Schizophrenia*. Toronto: University of Toronto Press, 1990. (This is a revised edition of the book by M. V. Seeman, et al.)

Johnson, J. *Hidden Victims—Hidden Healers*. New York: Doubleday, 1988. 2nd ed., paperback, by PEMA Publications, 1994.

Johnson, J. *Understanding Mental Illness*. Minneapolis: Lerner, 1989.

Jungbauer, J., and M. C. Angermeyer. "Living with a Schizophrenic Patient: A Comparative Study of Burden as It Affects Parents and Spouses." *Psychiatry* 65 (2002): 110–23.

Karp, D. A. *The Burden of Sympathy: How Families Cope with Mental Illness*. New York: Oxford University Press, 2001.

Keefe, R. and P. Harvey. *Understanding Schizophrenia*. New York: The Free Press, 1994.

Lamb, H. R. *Treating the Long-Term Mentally Ill*. San Francisco: Jossey-Bass, 1982.

Lefley, H. P., and D. L. Johnson, eds. *Families as Allies in Treatment of the Mentally Ill*. Washington, D.C.: American Psychiatric Press, 1990.

Levine, I. S., and L. R. Ligenza. "In Their Own Voices: Families in Crisis: A Focus Group Study of Families of Persons with Serious Mental Illness." *Journal of Psychiatric Practice* 8 (2002): 344–53.

McElroy, E., ed. *Children and Adolescents with Mental Illness: A Parents Guide*. Kensington, Md.: Woodbine House, 1988.

Marsh, D. T. *Families and Mental Illness: New Directions in Professional Practice*. New York: Praeger, 1992.

Marsh, D. T. *Serious Mental Illness and the Family*. New York: John Wiley, 1998.

Mendel, W. *Treating Schizophrenia*. San Francisco: Jossey-Bass, 1989.

Mueser, K. T., and S. Gingerich. *Coping with Schizophrenia: A Guide for Families*. Oakland, Calif.: New Harbinger, 1994.

Ray, D. *The Ghosts behind Him*. Prince George, B.C.: Caitlin Press, 1999.

Rollin, H., ed. *Coping with Schizophrenia*. National Schizophrenia Fellowship. London: Burnett Books, 1980.

Secunda, V. *When Madness Comes Home*. New York: Hyperion, 1997.

Vine, P. *Families in Pain: Children, Siblings, Spouses, and Parents of the Mentally Ill Speak Out*. New York: Pantheon, 1982.

Walsh, M. *Schizophrenia: Straight Talk for Family and Friends*. New York: William Morrow, 1985.

Wasow, M. *Coping with Schizophrenia: A Survival Manual for Parents, Relatives and Friends*. Palo Alto, Calif.: Science and Behavior Books, 1982.

Wasow, M. *The Skipping Stone: Ripple Effects of Mental Illness in the Family*. Palo Alto: Science and Behavioral Books, 1995.

Wechsler, J. *In a Darkness*. Miami: Pickering, 1988. Originally published in 1972.

Wilson, L. *This Stranger, My Son.* New York: New American Library, 1968.

Woolis, R. *When Someone You Love Has a Mental Illness.* New York: Perigee Books, 1992.

Patients' Viewpoint

Barham, P., and R. Hayward. "In Sickness and in Health: Dilemmas of the Person with Severe Mental Illness." *Psychiatry* 61 (1998): 163–70.

Carter, D. M., A. MacKinnon, and D. L. Copolov. "Patients' Strategies for Coping with Auditory Hallucinations." *Journal of Nervous and Mental Disease* 184 (1996): 159–64.

"Consumer-Survivors Share Awakening Insights." *Journal of the California Alliance for the Mentally Ill* 7 (1996): 32–58.

Cohen, A.N., A. B. Hamilton, E.R. J.D. Saks, et al. "How Occupationally High-Achieving Individuals With a Diagnosis of Schizophrenia Manage Their Symptoms." *Psychiatric Services* 68 (2017): 324–329.

Davidson, L., and D. Stayner. "Loss, Loneliness, and the Desire for Love: Perspectives on the Social Lives of People with Schizophrenia." *Psychiatric Rehabilitation Journal* 20 (1997): 3–12.

Davidson, L., M. Chinman, B. Kloos, et al. "Peer Support among Individuals with Severe Mental Illness: A Review of the Evidence." *Clinical Psychology: Science and Practice* 6 (1999): 165–87.

Frese, F. J. "Twelve Aspects of Coping for Persons with Schizophrenia." *Innovations and Research* 2 (1993): 39–46.

Frese, F. J., III, J. Stanley, K. Kress, et al. "Integrating Evidence-based Practices and the Recovery Model." *Psychiatric Services* 52 (2001): 1462–68.

Leete, E. "How I Perceive and Manage My Illness." *Schizophrenia Bulletin* 15 (1989): 197–200.

Leete, E. "The Treatment of Schizophrenia: A Patient's Perspective." *Hospital and Community Psychiatry* 38 (1987): 486–91.

Liberman, R. P., and A. Kopelowicz. "Teaching Persons with Severe Mental Disabilities to Be Their Own Case Managers." *Psychiatric Services* 53 (2002): 1377–79.

Siblings' Viewpoint

Brodoff, A. S. "First Person Account: Schizophrenia through a Sister's Eyes— The Burden of Invisible Baggage." *Schizophrenia Bulletin* 14 (1988): 113–16.

Conroy, P. *The Prince of Tides.* Boston: Houghton Mifflin, 1986. Paperback by Bantam Books, 1987.

Dering, K.F. *Shot in the Head: A Sister's Memoir, A Brother's Struggle.* Dundas, Ontario: Bridgeross, 2014.

Dickens, R. M., and D. T. Marsh, eds. *Anguished Voices: Siblings and Adult Children of Persons with Psychiatric Disabilities.* Boston: Center for Psychiatric Rehabilitation, 1994.

Friedrich, R. M., S. Lively, and L. M. Rubenstein. "Siblings' Coping Strategies and Mental Health Services: A National Study of Siblings of Persons with Schizophrenia." *Psychiatric Services* 59 (2008): 261–67.

Gerace, L. M., D. Camilleri, and L. Ayres. "Sibling Perspectives on Schizophrenia and the Family." *Schizophrenia Bulletin* 19 (1993): 637–47.

Greenberg, J. S., H. W. Kim, and J. R. Greenley. "Factors Associated with Subjective Burden in Siblings of Adults with Severe Mental Illness." *American Journal of Orthopsychiatry* 67 (1997): 231–41.

Hayner, K. K. "Kevin." *Journal of the California Alliance for the Mentally Ill* 11 (2000): 42–44.

Horwitz, A. V. "Siblings as Caregivers for the Seriously Mentally Ill." *Milbank Quarterly* 71 (1993): 323–39.

Hyland, B. *The Girl with the Crazy Brother.* New York: Franklin Watts, 1987.

Jewell, T. C. "Impact of Mental Illness on Well Siblings: A Sea of Confusion." *Journal of the California Alliance for the Mentally Ill* 11 (2000): 34–36.

Judge, M. "First Snow in Iowa." *Wall Street Journal,* December 12, 2009.

Lamb, W. *I Know This Much Is True.* New York: Regan Books, 1998. Paperback by HarperPerennial, 1999.

Landeen, J., C. Whelton, S. Dermer, et al. "Needs of Well Siblings of Persons with Schizophrenia." *Hospital and Community Psychiatry* 43 (1992): 266–69.

Marsh, D. T., N. F. Appleby, R. M. Dickens, et al. "Anguished Voices: Impact of Mental Illness on Siblings and Children." *Innovations and Research* 2 (1993): 25–34.

Marsh, D. T., R. M. Dickens, R. D. Koeske, et al. "Troubled Journey: Siblings and Children of People with Mental Illness." *Innovations and Research* 2 (1993): 13–23.

Moorman, M. *My Sister's Keeper.* New York: Norton, 1992.

Neugeboren, J. *Imagining Robert: My Brother, Madness and Survival.* New York: Morrow, 1997.

Pines, P. *My Brother's Madness.* Willimantic, CT: Curbstone Press, 2007.

Saylor, A. V. "Nannie: A Sister's Story." *Innovations and Research* 3 (1994): 34–37.

Simon, C. *Mad House: Growing Up in the Shadow of Mentally Ill Siblings.* New York: Doubleday, 1997.

Smith, M. J., and J. S. Greenberg. "The Effect of the Quality of Sibling Relationships on the Life Satisfaction of Adults with Schizophrenia." *Psychiatric Services* 58 (2007): 1222–24.

Smith, M. J., and J. S. Greenberg. "Factors Contributing to the Quality of Sibling Relationships for Adults with Schizophrenia." *Psychiatric Services* 59 (2008): 57–62.

Stålberg, G., H. Ekerwald, and C. M. Hultman. "Siblings of Patients with Schizophrenia: Sibling Bond, Coping Patterns, and Fear of Possible Schizophrenia Heredity." *Schizophrenia Bulletin* 30 (2004): 445–58.

Stewart, B. "My Sister's Unbelievable Mind." *New York Times Magazine*, May 5, 2002, pp. 60–62.

Swados, E. *The Four of Us: A Family Memoir.* New York: Farrar, Straus & Giroux, 1991. Paperback by Penguin Books, 1993.

Children of Parents with Schizophrenia Viewpoint

Bartok, M. *The Memory Place.* New York: Free Press, 2011.

Brasfield, L. *Nature Lessons.* New York: St. Martin's Press, 2003.

Caton, C.L.M., F. Cournos, A. Felix, et al. "Childhood Experiences and Current Adjustment of Offspring of Indigent Patients with Schizophrenia." *Psychiatric Services* 49 (1998): 86–90.

Crosby, D. "First Person Account: Growing Up with a Schizophrenic Mother." *Schizophrenia Bulletin* 15 (1989): 507–9.

Flynn, L. M. *Swallow the Ocean.* Berkeley: Counterpoint Press, 2008.

Higgins, J., R. Gore, D. Gutkind, et al. "Effects of Child-Rearing by Schizophrenic Mothers: A 25-Year Follow-up." *Acta Psychiatrica Scandinavica* 96 (1997): 402–4.

Holley, T. E., and J. Holley. *My Mother's Keeper: A Daughter's Memoir of Growing Up in the Shadow of Schizophrenia.* New York: Morrow, 1997. Reprinted in paperback, 1998.

Holman, V. *Rescuing Patty Hearst: Growing Up Sane in a Decade Gone Mad.* New York: Simon and Schuster, 2003.

Johanson, A.-L. "I Did Everything to Keep My Secret." *Good Housekeeping*, October 2001, pp. 141–45.

Kauffman, C., H. Grunebaum, B. Cohler, et al. "Superkids: Competent Children of Psychotic Mothers." *American Journal of Psychiatry* 136 (1979): 1398–1402.

Knuttsson-Medin, L., B. Edlund, and M. Ramklint. "Experiences in a Group of Grown-up Children of Mentally Ill Patients." *Journal of Psychiatric and Mental Health Nursing* 14 (2007): 744–52.

Lachenmeyer, N. *The Outsider: A Journey into My Father's Struggle with Madness.* New York: Broadway Books, 2000.

Lanquetot, R. "First Person Account: Confessions of the Daughter of a Schizophrenic." *Schizophrenia Bulletin* 10 (1984): 467–71.

Lanquetot, R. "First Person Account: On Being Daughter and Mother." *Schizophrenia Bulletin* 14 (1988): 337–41.

"Offspring." *Journal of the California Alliance for the Mentally Ill* 7 (1996).

Olson, L. S. *He Was Still My Daddy.* Portland, Ore.: Ogden Howe, 1994.

Östman, M., and L. Hansson. "Children in Families with a Severely Mentally

Ill Member: Prevalence and Needs for Support." *Social Psychiatry and Psychiatric Epidemiology* 37 (2002): 243–48.

Puffer, K. A. "The Intruder of the Mind." *Schizophrenia Bulletin* 36 (2010): 651–54.

Riley, J. *Crazy Quilt.* New York: Morrow, 1984.

Ross, R. G., and N. Compagnon. "Diagnosis and Treatment of Psychiatric Disorders in Children with a Schizophrenic Parent." *Schizophrenia Research* 50 (2001): 121–29.

Sanghera, S. *The Boy with the Topknot.* New York: Penguin Books, 2009. Originally titled *If You Don't Know Me by Now* when published in 2008 by Viking.

Sherman, M. D., and D. M. Sherman. *I'm Not Alone: A Teen's Guide to Living with a Parent Who Has a Mental Illness.* Edina, Minn.: Beavers Pond Press, 2006.

Steinem, G. "Ruth's Song (Because She Could Not Sing)." In W. Martin, ed., *Essays by Contemporary American Women.* Boston: Beacon Press, 1996, pp. 14–31.

Williams, A. S. "A Group for the Adult Daughters of Mentally Ill Mothers: Looking Backwards and Forwards." *British Journal of Mental Psychology* 71 (1998): 73–83.

Husband or Wife of Person with Schizophrenia Viewpoint

Angermeyer, M. C., R. Kilian, H.-U. Wilms, et al. "Quality of Life of Spouses of Mentally Ill People." *International Journal of Social Psychiatry* 52 (2006): 278–85.

"First Person Account: Life with a Mentally Ill Spouse." *Schizophrenia Bulletin* 20 (1994): 227–29.

Frese, P. "We All Make Accommodations." *Journal of the California Alliance for the Mentally Ill* 9 (1998): 6–8. This issue has ten other articles on schizophrenia written by spouses.

Jungbauer, J., B. Wittmund, S. Dietrich, et al. "The Disregarded Caregivers: Subjective Burden in Spouses of Schizophrenia Patients." *Schizophrenia Bulletin* 30 (2004): 665–75.

Mannion, E. "Resilience and Burden in Spouses of People with Mental Illness." *Psychiatric Rehabilitation Journal* 20 (1996): 13–23.

Nasar, S. *A Beautiful Mind: A Biography of John Forbes Nash, Jr., Winner of the Nobel Prize in Economics, 1994.* New York: Simon and Schuster, 1998. Paperback by Touchstone Books, 1999.

Seeman, M.V. "Bad, Burdened or Ill? Characterizing the Spouses of Women with Schizophrenia." *International Journal of Social Psychology* 59 (2012): 805–810.

12

Commonly Asked Questions

There is no disease more to be dreaded than madness. For what greater unhappiness can befall a man than to be deprived of his reason and understanding.

Richard Mead, Medical Precepts and Cautions, *1751*

Schizophrenia is like a movie that never ends. Even worse is the fact that you are in the movie. Just when you think you have seen it all, a new scene presents itself, with new questions.

The following are some of the questions patients and families frequently ask. For many, there are no simple answers, because each individual with schizophrenia and each family is a little different.

Does Schizophrenia Change the Underlying Personality?

For many years, based on my experiences in observing my sister and in working with hundreds of people afflicted with the disease, I suspected that it did not but could find no scientific study to verify my suspicions. For example, I remember one young man whose symptoms I helped to get under control using a combination of antipsychotic medications. His family, however, kept complaining that it was impossible to get him up in the morning and urged me to try different medications. After doing this for several months without success, I inquired whether the family had had difficulty getting him up before he got sick. "Oh yes," they said, "he would never get up then either, just like he doesn't get up now." That ended my medication changes and taught me a most useful lesson.

In the early 1990s an opportunity arose to ascertain whether schizophrenia does or does not change the underlying personality. We studied identical twins in which one had schizophrenia and the other was well. Since personality traits of identical twins are remarkably alike, by testing the personality traits of twins in which one is sick and one is well it should theoretically be possible to tell how much a person's personality has been changed by having schizophrenia. A total of twenty-seven identical twin pairs discordant for schizophrenia were tested.

The results were clear and unequivocal. On personality scales that measured traits such as happiness, nervousness, and satisfaction with social relationships, the twins with schizophrenia scored significantly lower, as would be expected from having the disease. However, on the remaining scales of personality traits there were remarkably few differences, and on many scales, such as adherence to traditional values and interest in risk-taking behavior, there were practically no differences. A pair of quiet, pious women were both still, quiet, and pious even though one had severe schizophrenia. A pair of hell-raising, risk-taking young men were both still raising hell and taking risks, even though one had schizophrenia. The underlying, core personality of the person with schizophrenia had been only minimally altered.

The fact that schizophrenia alters a person's underlying personality relatively little has been noted by other observers. The mother of one of the most severely affected women I have treated expressed it as follows: "The daughter I would have had—were it not for this evil illness—exists in embryo in the daughter I do have." The disease and the person are not the same; they can, and should, be separated.

Schizophrenia is an equal opportunity disease and randomly affects personality types from the most selfish and narcissistic to the most giving and altruistic. Once the person has schizophrenia, those underlying personality traits are still visible beneath the delusions, hallucinations, thinking disorders, and altered affect.

It is always tempting, of course, to attribute all undesirable personality traits in a person to the disease. I have known families who retrospectively idealized the personality of their family member before the person got schizophrenia when the reality was quite different. I have also known individuals with schizophrenia who used their disease as an excuse for all of their shortcomings and weaknesses when in fact they had had the same shortcomings and weaknesses prior to becoming sick.

It should be self-evident that schizophrenia also does not change the underlying personalities of mothers, fathers, brothers, or sisters. Family members come in all personality types and are not fundamentally changed by another family member having schizophrenia. Parents and siblings may be intrusive, helpful, rejecting, or loving, but such personality traits pre-exist the onset of schizophrenia in their family member. It was in fact the existence of undesirable personality traits in some parents of individuals with schizophrenia that formed the basis of family interaction theories of schizophrenia, reviewed in chapter 5; what these researchers failed to point out was that the undesirable personality traits in these families were neither more nor less common than they were in any other family. Schizophrenia is an equal opportunity disease for families as well as for individuals.

Are People with Schizophrenia Responsible for Their Behavior?

One of the most challenging problems for individuals with schizophrenia, their families, mental illness professionals, and judges and juries is to assess how much control a person with schizophrenia has over his/her symptoms and behavior. Most individuals have some control and can be held at least partly responsible, but the degree varies widely from individual to individual and, in a single individual, from week to week. Many patients, for example, can suppress with great effort their auditory hallucinations or bizarre behavior for brief periods but not for long periods. The dilemma of responsibility was nicely expressed by Dr. John Wing, a leading schizophrenia researcher in England:

> Part of the peculiar difficulty in managing schizophrenia is that it lies somewhere between conditions like blindness which, though severely handicapping, do not interfere with an individual's capacity to make independent judgments about his own future, and conditions like severe mental retardation, in which it is clear that the individual will never be able to make such independent judgments. There is frequently a fluctuating degree of insight and of severity.

What should be done, for example, when your son with schizophrenia insists on suddenly disrobing in front of visiting Aunt Agatha? In some cases he may be responding to command hallucinations that are telling him that if he does not do so the world will end and he will be responsible. In other cases his disrobing may represent a complex mixture of confused thinking and resentment against some real or imagined slight by someone who looks like Aunt Agatha. In still other cases his disrobing may represent a consciously hostile gesture toward Aunt Agatha or toward his family. Some individuals with schizophrenia, just like some individuals who do not have schizophrenia, are very skilled at using their symptoms to manipulate those around them to get what they want. Some patients who are placed where they do not want to live, for example, know exactly what to do behaviorally to ensure that they will be returned to the hospital or wherever they were living previously. And I have had many patients improve and tell me explicitly, "Doc, I'm a little better, but I'm not well enough to go to work."

How can you tell how much responsibility the person with schizophrenia has for his or her behavior? Family members, friends, and mental illness professionals who have known the person for a long period of time are most capable of making such assessments because they know the person's underlying personality traits. In the case cited above, the family should sit down with the person after Aunt Agatha has gone and calmly review what happened, why it happened, how it might be prevented in the future, the consequences of such behavior for the person's living at home, and the legal consequences for disrobing in public. It is often useful to include the patient's psychiatrist, counselor, social worker, or case manager in such discussions.

The question of responsibility for behavior for persons with schizophrenia becomes even more convoluted when the person is charged with a crime. In such cases the person may be declared incompetent to stand trial and involuntarily committed to a mental hospital, or he/she may be brought to trial. In such cases the insanity defense is often invoked for persons with schizophrenia.

The insanity defense dates back to the thirteenth century, when it was known as the "wild beast test" (insofar as persons are like wild beasts, they cannot be held accountable). In England in the nineteenth century it was modified in the M'Naghten case to the "right or wrong test" (insofar as persons do not know right from wrong, they cannot be held accountable). In the United States in recent years this has been replaced in many states by the "product test" (insofar as their acts were a product of a mental disease, persons cannot be held accountable) or by various modifications and compromises between the "right or wrong test" and the "product test." Most of these incorporate a volitional element, stating that the person acted on an "irresistible impulse."

Among the arguments favoring the insanity defense for persons accused of crimes is the fact that it protects them from being simply convicted and punished as if they had been fully responsible. Thus, a person with schizophrenia who steals a car with the key in it because he thought it was his car or because voices told him to do so is not treated in the same way as a car thief who steals it to sell to others.

Arguments against use of the insanity defense are impressive, and many people have suggested that it be abolished. Deciding whether a person's behavior is a "product" of his or her mental illness is an exceedingly difficult and subjective task. As one observer has noted, "Almost all crimes, by definition, involve transgressions of societal norms that could be called insane." And in terms of an "irresistible impulse," it has been noted that "the line between an irresistible impulse and an impulse not resisted is probably no sharper than that between twilight and dusk." Such judgments are made even more difficult by the fact that they are retrospective. Who can really know what was in a person's mind when a criminal act was being committed months before he or she came to trial?

Many proposals to change the insanity defense have included a two-part trial in which the issues of guilt for the crime and extenuating circumstances (including insanity) would be separated. In the first part the only question addressed would be whether or not the accused actually committed the crime. If the person were found guilty, *then* psychiatrists and other witnesses would be allowed to testify on the person's mental state and other extenuating circumstances; this testimony would be used to help decide where the person should be sent (prison or psychiatric hospital) and for how long.

If the second part of the trial specifically addressed the question of responsibility, such a system would be a definite improvement over the current legal quagmire engendered by the insanity defense. The insanity defense as currently practiced includes an assumption that persons are either responsible or not responsible for their actions. Sane persons are considered to be responsible, insane persons to be not responsible; it is an all-or-nothing determination. Such simplistic thinking, however, contradicts the experience of everyone who has ever lived with someone with schizophrenia. People with schizophrenia sometimes are fully responsible for their behavior and sometimes are not at all responsible; in the majority of cases, however, the truth is somewhere in between.

Does Schizophrenia Affect the Person's IQ?

Neuropsychological abnormalities occur commonly in individuals with schizophrenia, as was discussed in chapter 5. But one specific aspect of neuropsychological function—intelligence—is of special concern to both individuals afflicted with schizophrenia and their families. Ours is, after all, a society obsessed with IQ.

In discussing IQ and schizophrenia, it is important to remember what IQ measures. Most IQ tests measure some combination of reading, reasoning, and mathematical skills, which are assessments of specific types of brain function. IQ tests do not measure experience, common sense, or wisdom. And they certainly do not tell you how much of the person's IQ he/she uses on a day-to-day basis. I once had a "normal" relative, for example, who had an IQ of 160; on most days he appeared to use about half of it and was practically devoid of common sense and wisdom.

Recent studies of IQ and schizophrenia have established the following:

1. As a rule, many but not all, individuals with schizophrenia have a small loss of IQ (i.e., approximately 8 to 10 points), which occurs early in life, many years before they develop their illness. This has been demonstrated in European studies that measured the IQ of large numbers of children, then later ascertained which of the children developed schizophrenia. This loss of IQ is probably associated with the same brain damage that caused the schizophrenia.

2. There are major exceptions to this rule. In a study in Finland, for example, a disproportionate number of boys who had excellent school grades later developed schizophrenia. One also thinks of John Nash, who accomplished mathematical feats in his early twenties, for which he was later awarded a Nobel Prize, but who in his late twenties developed schizophrenia.

3. For individuals who develop schizophrenia in childhood, there is also a small loss of IQ because their illness interferes with learning and their ability to acquire new information.

4. Studies are inconclusive about whether or not, once a person has developed schizophrenia in adulthood, there is any additional loss of IQ. It probably depends on the severity of the schizophrenia. On average, however, such a loss of IQ in adulthood is very small.

Should People with Schizophrenia Drive Vehicles?

Remarkably little has been written about whether individuals with schizophrenia should drive motor vehicles, despite the fact that patients, their families, and insurance companies face this problem regularly. In a 1989 study of this problem, it was reported that only 68 percent of outpatients with schizophrenia drive compared to 99 percent of nonpsychiatrically ill controls. Even those patients who did drive did so far less than the controls. Most important, mile for mile, the drivers with schizophrenia had an accident rate that was twice as high as the controls. Two earlier studies had not found a higher accident rate among drivers with schizophrenia.

Should individuals with schizophrenia drive motor vehicles? Driving a vehicle utilizes three separate skills: (1) planning trips and making decisions about crowded roads and darkness; (2) tactical decisions involving judgment and paying attention, such as knowing when to pass another vehicle; and (3) operational coordination, such as being able to quickly put on the brakes. Individuals with schizophrenia are least likely to have problems with operational coordination, although some slowing of movements may be a side effect of antipsychotic drugs. However, some individuals with schizophrenia are clearly impaired in their planning and/or tactical decisions, and this should be self-evident from their planning, judgment, and ability to pay attention in other areas of their lives.

In summary, the majority of individuals with schizophrenia can and do drive. However, those whose planning and/or tactical decisions are clearly impaired should not drive. The assessment of which individuals with schizophrenia should drive and which should not is similar to the assessment made for individuals who are elderly. For some patients whose ability to drive is dependent on taking antipsychotic medication, it would seem reasonable to make their driving license conditional on taking medication, much as is done for some people with epilepsy.

How Do Religious Issues Affect People with Schizophrenia?

People with schizophrenia, like other people, have a need to relate to a god or philosophical worldview that allows them to place themselves and their lives within a larger context. For individuals with schizophrenia this can be particularly problematical for many reasons. For one thing, the onset of the disease often occurs during the same period of life when religious and philosophical beliefs are in great flux, thus making resolution extremely difficult. Another complicating factor is that many persons with this disease undergo intense heightened awareness, or "peak experiences" (as described in chapter 1), during the early stages of their illness and conclude that they have been specially chosen by God. When auditory hallucinations are experienced, these usually reinforce such a belief. Still another impediment to resolution of religious concerns is the person's inability to think metaphorically and in symbols, which most formalized religious belief systems require. It is therefore not surprising that religious concerns continue to be important for many persons with this disease throughout the course of their illness. One recent study, in fact, reported that 30 percent of individuals with schizophrenia reported "an increase in their religiousness after the onset of illness."

Delusions of a religious nature are extremely common, and can be found in almost half of all people with schizophrenia. It is also known that members of the clergy are frequently consulted by individuals with schizophrenia; in one study it was found that "the clergy are as likely as mental health professionals to be sought out by individuals from the community who have serious psychiatric disorders." Many clergy are knowledgeable and helpful in such situations. Unfortunately, however, many others are not current regarding what is known about serious mental illnesses and erroneously tell mentally ill persons or their families that the illness has been caused by sin. Such a message can, of course, be very destructive and make an already bad situation much worse.

Occasionally individuals with schizophrenia resolve their religious concerns by joining a religious cult of one kind or another. The variety of available cults is wide and includes the Unification Church ("Moonies"), Hare Krishna, Divine Light Mission, Jesus People, Scientology, and many smaller groups. A study reported that 6 percent of the members of the Unification Church and 9 percent of the members of the Divine Light Mission had been previously hospitalized for psychiatric problems. However, psychiatrists who have studied such groups believe that most of these previously hospitalized members were severely neurotic. The groups themselves tend to exclude seriously disturbed individuals as too disruptive to the closely cooperative living and working conditions demanded by the groups.

For individuals with schizophrenia who are accepted into these cults, there may be some advantages. A highly structured belief system and lifestyle are inherent in such groups, as is also a sense of belonging and community. These in turn lead to increased self-esteem for the member. Some cults also value unusual religious experiences, and in such settings a person with schizophrenia may feel more comfortable with his/her "peak experiences" or auditory hallucinations.

The cults also pose potential dangers, however. Many such groups emphasize the desirability of not taking any drugs; patients who are doing nicely on maintenance medication may be encouraged to stop the drug, with resultant relapse. The groups may also encourage the person to deny the reality of his or her illness, casting problems such as delusional thinking and auditory hallucinations into the mold of spiritual shortcomings rather than acknowledging that they are products of a brain disease. Some groups may also encourage paranoid thinking in persons who are already inclined in that direction, as there is often a siege mentality in the cults, a "we-they" feeling that the world is out to persecute them as a group. Finally, a few religious cults may exploit the money or property of members with schizophrenia, as they sometimes do that of other members.

Should You Tell People That You Have Schizophrenia?

The question of whether or not to tell people that you have schizophrenia is a difficult one, especially when the person is a prospective date or employer. Increasingly, however, the answer is "yes." Some issues to consider in thinking about the problem are: Is the person likely to find out anyway? How sophisticated is the person likely to be about mental illness? If I withhold this information, will the person be able to trust me on other issues? How difficult is it for me to interact with the person knowing that I have not told him/her?

Since the early 1980s there has been a dramatic increase in open discussion of schizophrenia by both patients and their families. The Americans with Disabilities Act affords some theoretical protection against discrimination by employers, but how effective this is in actuality is less clear. There are still occasions, however, when it is better not to disclose the fact that you have schizophrenia. On such occasions Dr. Frederick Frese, a psychologist who had schizophrenia, suggests "that you respond by saying you are a writer, an artist, a (mental health) consultant, or perhaps that you freelance, depending on how you have been spending your time. None of these responses are lies, per se, but they leave considerable latitude for interpretation and they do not require that you have a specific employer or work location."

Genetic Counseling:
What Are the Chances of Getting Schizophrenia?

Almost every brother, sister, son, daughter, nephew, or niece of a person with schizophrenia has at one time or another wondered about the chances of themselves or their children developing schizophrenia. Furthermore, since an increasing number of individuals with schizophrenia are now having children, genetic counseling is increasingly important.

One might suppose that information on the risk of developing schizophrenia in relatives of affected individuals would be accurate, widely available, and generally agreed upon by the experts. One would be wrong. As discussed in chapter 5, opinions regarding the relative importance of genetic factors in the causation of schizophrenia vary widely and inevitably color genetic counseling. Some of what appears to be a genetic transmission may not be truly genetic at all, but rather the familial transmission of an infectious agent. A researcher who believes that genetic factors are the most important antecedents of schizophrenia will give comparatively conservative advice regarding reproduction among relatives, while a researcher who believes that genetic factors are less important will be likely to give less conservative advice.

In thinking about one's chances of getting schizophrenia, it is useful to keep in mind some general observations:

1. Genes certainly play some role, but the magnitude of that role is not nearly as clearly established as most geneticists would have you believe.

2. A majority of individuals who develop schizophrenia—63 per-

cent—do not have any family history of schizophrenia in first-degree (parents and siblings) or second-degree (grandparents, aunts, and uncles) relatives.

3. The more relatives you have with schizophrenia, the higher your risk is of developing it. From a practical point of view this means that if your sister is your only close relative with schizophrenia, your own risk is very low. If, on the other hand, your uncle and sister both have schizophrenia, then your risk is higher. And if you are unfortunate enough to come from one of the relatively rare families that are heavily loaded with the disorder (e.g., mother, aunt, grandfather, and two siblings affected), then your own risk is substantially higher and you should give serious consideration to the question of having children.

4. Many risk-figures that are found in psychiatric textbooks are worst-case scenarios and are based on older studies with questionable methodology. For example, the risk of developing schizophrenia if both parents are affected is usually said to be 46 percent. Two more recent studies, however, reported the risk to be 28 and 29 percent, and a consensus risk appears to be approximately 36 percent. Similarly, the risk of developing schizophrenia in the second twin of identical twins is traditionally said to be 48 percent, but that number depends on the use of selected twin samples and a type of double-counting called probandwise rates. When unselected twin samples and single-counting (pairwise) rates are used, the chances of the second identical twin developing schizophrenia is found to be 28 percent and, in the most recent (2018) study, only 15 percent.

5. The risks of developing schizophrenia can be viewed as a glass half empty or half full. For a brother or sister of an affected sibling the probability of developing schizophrenia is 9 percent, but the risk of *not* developing it is 91 percent. For a child when one parent is affected, the probability of developing schizophrenia is 13 percent but the probability of *not* developing it is 87 percent. Even for identical twins the probability of the second twin *not* developing schizophrenia is 72 percent. (Note: The estimate of risk numbers used here differ slightly from those given in chapter 5 because they were taken from a different study.)

WHAT ARE MY CHANCES OF GETTING SCHIZOPHRENIA?	
If nobody in my family (first- or second-degree relative) has it	1 percent
If my half-brother or half-sister has it	4 percent
If my full brother or full sister has it	9 percent
If my mother or father has it	13 percent
If both my mother and father have it	36 percent
If my identical twin has it	28 percent
If my aunt or uncle has it	3 percent
If my grandfather or grandmother has it	4 percent

6. Schizophrenia is only one of many disorders for which there is some genetic risk. Creating life is, and always has been, a genetic lottery. Knowing the odds in the game will not make the decision for you but will allow you to choose more intelligently.

Why Do Some Adopted Children Develop Schizophrenia?

When families who have a family member with schizophrenia gather together, they often find that in a surprising number of cases, the affected individual had been an adopted child. Why should adopted children develop schizophrenia more often than expected?

The reason is, of course, that a disproportionate number of children who are available to be adopted had mothers, and often fathers as well, who had schizophrenia or bipolar disorder. The parents are unable to care for the child and so he or she is put up for adoption. In earlier years, when it was thought that bad parenting was the principal cause of schizophrenia, it was not thought to be important to tell the adopting parents about this background, so many adoption agencies did not do so.

It is now known that genes confer the same risk, whether the child is adopted or not. A child whose mother and father both had schizophrenia will have approximately a one-third risk of developing the disease, regardless of whether he or she is adopted. In recent years, it has become much more common for adoption agencies to give prospective parents a more complete and truthful history.

A good account of a couple who adopted a child who developed schizophrenia and then sued the adoption agency for not disclosing the child's background was published in 1999 (see "Recommended Further Reading"). This is one of the first things published on this surprisingly common but little discussed phenomenon.

What Will Happen When the Parents Die?

One of the most troubling problems for families with a family member with schizophrenia is what will happen after the family members who are providing the person's care die. Typically it is a mother and father who provide much of the care needed by an ill son or daughter, although in other cases the same problem may arise for an aging or sick person who is providing care for an ill sibling. In the old days such care was transferred to the extended family or the state hospital. Now, however, the extended family has disappeared and the state hospital will simply discharge the person with schizophrenia to live in the community. The specter of their family member ending up living in public shelters and on the streets haunts many families.

Guardianship is one mechanism used by families to ensure care for the family member and safeguard his or her assets after the death of the well family members. The guardian may be either a relative or friend of the patient or, if none is available or appropriate, another person selected by the judge. The appointment of a guardian occurs most frequently when the patient owns large amounts of money or property or is likely to inherit some. Guardianship is a legal relationship authorizing one person to make decisions for another and is based on the same *parens patriae* tenet of English law that permits involuntary hospitalization. When the guardian has jurisdiction only over the property of the patient, it is frequently referred to as a conservatorship. When both property and personal decisions are involved it is called a guardianship.

Guardianship (and conservatorship) laws are remarkably outmoded in most states. In many instances no distinction is made between personal and property decisions, and a guardian automatically is granted decision-making permission for both. Personal decisions affected by a guardianship may include where the patient may reside, the right to travel freely, and the right to consent to medical or psychiatric treatment; property decisions may include the right to sign checks or withdraw money from a bank account. Most guardianship laws are all-or-nothing affairs and fail to take into account the ability of patients to manage some areas of their lives but not others. The laws are often extremely vague: the law in California, until recently changed, said that a guardian could be appointed for any "incompetent person . . . whether insane or not . . . who is likely to be deceived or imposed upon by artful and designing persons." This could include most of us! The actual appointment of a guardian is usually done without legal due process and without the person present; nor is there periodic review to determine whether the guardianship is still necessary.

Another mechanism used by some families to plan for the future are nonprofit organizations founded by groups of families. These organizations will accept responsibility for the ill family member after the death of the well family members. For many years, such organizations were utilized by families with mentally retarded members; more recently, groups under NAMI have been setting them up on a local level. For example, in Virginia, Maryland, and several other states, there is the Planned Lifetime Assistance Network (PLAN), with family members serving on the organization's board of directors. A person who joins pays a membership fee and annual dues, then develops a plan of care for the family member with schizophrenia to be activated after the death of other family members. At that time the professional staff and volunteers of PLAN will assume the responsibilities previously provided by the family, including visiting the person regularly, maintaining contact with the person's doctor or case manager, paying the person's bills, acting as payee for SSI payments, and assuming other fiscal or supervisory functions as needed.

Planning for the future of relatives with schizophrenia is essential both for their well-being and for your own peace of mind. However, understanding benefits, assets, wills, trusts, estate taxes, and everything that goes with them is a major undertaking for nonlawyers. Some state NAMI groups have prepared relevant material (e.g., a booklet by Jean Little titled "Take Me to Your Lawyer," published by NAMI New York State in 1991). A very helpful publication is a book by attorney L. Mark Russell et al., *Planning for the Future: Providing a Meaningful Life for a Child with a Disability after Your Death.*

Recommended Further Reading

Belkin, L. "What the Jumans Didn't Know about Michael." *New York Times Magazine,* March 14, 1999, pp. 42–49.

DiLalla, D. L., and I. I. Gottesman. "Normal Personality Characteristics in Identical Twins Discordant for Schizophrenia." *Journal of Abnormal Psychology* 104 (1995): 490–99.

Edlund, M. J., C. Conrad, and P. Morris. "Accidents among Schizophrenic Outpatients." *Comprehensive Psychiatry* 30 (1989): 522–26.

Hatfield, A. B. "Who Will Care When We Are Not There?" *Journal of the California Alliance for the Mentally Ill* 11 (2000): 60–61.

Huguelet, P., S. Mohr, C. Betrisey, et al. "A Randomized Trial of Spiritual Assessment of Outpatients with Schizophrenia: Patients' and Clinicians' Experience." *Psychiatric Services* 62 (2011): 79–86.

Journal of the California Alliance for the Mentally Ill 8 (1997). This entire issue is devoted to spirituality and mental illness.

Khandaker, G. M., J. H. Barnett, I. R. White, et al. "A Quantitative Meta-Analysis of Population-based Studies of Premorbid Intelligence and Schizophrenia." *Schizophrenia Research* 132 (2011): 220–27.

Kirov, G., R. Kemp, K. Kirov, et al. "Religious Faith after Psychotic Illness." *Psychopathology* 31 (1998): 234–45.

Lefley, H. P., and A. B. Hatfield. "Helping Parental Caregivers and Mental Health Consumers Cope with Parental Aging and Loss." *Psychiatric Services* 50 (1999): 369–75.

Pies, R. "A Guy, a Car: Beyond Schizophrenia." *The New York Times.* May 4, 2009.

Russell, L. M., A. E. Grant, S. M. Joseph, et al. *Planning for the Future: Providing a Meaningful Life for a Child with a Disability After Your Death,* 3rd ed. Evanston, Ill.: American Publishing, 1995.

Tepper, L., S. A. Rogers, E. M. Coleman, et al. "The Prevalence of Religious Coping among Persons with Persistent Mental Illness." *Psychiatric Services* 52 (2001): 660–65.

Torrey, E. F. "Are We Overestimating the Genetic Contribution to Schizophrenia?" *Schizophrenia Bulletin* 18 (1992): 159–70.

Waterhouse, S. *Strength for His People: A Ministry for Families of the Mentally Ill.* Amarillo, Tex.: Westcliff Bible Church (Box 1521, Amarillo, TX 79105).

Zammit, S., P. Allebeck, A. S. David, et al. "A Longitudinal Study of Premorbid IQ Score and Risk of Developing Schizophrenia, Bipolar Disorder, Severe Depression, and Other Nonaffective Psychoses." *Archives of General Psychiatry* 61 (2004): 354–60.

13

Schizophrenia in the Public Eye

But the brilliance, the versatility of madness is akin to the resourcefulness of water seeping through, over and around a dike. It requires the united front of many people to work against it.

F. Scott Fitzgerald, Tender Is the Night, *1934*

Schizophrenia has come out of the closet. Slowly, reluctantly, and shyly at first, the disease has increasingly entered the public arena. In 1960 many individuals with schizophrenia denied that anything was wrong except, perhaps, "a case of nerves." In 1980 individuals with schizophrenia would whisper to those they trusted that they had, indeed, been given this label. By 2000 individuals with schizophrenia were regularly, even proudly, identifying themselves in public meetings and on national television. It has been a remarkable change over the past half century.

The major breakthroughs into the public arena began in the early 1980s. The public television series *The Brain* included an excellent segment on schizophrenia produced by DeWitt Sage. Phil Donahue followed with three separate shows discussing the disease; this was the first time most people had heard the term "schizophrenia" mentioned on a major network or seen people who had schizophrenia discussing it. Now schizophrenia has become so commonplace on television that in 1998 Oprah Winfrey featured a book about schizophrenia, Wally Lamb's *I Know This Much Is True*, on her show. And in March 2000 a television series, *Wonderland*, featured individuals with schizophrenia in a psychiatric emergency room; the program generated considerable public controversy but survived just two episodes because of low viewership.

The progress in television has been mirrored by the movies. Except for Ingmar Bergman's films, such as his stunning 1961 *Through a Glass Darkly*, almost no serious movies were made about schizophrenia until the 1990s. Since that time, many have been released, some of which are reviewed below.

In literature, there has been an occasional depiction of "insanity" by major writers over the past two centuries, but few people have connected these to the contemporary concept of schizophrenia. Many of these older portrayals deserve to be more widely known and are summarized below. With rare exceptions, such as Mark Vonnegut's 1975 *The Eden Express*, there were almost no books written by individuals with schizophrenia or by their families until the 1980s. Now they are numerous.

Schizophrenia in the Movies

The serious depiction of schizophrenia in cinema is a recent phenomenon. There have, of course, been insane characters in movies for as long as movies have been made. These characters, however, were until recently merely caricatures, used as props for humor (e.g., *Dr. Dippy's Sanitarium* in 1906) or horror (e.g., *Maniac Barber* in 1902). As the century progressed and Hollywood fell increasingly under the spell of Freudian psychoanalysis, insane characters were also used as props to display the talents of omniscient and wise psychiatrists, as depicted in *David and Lisa* (1962). It was only later that Hollywood's psychiatrists fell from grace, as shown in such movies as *Dressed to Kill* (1980) and *Frances* (1982).

Another common way of representing insane persons in films in the 1960s and 1970s was to depict them as not really insane at all but as rather more sane than the purportedly normal people around them. *King of Hearts* (1966) was an enormously popular film in which the inmates leave their asylum and take over a war-deserted town. Their sane behavior is contrasted with the insanity of the ongoing war, and in the end Alan Bates, as Private Plumpick, decides to leave the army and join the inmates.

The theme of *One Flew over the Cuckoo's Nest* (1975) was similar, with the inmates of the asylum shown as more normal than Nurse Ratched and her staff. Jack Nicholson as Randle McMurphy is finally defeated by a lobotomy but not before he has shown his fellow inmates the road to freedom. *Cuckoo's Nest* was, in the words of one reviewer, "the quintessential film for the counterculture: the mental institution as a metaphor for the abuse of authority."

Serious attempts to portray individuals with schizophrenia began with Ingmar Bergman's film *Through a Glass Darkly* in 1961, but such attempts were rare until recent years. The following are synopses of some of these films. Most are available for rent or sale over the Internet. The best of them, in my opinion, are *Through a Glass Darkly; Clean, Shaven; Angel Baby;* and *People Say I'm Crazy.*

Through a Glass Darkly, 1961. Directed by Ingmar Bergman. In Swedish with English subtitles. B&W. This is a brilliant movie, one of Bergman's finest. Karin (Harriet Andersson), married to a physician (Max von Sydow), has returned from the hospital in a remission from her illness after having been treated with ECT. Gradually her schizophrenia returns, including symptoms of acuteness of hearing and auditory hallucinations. The depiction of her symptoms, as she finds herself repeatedly lured into an upstairs room where voices invite her to step behind the wallpaper and await the coming of God, and her description of her hallucinations to her teenage brother are very moving. The voices, she says, are not dreams but real, and she is exhausted from struggling against them. Her family watches helplessly as she slowly deteriorates, and at the end of the film she returns to the hospital. Starkly filmed in black and white on a desolate seacoast, the film won an Academy Award for Best Foreign Language Film in 1961.

Repulsion, 1965. Directed by Roman Polanski. B&W. This classic horror film, by the director of *Rosemary's Baby*, is a superb portrayal of a young woman slipping progressively into schizophrenia. In one of her earliest and best roles, Catherine Deneuve plays a beautiful but withdrawn beautician who accurately shows such early symptoms of psychosis as distractibility, acuteness of hearing, and compulsive traits. Slowly, her symptoms become worse, and hallucinations take over her life, leading up to murder. The film is not for the faint-hearted and is frequently compared to Alfred Hitchcock's *Psycho*. However, it is worth seeing for the performance of Catherine Deneuve alone.

Clean, Shaven, 1993. Directed by Lodge Kerrigan. Spare, bleak, and mean, this film is not for the faint of heart. Film critic Roger Ebert calls it a "must see" for anyone with a serious interest in schizophrenia, and indeed, it is the most vivid cinematic portrait to date of the "view from the inside." Peter Winter (Peter Greene), just released from a psychiatric hospital, is desperate to find his daughter, who was given up for adoption by Peter's mother during his confinement. ("Do you know what it's like to see your son deteriorate?" Mrs. Winter explains: "When he was growing up, he was a quiet boy, but he was happy. Then all of a sudden he changed. I won't have that same thing happen to her.") Plagued by voices and fears that are palpable to the viewer, Peter smashes in or covers any glass that reflects his image or allows others to look in, including the rearview mirrors and side windows of his car. Haunted by memories that are presumably false, he frantically flees the siren of a police car that never materializes. In an effort to rid himself of the receiver he believes was implanted in the back of his head and the transmitter he believes is in his finger, he gouges his scalp with scissors and tears off a fingernail. Convinced he has extricated the transmitter, he explains: "I feel better. I think clearer. I still have to get the receiver out of my head. If I could just slow down a little bit, I know I could come up with a solution." The film raises troubling questions that its eighty minutes don't have time to answer: What was the course of Peter's illness, and what treatment did he receive? What are we to assume from his mother's distant behavior upon his return? A cacophony of sounds—buzzing wires, radio static, voices spewing profanity—and disordered images contribute to our uncertainty but also help us better understand the turmoil in Peter's brain. The film won the Best First Feature award for 1993 at the Chicago International Film Festival and was presented at the 1994 Cannes Film Festival.

Benny and Joon, 1993. Directed by Jeremiah Chechik. A beautifully filmed but unrealistic story about a brother who is the sole caretaker of his kid sister, who has schizophrenia. Benny (Aidan Quinn) owns an auto repair shop; Joon (Mary Stuart Masterson) stays at home and paints, except when the urge hits her to set fire to something or don scuba gear and direct traffic. Along the way, she loses a poker bet and "wins" another player's eccentric cousin Sam (Johnny Depp), whose whimsical pantomimes à la Buster Keaton and Charlie Chaplin charm her. While the film addresses such issues as noncompliance with medication and disputes over independent living arrangements, the bad times are never too severe or long-lasting. As film reviewers Mick Martin and Marsha Porter point out: "[Although] most viewers will enjoy this bittersweet comedy . . . folks coping with mental illness in real life will be offended by yet another film in which the problem is sanitized and trivialized."

The Saint of Fort Washington, 1994. Directed by Tim Hunter. More about homelessness than schizophrenia per se, this film nevertheless touches on issues of importance to those cut off from their families and society by their symptoms. Matthew (Matt Dillon), a young man suffering from schizophrenia, is forced out of his cheap hotel room by a wrecker's ball. When Social Services directs him to the Fort Washington Shelter for men, he finds himself vulnerable to the criminal elements residing there. Jerry (Danny Glover), a Vietnam vet who has gradually lost his business, his home, and his family, rescues Matthew, and together the two struggle to find work, food, and shelter on the street. The film falls far short in its depiction of Matthew's schizophrenia and attributes too much success to Jerry's attempts to talk Matthew out of his hallucinations. Furthermore, Matt Dillon seems unsure how an individual with schizophrenia should act. But the film does address some of the problems peculiar to the homeless mentally ill, including the vagaries of a mental health system that can't provide assistance to someone with no address.

Angel Baby, 1995. Directed by Michael Rymer. The winner of seven Australian Film Institute awards for 1995, this film is a sensitive, realistic portrayal of love between two people with schizophrenia. Harry (John Lynch) is a regular at a local clubhouse. From the moment he sees Kate (Jacqueline McKenzie), he is smitten. He pursues and she responds. To the distress of his family, Harry moves out of his brother's home and Kate leaves her halfway house to move into an apartment together. Harry takes a job as a computer programmer and Kate does the neighbors' laundry, and their life is marginally successful until Kate becomes pregnant and they both stop taking their medication. Largely unnoticed in the United States, this film deals frankly with many important issues affecting those who suffer from serious mental illness: sexual relations, independent living arrangements, relationships with family members, noncompliance with medication, pregnancy, stigma, and suicide. Since a copy of *Surviving Schizophrenia* is shown in the movie, it ranks very high on my list!

Shine, 1996. Directed by Scott Hicks. This highly successful movie, which garnered seven Academy Award nominations, depicts Australian pianist David Helfgott, afflicted with a severe mental disorder not named in the film but obviously schizophrenia. Geoffrey Rush as Helfgott gives a sterling performance portraying a gifted artist with continuing symptoms of his illness, and the movie is worth seeing for this alone. Unfortunately, those making the movie were three decades behind in their knowledge of the disease, and the movie implies that Helfgott's illness was

caused by his having been cruelly treated in childhood by his father (Armand Mueller-Stahl), a charge that has been emphatically
refuted by Helfgott's older sister. Following the film's success,
Helfgott was taken on a recital tour of the United States, which
impressed some critics as pure exploitation. For example, Terry
Teachout of the *New York Daily News* wrote: "Two centuries ago,
nice people went to asylums on Sunday, and gawked at the inmates. But times have changed. Today, we let the inmates out
of the asylums and encourage them to live 'normal' lives. Some
preach strange religions on street corners; others give concerts at
Avery Fisher Hall, and nice people pay $50 a head to watch them,
and call it progress."

Pi, 1998. Directed by Darren Aronofsky. B&W. This disturbing film deals with the complex relationship between insanity and
genius. Max Cohen (Sean Gullette) is a brilliant, reclusive mathematician who earned his Ph.D. at age twenty. Convinced that
everything in nature can be explained by mathematical patterns,
he becomes obsessed with a 216-digit series in the expansion of
pi that he believes holds a secret about the universe. His work,
however, is stymied by computer crashes that destroy his data and
by excruciating headaches that climax in auditory and visual hallucinations from which he can find no relief. Like *Clean, Shaven*,
this film seeks to portray psychosis from the inside, leaving the
viewer uncertain where Max's paranoia ends and reality begins.
Even holed up in his apartment behind triple locks and a dead
bolt, he is pursued by Wall Street brokers who are convinced he's
found a pattern in the stock market, Jewish mystics who believe
he can tell them the true name of God, and visions of his own
brain on the steps of a subway station. The film won the Sundance
Film Festival's Directing Award for 1998.

A Beautiful Mind, 2001. Directed by Ron Howard. Based on
Sylvia Nasar's book with the same title, this is an excellent description of what it is like to have schizophrenia. It depicts the life
of mathematician John Nash, who received a Nobel Prize for work
done before the onset of his illness. Russell Crowe is outstanding

in conveying the psychiatric pain experienced by Nash. Jennifer Connelly, in an Oscar-winning performance as Nash's wife, poignantly demonstrates how difficult this disease is for family members. The importance of medication in recovery is appropriately stressed. And, best of all, no mention whatsoever is made of Nash's mother or his childhood. This is surely a breakthrough movie for a film industry that has been immersed in psychoanalytic theory for sixty years. The screenwriter, director, and producer deserved their Academy Awards for ignoring their psychoanalysts, if for no other reason.

Revolution #9, 2002. Directed by Tim McCann, Exile Productions, 51 Kinney St., Piermont, NY 10968. This is an excellent portrayal of the first psychotic break of a young man with schizophrenia. Michael Risley is convincing as a young man who slowly succumbs to his increasingly prominent delusional system. His fiancée, played by Adrienne Shelly, tries to get him treated and finds that the psychiatric care system is even more dysfunctional than the patients it is supposed to help. Supporting actors are equally genuine in their reactions to the young man's illness. The movie is the real-life antidote to *A Beautiful Mind* and reminds us that death by suicide is a much more common outcome of schizophrenia than winning a Nobel Prize. The film played briefly in New York, Chicago, and Los Angeles, where it received very favorable reviews. It was also lauded at film festivals in Toronto and Telluride and received the 2003 Media Award from the American College of Neuropsychopharmacology.

Spider, 2002. Ralph Fiennes plays a man with schizophrenia who has just been released from a psychiatric hospital after two decades, to live in a rundown halfway house in London. Fiennes's acting is brilliant, all the more so since he says almost nothing. He has nicotine-stained fingers and a secret language and wears four shirts. But *The Sound of Music* this is not; one review called it "bone-chillingly bleak . . . as harrowing a portrait of one man's tormented isolation as the commercial cinema has produced." And that's the good news. The bad news is that the movie incorporates traditional Freudian themes in its portrayal of the origin of schizophrenia. With Oedipus as a major, if invisible, character, the movie looks as if it was made in the 1960s. It is a shame to waste such brilliant acting on such an outmoded storyline.

People Say I'm Crazy, 2003. This is an extraordinary film, directed by John Cadigan, an artist who has schizophrenia, and Katie Cadigan, his sister. The goal of the film, as John explains, is "to show the world what it's like to be inside my brain." John is remarkably articulate in describing his paranoid ideas, anxiety, depression, difficulty in thinking clearly, and general mental pain due to his affliction with the disease. John did much of his own filming of himself, which is a major reason for the film's success; the viewer truly does see the world from John's perspective. The film has won many awards, including at the Chicago and Vancouver film festivals, and received NAMI's Outstanding Media Award in 2004. If I were to select a single movie to show to high school or college students to educate them about schizophrenia, this would be it. The film is available online at www.peoplesayimcrazy.org.

Out of the Shadow, 2004. This is a documentary produced and directed by Susan Smiley and is strongly recommended. It is a powerful story about Susan and her sister, raised by their mother, who had paranoid schizophrenia. Childhood pictures and home movies are mixed with interviews of the two sisters, their mother, and the father who left them. The central story follows Millie, the mother, through a relapse, her seventeenth hospitalization, and then stabilization in a group home. Millie says it best when she describes her own brain: "I think the circuitry missed a connection or something." The movie was widely praised at the Vancouver, Durango, and Rocky Mountain Women's film festivals, the Discovery Channel Documentary Festival, and was shown on PBS. It is available from Vine Street Pictures, P.O. Box 662120, Los Angeles, CA 90066, and online at www.outoftheshadow.com.

The Soloist, 2009. This movie was based on the true story of *Los Angeles Times* reporter Steve Lopez, played by Robert Downey, Jr., who befriends a homeless man with schizophrenia named Nathaniel Ayers, played by Jamie Foxx. One day, Lopez hears Ayers playing the violin on the street. Impressed, he gets to know Ayers and discovers that Ayers had been a musical child prodigy and attended the Juilliard School for two years before becoming sick. The movie follows Lopez's attempts, both eventually successful, to get Ayers into his own apartment and reconnected to his family. The movie was criticized for its weak storyline and got mixed reviews. Its depiction of auditory hallucinations and chaotic thinking are realistic. However, it fails to resolve the issue of treatment, which Ayers predictably refuses, and Lopez respects his refusal. The viewer is left with an unsettling question: What might have happened if Ayers had been treated for his schizophrenia?

Schizophrenia in Literature

Descriptions of schizophrenia are now widely represented in both medical and popular literature. Medical journals, such as *Schizophrenia Bulletin* and *Psychiatric Services,* regularly carry accounts of the illness written by those who have been afflicted. Popular journals do likewise; Susan Sheehan's superb account of schizophrenia was originally carried in *The New Yorker* and later published as *Is There No Place on Earth for Me?* This book, and many other books on schizophrenia, are summarized in appendix A. The literature now available on schizophrenia includes an abundance of riches, providing many choices for those who wish to learn more about the disease.

This was not always the case. Until approximately 1980, the subject of schizophrenia was confined mostly to textbooks of psychiatry. Within general literature, however, there were also occasional descriptions of "mad" or "insane" persons who had symptoms of schizophrenia. Some of these descriptions are both instructive and entertaining, and a selection of them is included below. Most are from the English language, although others exist in other languages. Such accounts enrich our understanding of this disease.

One early example was Honoré de Balzac's short story "Louis Lambert," written in 1832 in French. Even in translation, it is an extraordinary story, and an excerpt from it is included at the end of chapter 1. Other selections from literature prior to 1950 that depict individuals with symptoms of schizophrenia include the following:

"Diary of a Madman" by Nicolai Gogol, 1834. One of Gogol's earliest stories, this has been called "one of the oldest and most complete descriptions of schizophrenia." The protagonist, a Russian civil servant, develops a delusion that he is the King of Spain. As the story evolves, he exhibits ideas of reference, increasingly disordered thinking, bizarre behavior, and auditory hallucinations in hearing two dogs talking to each other in Russian. In his later years, Gogol himself became extremely depressed and preoccupied with religion.

"Berenice" by Edgar Allan Poe, 1835. Poe's descriptions have been widely praised for their realism. In this short story, the narrator, Egaeus, suffers from schizophrenia characterized by a fixed delusion, previously called monomania. When he becomes engaged to his cousin Berenice, he fixates on her teeth, believing that his possession of them will restore him to reason: "Then came the full fury of my *monomania*, and I struggled in vain against its strange and irresistible influence. In the multiplied objects of the external world I had no thoughts but for the teeth. For these I longed with a phrenzied desire." In the end, as if in nightmare that he later only vaguely remembers, Egaeus, believing Berenice to be dead from an epileptic seizure, extracts her teeth and puts them in a box.

"A Madman's Manuscript" in *The Pickwick Papers* by Charles Dickens, 1837. Charles Dickens was fascinated by insanity, was close friends with several prominent psychiatrists, had many medical books on insanity in his personal library, and visited asylums whenever he had the opportunity. "A Madman's Manuscript" is a strange tale, told in the first person by an asylum inmate who is being laughed at by visitors peering into his cell. Rather than being humiliated, he delights in his status:

> Yes!—a madman's! How that word would have struck to my heart, many years ago! . . . I like it now though. It's a fine name. Show me the monarch whose angry frown was ever feared like the glare of a madman's eye—whose cord and axe were ever half so sure as a madman's grip. Ho! ho! It's a grand thing to be mad! To be peeped at like a wild lion through the iron bars—to gnash one's teeth and howl, through the long still night, to the merry ring of a heavy chain—and to roll and twine among the straw, transported with such brave music. Hurrah for the madhouse! Oh, it's a rare place!

Jane Eyre by Charlotte Brontë, 1847. When Jane Eyre takes the position of governess at Thornfield Hall, she is both frightened and intrigued by noises she hears coming from the attic. But it is not until her wedding day that she actually sees Bertha Rochester, whose existence and insanity have been kept a secret by her husband for ten years. Brontë's description of Mrs. Rochester is of a dangerous wild animal:

> In the deep shade, at the farther end of the room, a figure ran backwards and forwards. What it was, whether beast or human being, one could not, at first sight, tell: it grovelled, seemingly, on all fours; it snatched and growled like some strange wild animal: but it was covered with clothing, and a quantity of dark, grizzled hair, wild as a mane, hid its head and face.

When Brontë was criticized for her brutish depiction of Mrs. Rochester, she responded that she was merely reflecting the reality of some cases of madness "in which all that is good or even human seems to disappear from the mind and a fiend-like nature replaces it."

David Copperfield by Charles Dickens, 1850. When David runs away from London to seek refuge with his Aunt Betsey in Dover, he is introduced to her permanent houseguest, Mr. Dick, who clearly has symptoms of schizophrenia. His primary symptom is a belief that thoughts are being inserted into his head, considered by many psychiatrists to be an almost certain sign of this disease. Mr. Dick believes the thoughts have come from the head of King Charles I and that they were transferred to him when the king was beheaded in 1649. That the king's demise was so far in the past seems to trouble Mr. Dick more than the motives of those inserting the thoughts: "'Well,' returned Mr. Dick, scratching his ear with his pen, and looking dubiously at me. '. . . I don't see how that can be. Because, if it was so long ago, how could the people about him have made that mistake of putting some of the trouble out of *his* head, after it was taken off, into *mine*?'"

Bartleby the Scrivener by Herman Melville, 1853. Bartleby's illness is a classic example of the type of schizophrenia in which the negative symptoms predominate. He has what used to be called "simple" schizophrenia. As the narrator notes, "his eccentricities are involuntary" and he "was the victim of [an] innate and incurable disorder." The man who hires him as a scrivener (law-copyist) and who tries unsuccessfully to help him finally concludes that "he is a little deranged." Bartleby's behavior slowly deteriorates as the story progresses, and he is overtaken by apathy and an inability to act. His affect is completely flat as he refuses all offers of help, repeating politely but firmly: "I would prefer not to make any change." At the end of the story, Bartleby is put in prison as a vagrant and there he dies, with "his knees drawn up, and lying on his side, his head touching the cold stones" of the prison wall.

"Ward No. 6" by Anton Chekhov, 1892. Chekhov's talents as a writer and a physician came together in his moving portrayal of Ivan Dmitritch, who suffers from paranoid schizophrenia. He is a lonely man with no family or friends, and as a teacher he has a hard time getting along with his colleagues and his students. One autumn day, he encounters convicts on the road. In the past, he felt compassion; now, paranoid thoughts begin: "At home he could not get the convicts or the soldiers with their rifles out of his head all day . . . at night he could not sleep, but kept thinking that he might be arrested, put into fetters, and thrown into prison. . . . Everyone who passed by the windows or came into the yard seemed to him a spy or a detective." In the spring, when the snow melts, an old woman and boy are found dead. Worrying that others will suspect him, Ivan hides in his landlady's cellar but runs away when workmen come to the house, fearing they are policemen in disguise. When he is stopped and brought home, his landlady calls for a doctor. Ivan is taken to the hospital, where he is put on the ward for patients with venereal disease. When he disturbs the other patients there, he is taken to Ward No. 6, the psychiatric ward.

Mrs. Dalloway by Virginia Woolf, 1925. Virginia Woolf herself had manic-depressive illness, but Septimus Warren Smith in *Mrs. Dalloway* is depicted as having classic symptoms of schizophrenia. These include a heightening of the senses, alterations in bodily boundaries, and paranoid delusions:

> But they beckoned; leaves were alive; trees were alive. And the leaves being connected by millions of fibres with his own body, there on the seat, fanned up and down; when the branch stretched he, too, made that statement. The sparrows fluttering, rising, and falling in jagged fountains were part of the pattern; the white and blue, barred with black branches. Sounds made harmonies with premeditation; the spaces between them were as significant as the sounds. A child cried. Rightly far away a horn sounded. All taken together meant the birth of a new religion— . . .

Faced with separation from his wife and life in a "home," he climbs out the window of his boardinghouse, hesitates momentarily on the sill, and then flings himself down, impaling himself on the rusty spikes of the railing below.

The Waves by Virginia Woolf, 1931. In this novel, one of Woolf's most experimental, each of six characters is revealed through a series of soliloquies. One character, Rhoda, like many individuals with schizophrenia, is unable to sort and interpret incoming stimuli and so often responds inappropriately. She is similarly stymied in society: "Other people have faces; . . . they are here. . . . The things they lift are heavy. . . . They laugh really; they get angry really; while I have to look first and do what other people do when they have done it. . . . I attach myself only to names and faces; and hoard them like amulets against disaster. . . . Alone, I often fall down into nothingness. . . . Month by month things are losing their hardness; even my body now lets the light through; my spine is soft like wax near the flame of the candle. . . . Every time the door opens I am interrupted. I am not yet twenty-one. I am to be broken. I am to be derided all my life."

"Silent Snow, Secret Snow" by Conrad Aiken, 1932. Conrad Aiken's father and sister both developed insanity, and Aiken lived his entire life in the fear that he was destined for the same fate. "Silent Snow, Secret Snow" is an account of the onset of schizophrenia in a twelve-year-old boy whose auditory and visual hallucinations entice him to withdraw from the world around him. Paul's symptoms begin with a muffling of sound, "a sense as of snow falling about him, a secret screen of new snow between himself and the world." Later, his illness takes on an aspect of paranoia and his hallucinations become more vivid: his mother's entrance into his room is seen as something alien and hostile, and the snow laughs and calls to him: "Lie down. Shut your eyes, now—you will no longer see much—in this white darkness who could see, or want to see? We will take the place of everything."

Save Me the Waltz by Zelda Fitzgerald, 1932. Like her husband's novel *Tender Is the Night,* Zelda Fitzgerald's *Save Me the Waltz* is a thinly disguised description of her experience with schizophrenia and her family's reaction to her illness. Written in 1932, shortly after her second breakdown, the novel describes a young woman's delirium after she is hospitalized for what is said to be blood poisoning:

The walls of the room slid quietly past, dropping one over the other like the leaves of a heavy album. They were all shades of gray and rose and mauve. There was no sound when they fell. . . .

Meaningfully the nurses laughed together and left her room. The walls began again. She decided to lie there and frustrate the walls if they thought they could press her between their pages like a bud from a wedding bouquet.

Tender Is the Night by F. Scott Fitzgerald, 1934. After the success of *The Great Gatsby,* F. Scott Fitzgerald proposed a new idea to his editor. Even as he started the new project, however, Zelda began showing signs of illness, and in spring 1930 she had her first breakdown. Fitzgerald began anew, and the result was *Tender Is the Night,* in which the main characters' lives—Nicole Diver's illness and her husband, Dick's, reaction to it—so closely parallel the Fitzgeralds' experiences that it is often difficult to separate the fictional story from the real one. Scott writes to Zelda's doctor: ". . . my great worry is that time is slipping by, life is slipping by. . . . If she were an anti-social person who did not want to face life and pull her own weight that would be one story, but her passionate love of life and her absolute inability to meet it seems so tragic that it is scarcely to be endured." In the book, Dick tries to contain Nicole's illness but is unsuccessful. He says: "It was necessary to treat her with active and affirmative insistence, keeping the road to reality always open, making the road to escape harder going. But the brilliance, the versatility of madness is akin to the resourcefulness of water seeping through, over and around a dike. It requires the united front of many people to work against it."

"I Am Lazarus" by Anna Kavan, 1940. Anna Kavan was twice confined to mental hospitals in Switzerland and England. In "I Am Lazarus," Thomas Bow, twenty-five, is confined to a clinic where he has been receiving insulin shock treatment for "advanced dementia praecox." A visiting doctor finds him apparently cured but with an "inexpressive face and . . . curious flat look of the eyes." He takes no notice of those around him: "What had he to do with talking? All around the table were different colored shapes whose mouths opened and closed and emitted sounds that meant nothing to him."

"The Headless Hawk" by Truman Capote, 1946. Truman Capote was only twenty-two when he wrote this short story about a young woman with schizophrenia. Vincent firsts meets D.J. when she tries to sell him her self-portrait: a figure dressed in a monk-like robe, reclining on a vaudeville trunk, with her severed head lying bleeding at her feet. Although he finds her odd, with lips that tremble "with unrealized words as though she had possibly a defect of speech" and a mind "like a mirror reflecting blue space in a barren room," he is attracted to her. In the end, however, he is overwhelmed by her paranoid delusions about a man. *"Sometimes he's not a man at all—she'd told him . . . —sometimes he is something very different: a hawk, a child, a butterfly . . . I knew he was going to murder me. And he will. He will."*

Schizophrenia, Creativity, and Famous People

An oft-debated question around firesides and pubs is whether there is a relationship between creativity and schizophrenia. John Dryden reflected the views of many people when he wrote three hundred years ago, "Great wits are sure to madmen near allied." Since then we have moved a little closer to a definitive answer to this question.

It is known that the creative person and the person with schizophrenia share many cognitive traits. Both use words and language in unusual ways (the hallmark of a great poet or novelist), both have unusual views of reality (as great artists do), both often utilize unusual thought processes in their deliberations, and both tend to prefer solitude to the company of others. When creative persons are given traditional psychological tests, they manifest more psychopathology than noncreative persons, and creative persons are often viewed as eccentric by their friends. Conversely, when people with nonparanoid schizophrenia are given traditional tests of creativity they score very high (people with paranoid schizophrenia do not). Both creative people and people with schizophrenia have been reported to have fewer dopamine-2 receptors in the brain's thalamus, according to a recent neuroimaging study; this may provide a biological base for the similarity.

Several surveys have shown that highly creative persons are not themselves more susceptible to schizophrenia. However, one study has suggested that the immediate relatives of creative persons may be more susceptible to schizophrenia. As a case in point one thinks of Robert Frost, whose aunt, son, and perhaps daughter all developed schizophrenia. In addition, Albert Einstein's son developed schizophrenia, as did the daughters of Victor Hugo, Bertrand Russell, and James Joyce.

James Joyce is a particularly interesting study in psychopathology. A biography on him noted his "keen pleasure in sounds," his periods of depression, intermittent alcohol abuse, and at least one episode of mania during which "he could not sleep for six or seven nights . . . he felt as if he were wound up and then suddenly shooting out of water like a fish. During the day he was troubled by auditory hallucinations." A psychiatrist who studied Joyce's writings concluded that he was a schizoid personality with paranoid traits and claimed that "*Finnegans Wake* must ultimately be diagnosed as psychotic." Joyce's only daughter, Lucia, was diagnosed with classical schizophrenia at age twenty-two, treated by Jung, and spent the rest of her life in mental hospitals. It was noted that "Joyce had a remarkable capacity to follow her swift jumps of thought, which baffled other people completely."

There is, however, one fundamental difference between the creative person and the person with schizophrenia. The creative person has his/her unusual thought processes under control and can harness them in the creation of a product. The person with schizophrenia, on the other hand, is at the mercy of disconnected thinking and loose associations which tumble about in cacophonic disarray. The creative person has choices, whereas the schizophrenia sufferer does not.

The list of creative individuals who are thought to have had schizophrenia or schizoaffective disorder is remarkably short; this is not surprising when one considers how thinking disorders interfere with a person's ability to work. Individuals who apparently suffered from schizophrenia include Buddy Bolden, known as the founder of jazz; Tom Harrell, a renowned jazz musician and composer; Roger

Keith "Syd" Barrett, a founder of the rock band Pink Floyd; Peter Green, guitarist and founder of the band Fleetwood Mac; and Harold Humes, who founded *The Paris Review* and was regarded as a promising young writer before he became sick. But the five best-known creative people who became afflicted with schizophrenia are the following:

Antonin Artaud, a writer and actor, was a major figure in the French Surrealist movement from 1924 to 1927. He exhibited occasional symptoms of schizophrenia during those years, but in 1937, at age forty-one, he was hospitalized and spent much of his remaining life confined in Paris, Rouen, and Rodez. His *Letters from Rodez* describe his sickness, as in this 1943 letter to a friend:

> . . . this sickness has to do with the scandal of the horrible plot of which I am the victim and which you know about in the privacy of your soul and your conscience; for you have suffered from it horribly yourself. You have seen the hordes of demons which afflict me night and day, you have seen them as clearly as you see me. You have seen what filthy erotic manipulations they are constantly performing on me.

In 1993 a movie was released about Artaud's later years (*My Life and Times with Antonin Artaud*). It depicts his paranoid symptoms but focuses mostly on his drug abuse and is not especially helpful in understanding his illness.

Ralph Blakelock was a prominent American landscape artist whose paintings just prior to World War I sold for more than had ever before been paid to a living American artist. By then, however, Blakelock had been diagnosed with dementia praecox and hospitalized for more than a decade in the state psychiatric hospital at Middletown, New York.

The onset of Blakelock's overt symptoms was in his early forties, although he had previously been regarded as very strange by his family and friends. He had paranoid and grandiose delusions (e.g., he claimed to be the Duke of York) as well as mood swings and episodes of mania. In today's diagnostic system, he would probably be diagnosed as having schizoaffective disorder. Regarding his illness, Blakelock wrote (without punctuation): "If I am insane I am not conscious of it I am not a paranoiac I am not in the period of senility nor aged dotage. For I can whistle and sing."

When Blakelock died in 1919, he was America's best-known artist, more so than Whistler, Homer, or Sargent, and President Woodrow Wilson sent a message of condolence. In 2003, an excellent biography of Blacklock was published: Glyn Vincent, *The Unknown Night: The Madness and Genius of R. A. Blakelock, An American Painter* (New York: Grove Press). The effects of his illness are sadly chronicled, including how Blakelock and his family were cheated out of most of the earnings from his art.

Ivor Gurney was a promising English composer and poet when he was struck down by what most Gurney scholars have labeled as schizophrenia. A recent biography casts some doubt on this diagnosis and suggests that manic-depressive illness may have been the problem. He had studied under Ralph Vaughan Williams, but by age twenty-three was already complaining that "his brain won't move as he wishes it to." In 1917, at age twenty-seven, Gurney had his first psychotic break, during which he believed he was being visited by Beethoven: "I felt the presence of a wise and friendly spirit; it was old Ludwig van all right . . . Bach was there but does not care for me." His illness worsened and he became convinced that "electrical tricks" were being played on him. "He would sit with a cushion on his head to guard against electric waves coming from the wireless [radio] . . . He has had such pains in the head that he felt he would be better off dead." Finally, at age thirty-two, he was permanently hospitalized in the London Mental Hospital in Kent and there he spent the next fifteen years, continuing to write poetry, such as these lines from the poem "To God":

> *Why have you made life so intolerable*
> *And set me between four walls, where I am able*
> *Not to escape meals without prayer, for that is possible*
> *Only by annoying an attendant. And tonight a sensual*

Hell has been put upon me, so that all has deserted me
And I am merely crying and trembling in heart
For Death, and cannot get it. And gone out is part
Of sanity. And there is dreadful Hell within me.

At age forty-seven, still hospitalized, he died from tuberculosis.

John Nash was awarded the Nobel Prize for Economics in 1994 for work he had done at age twenty-one on mathematical game theory. *Fortune* magazine had called him "America's young star" at that time. In his late twenties, however, he developed a type of schizophrenia characterized by paranoid and grandiose delusions. He believed that "his career was being ruined by aliens from outer space" and that "he was scheduled to become Emperor of Antarctica" as part of a new world government. For more than twenty years he wandered between hospitals and lived with family members, supported mostly by his wife. Then, in his fifties, Nash's condition improved. When he received the Nobel Prize, the White House invited him for a visit. His life and illness have been nicely chronicled by Sylvia Nasar in *A Beautiful Mind* (see appendix A).

Vaslav Nijinsky was the most famous dancer in the years preceding World War I and, some have said, the greatest dancer who ever lived. His leaps were astounding, as he was said to be the only dancer who could, while in the air, cross his feet back and forth ten times. At age twenty-nine, he was diagnosed with schizophrenia and was intermittently hospitalized for the remainder of his life. He was markedly delusional, catatonic, and at times exhibited a word-salad thought disorder. He was treated by Alfred Adler and Manfred Bleuler, and Nijinsky's wife also consulted Freud and Jung. Nijinsky was also among the first to be treated by insulin coma therapy, which is no longer used. In his diary, he wrote:

I love life and want to live, to cry but cannot—I feel such a pain in my soul—a pain which frightens me. My soul is ill. My soul, not my mind. The doctors do not understand my illness.

In Paris, at the height of his career, the newspapers had labeled Nijinsky "God of the Dance." Nijinsky signed his diary entry, "God and Nijinsky."

One additional artist who is sometimes said to have had schizophrenia was Vincent van Gogh. Van Gogh has been given many other retrospective diagnoses by medical historians, including manic-depressive illness, brain syphilis, porphyria, and heavy metal poisoning from his paints. His symptoms included paranoid delusions, auditory and visual hallucinations, mutism, depression, and periods of great energy. Although there is a tendency to romanticize his psychosis and view it as partially responsible for his great art, van Gogh's own letters make explicit how painful and unpleasant it was. He ultimately committed suicide after painting for just ten years. From St.-Rémy he wrote to his brother, Theo: "Oh, if I could have worked without this accursed disease—what things I might have done."

In contrast to schizophrenia, manic-depressive illness lends itself to creativity because of the high energy level and rapid thought processes experienced by many people with this disease. The list of people suspected of having manic-depressive illness among creative individuals includes Handel, Berlioz, Schumann, Beethoven, Donizetti, Gluck, Byron, Shelley, Coleridge, Poe, Balzac, Hemingway, Fitzgerald, Eugene O'Neill, and Virginia Woolf.

The Problem of Stigma

People with schizophrenia and their families have to live with an extraordinary amount of stigma. Schizophrenia is the modern-day equivalent of leprosy, and in the general population the level of ignorance about schizophrenia is appalling. A 1987 survey among college freshmen found that almost two-thirds mistakenly believed that "multiple personalities" were a common symptom of schizophrenia, whereas less than half were aware that hallucinations are a common symptom. A 1986 poll found that 55 percent of the public did not believe that mental illness existed, and only 1 percent realized that mental illness is a major health problem. Other surveys have reported that many people continue to believe that schizophrenia and other severe psychiatric disorders are caused by sin or weakness of character.

There is good news and bad news regarding stigma. The good news is that the emergence of schizophrenia into the public eye has led to a marked increase in public understanding of the disease. Unlike in the past, the majority of Americans now accept the fact that schizophrenia is a brain disease, not God's punishment. One would have predicted that such increased understanding would significantly decrease stigma against those with the disease.

The bad news is that stigma against individuals with schizophrenia did not lessen in recent decades but actually got worse. This was documented in a 1996 survey that compared public attitudes in 1950 and 1996 and reported that the public in 1996 viewed individuals with schizophrenia as considerably more violent than in the past. Indeed, it reported that the proportion of respondents "who described a mentally ill person as being violent increased by nearly 2½ times between 1950 and 1996." This was noted in the 1999 *Report on Mental Health of The United States Surgeon General:*

> Why is stigma so strong despite better public understanding of mental illness? The answer appears to be fear of violence: people with mental illness, especially those with psychosis, are perceived to be more violent than in the past. . . . In other words, the perception of people with psychosis as being dangerous is stronger today than in the past.

Since the 1999 Surgeon General's report, this trend has continued—the general public increasingly understands that schizophrenia is a disease of the brain, but at the same time stigma against people with schizophrenia has increased. A 2006 follow-up to the 1996 survey cited above reported that stigma against mentally ill persons had increased during the 11-year period. Specifically, "significantly more respondents in the 2006 survey than the 1996 survey reported an unwillingness to have someone with schizophrenia as a neighbor . . . Our most striking finding is that stigma among the American public appears to be surprisingly fixed, even in the fact of anticipated advances in public knowledge." Similarly, a 2016 study of news media stories about mental illness for 1995–2004 compared to 2005–2014 reported that the mention of stigma or discrimination in the stories increased from 23 percent to 28 percent. It is now clear that the hopes of the past— that education about schizophrenia would lead to decreased public stigma—is a vain hope.

It is not a lack of education that is driving the stigma, but rather high-profile violent acts committed by a small number of people with schizophrenia, almost all of whom were not being treated at the time. For example, a study using university volunteers demonstrated that reading a newspaper article reporting a violent crime committed by a mental patient led to increased "negative attitudes toward people with mental illnesses." In Germany, following highly publicized attacks on prominent officials by individuals with severe mental illnesses, there was a measurable "marked increase in desired social distance from mentally ill people immediately following [the] violent attacks." The increased social distance and consequent stigma slowly decreased over time but had not returned to baseline two years later.

A similar study in 2012 of 1,797 Americans assessed the effects of a news story about "a mass shooting by a person with a history of serious mental illness" on the attitude of the public. The news story significantly increased negative attitudes to, and stigma against, mentally ill persons; the authors concluded that such stories "appear to play a critical role in influencing negative attitudes towards persons with serious mental illness." And in the 2016 study that compared news stories in 1995–2004 with stories in 2005–2014, "the proportion of newspaper stories about interpersonal violence related to mental illness that appeared on the front page increased from 1 percent in the first decade of the study to 18 percent in the second decade." The latter, of course, was the decade when the mass killings at Virginia Tech, Tucson, Aurora, and Newtown all took place. Thus the faces of schizophrenia that have now become firmly embedded in the public mind are the wide-eyed grin of Jared Loughner, who killed 6 in Tucson, and the psychotic-looking, orange-haired visage of James Holmes, who killed 12 in Aurora.

The people who suffer for this increasing stigma are, of course, all of those who have a mental illness, especially schizophrenia and other serious mental illnesses. Each public tragedy that is caused by someone with a mental illness makes life more difficult for everyone else with a mental illness. For example, in 1999, when a man with schizophrenia killed two people in a church library in Salt Lake City, "within hours Valley Mental Health began getting calls from frightened clients. Clients were just sobbing," said a spokesperson. "They were afraid that the public would want to retaliate against them." Such events are said to "set back years" ongoing efforts to destigmatize mental illness in the minds of the public.

Suggestions for how such stigma can be effectively decreased will be discussed in chapter 15.

Recommended Further Reading

Journal of the California Alliance for the Mentally III 4(1) 1993. This entire issue is on mental illness in the media.

McGinty, E. E., A. Kennedy-Hendricks, S. Chosky, et al. "Trends in News Media Coverage of Mental Illness in the United States: 1995-2015." *Health Affairs* 35 (2016): 1121–29.

Nasar, S. *A Beautiful Mind: A Biography of John Forbes Nash, Jr., Winner of the Nobel Prize in Economics, 1994.* New York: Simon & Schuster, 1998.

Pescosolido, B. A., J. K. Martin, J. S. Long, et al. "'A Disease Like Any Other?' A Decade of Change in Public Reactions to Schizophrenia, Depression, and Alcohol Dependence." *American Journal of Psychiatry* 167 (2010): 1321–30.

Pescosolido, B. A., J. Monahan, B. G. Link, et al. "The Public's View of the Competence, Dangerousness, and Need for Legal Coercion of Persons with Mental Health Problems." *American Journal of Public Health* 89 (1999): 1339–45.

Phelan, J. C., B. G. Link, A. Stueve, et al. "Public Conceptions of Mental Illness in 1950 and 1996: What Is Mental Illness and Is It to Be Feared?" *Journal of Health and Social Behavior* 41 (2000): 188–207.

Thornicroft, G. *Shunned: Discrimination Against People with Mental Illness* (Oxford: Oxford University Press, 2007).

Torrey, E. F. "Stigma and Violence: Isn't It Time to Connect the Dots?" *Schizophrenia Bulletin* 37 (2011): 892–96.

Vincent, G. *The Unknown Night: The Genius and Madness of R. A. Blakelock, An American Painter.* New York: Grove Press, 2003.

Wahl, O. F. "Mental Health Consumers' Experience of Stigma." *Schizophrenia Bulletin* 25 (1999): 467–78.

14

Dimensions of the Disaster

Schizophrenia is to psychiatry what cancer is to medicine: a sentence as well as a diagnosis.

W. Hall, G. Andrews, and G. Goldstein, Australian and New Zealand Journal of Psychiatry, *1985*

Schizophrenia has been called "one of the most sinister words in the language." It has a bite to it, a harsh grating sound that evokes visions of madness and asylums. It is not fluid like *démence*, the word from which "dementia" comes. Nor is it a visual word like *écrasé*, the origin of "cracked," meaning that the person is like a cracked pot. Nor is it romantic like "lunatic," meaning fallen under the influence of the moon (which in Latin is *luna*). "Schizophrenia" is a discordant and cruel term, just like the disease it signifies.

Our treatment of individuals with this disease has, all too often, also been discordant and cruel. It is, in fact, the single biggest blemish on the face of contemporary American medicine and social services;

when the social history of our era is written, the plight of persons with schizophrenia will be recorded as having been a national scandal. Consider the dimensions of the disaster.

1. *There are at least four times as many people with schizophrenia who are homeless than there are in public psychiatric beds.* Studies of homeless individuals in the United States have estimated their total number to be between 250,000 and 550,000. A median estimate of 400,000 is consistent with the data from most of the studies. Studies have also reported that approximately one-third of homeless individuals are seriously mentally ill, the vast majority of them with schizophrenia. It is likely, therefore, that on any given day at least 100,000 persons with schizophrenia are living in public shelters and on the streets. By contrast, there are only about 35,000 public psychiatric beds remaining in state and county hospitals in the United States. Approximately 25,000 of these beds are filled by individuals with schizophrenia on any given day. There are therefore at least four times the number of people with schizophrenia who are homeless than there are in public psychiatric beds.

2. *There are ten times as many people with schizophrenia in jails and prisons than there are in public psychiatric beds.* In 2012 there were more than 2.3 million individuals in jails and prisons in the United States. A study by the U.S. Department of Justice reported that 15 percent of those in state prisons, 10 percent in federal prisons, and 24 percent in jails had a psychotic disorder, totaling approximately 383,400 individuals. Although there are other causes of psychotic disorders, studies would suggest that at least 250,000 of these individuals have schizophrenia. Thus there are ten times as many people with schizophrenia in jails and prisons than there are in public psychiatric beds.

3. *There are increasing episodes of violence committed by individuals with schizophrenia who are not being treated.* Individuals with schizophrenia who take medications are not more violent than the general population. However, as discussed in chapter 10, recent studies have shown that some individuals with schizophrenia who are not taking medication *are* more violent. In one study 9 percent of individuals with schizophrenia who were living in the community had used a weapon in a fight in the preceding year. In another study "27 percent of re-

leased male and female patients report at least one violent act within a mean of four months after [hospital] discharge." Assaults against family members by individuals with schizophrenia have also risen sharply; a 1991 survey of the members of the National Alliance for the Mentally Ill reported that 11 percent of the seriously mentally ill family members had physically harmed another person within the previous year. A Department of Justice study reported that there are almost one thousand homicides a year committed by individuals with "a history of mental illness"; media accounts suggest that the majority of these have been diagnosed with schizophrenia. Drug and alcohol abuse and noncompliance with medications both appear to be important factors in increasing violent behavior in this population.

4. *Individuals with schizophrenia are increasingly being victimized by others.* Most crimes against individuals with schizophrenia are not reported; those instances that are reported are often ignored by officials. Purse snatchings and the stealing of disability checks are common, but rapes and even murders are not rare. In Los Angeles a study of board-and-care home residents, the majority of whom had schizophrenia, reported that one-third of them had been robbed and/or assaulted in the preceding year. In New York a study of twenty women with schizophrenia reported that half of them had been raped at least once, and five had been raped more than once. In Des Moines, Van Mill, a homeless man diagnosed with schizophrenia, was beaten to death by three men, then dumped into a children's wading pool. See also chapter 10.

5. *Housing for many individuals with schizophrenia is often abysmal.* Because of pressure from state departments of mental health to discharge patients from state hospitals, seriously mentally ill individuals are frequently placed into housing that would not be considered fit for anyone else. For example, the police removed twenty-one "ex-mental patients" living in New York City board-and-care homes "amid broken plumbing, rotting food and roaches. . . . The police found the decaying corpse of a former patient lying undisturbed in one home inhabited by six other residents." In 1990 the *New York Times* headlined: MENTAL HOMES ARE WRETCHED, A PANEL SAYS. In Mississippi "9 ex-patients" were found in a primitive shed with "no toilet or running water" and "guarded by two vicious dogs" to ensure that they did not run away.

6. *Many individuals with schizophrenia revolve between hospitals,*

jails, and shelters. Because of the failure of mental health professionals to provide medications and ensure aftercare for discharged patients, many individuals with schizophrenia undergo a revolving door of admissions and readmissions to hospitals, jails, and public shelters. In Illinois 30 percent of patients discharged from state psychiatric hospitals are rehospitalized within thirty days. In New York 60 percent of discharged patients are rehospitalized within a year. A study of readmissions to state psychiatric hospitals found patients with schizophrenia who had been readmitted as many as one hundred twenty-one times. A jail survey identified individuals with schizophrenia who had been jailed as many as eighty times. Between hospitalizations and jailings these individuals consume inordinate amounts of police and social service time and resources. Studies in Ohio and California in the 1990s reported that law-enforcement officials responded to more "mental health crisis" calls than robbery calls. In New York City in 1976 the police responded to approximately 1,000 calls regarding "emotionally disturbed persons"; in 1998 the police responded to 24,787 such calls.

7. *Schizophrenia is remarkably neglected by mental health professionals.* Despite an increase in total psychiatrists, psychologists, and psychiatric social workers from approximately 9,000 in 1940 to more than 200,000 in 1998, schizophrenia has been remarkably neglected by these professionals. For example, a study published in 1994 reported that only *3 percent* of all patients seen by psychiatrists in private office practice had a diagnosis of schizophrenia. One major reason for the failure of mental health professionals to treat patients with schizophrenia is the shockingly poor preparation they receive in their training programs. State psychiatric hospitals frequently must fill their positions with poorly trained and/or incompetent professionals; indeed, Wyoming State Hospital in the 1980s went for almost a year without a single psychiatrist on its staff. Many Community Mental Health Centers (CMHCs), originally conceived and funded to provide care for seriously mentally ill individuals being discharged from psychiatric hospitals, merely evolved into counseling centers to do personality polishing for the "worried well." Some CMHCs also built swimming pools with federal funds and paid their administrators handsomely. In 1989 three administrators at a Utah CMHC were charged with 117 counts of felony theft for paying themselves $3.6 million over five years. In 1990

the executive director of a CMHC in Fort Worth was indicted on four counts of felony theft. These stolen funds are but a fraction of the resources that were originally intended for individuals with serious mental illnesses such as schizophrenia but which have been diverted, legally or illegally, to other purposes.

8. *At least 40 percent of all individuals with schizophrenia are receiving no treatment at any given time.* A report from the National Institute of Mental Health Epidemiologic Catchment Area (ECA) survey revealed that only 60 percent of individuals with schizophrenia receive any psychiatric or medical care within a one-year period. At any given time, therefore, at least 40 percent are receiving no treatment. A community survey in Baltimore found that half of all persons with schizophrenia were receiving no treatment for their illness. A major reason for this remarkably low treatment rate has been changes in laws making involuntary hospitalization and treatment more difficult to effect for individuals who, because of their brain dysfunction, have no awareness of their need for treatment. Sadly misguided civil rights lawyers and "patient advocates" regularly defend the individual's right to be psychotic; the thinking of the lawyers and advocates is more thought-disordered than the people they are defending. For example, in Wisconsin a public defender argued that an individual with schizophrenia who was mute and eating his feces was not a danger to himself; the judge accepted the defense and released the man.

The disastrous care and treatment of individuals with schizophrenia is not unique to the United States, although it is probably worse in this country than in most other developed nations. Many Canadian provinces are proceeding with deinstitutionalization along the same lines as those pioneered by the United States, and conditions in Ontario have especially deteriorated. England has had a series of homicides by discharged patients who were not receiving treatment, and mentally ill homeless individuals have increased markedly in Australia and France. Italy passed a law in 1978 prohibiting new admissions to psychiatric hospitals and, except in Verona and Trieste, where community treatment facilities are good, the "Italian experiment" as it is known has been a failure. Japan puts individuals with schizophrenia into private hospitals, which are often owned by the doctors them-

---

FACT SHEET ON SCHIZOPHRENIA

· Approximately 2.6 million Americans have schizophrenia in any given year. That is 8 persons out of every 1,000.

· At least 40 percent of them are not receiving treatment at any given time. Thus, there are over 1 million individuals with schizophrenia who are not being treated.

· There are at least four times more individuals with schizophrenia who are homeless, living on the streets and in shelters, as there are in all public psychiatric beds.

· There are ten times more individuals with schizophrenia in jails and state prisons than there are in all public psychiatric beds.

· There are increasing episodes of violence committed by individuals with schizophrenia who are not being treated. This is the single biggest cause of stigma against individuals with this diagnosis.

· Individuals with schizophrenia are increasingly the victims of crimes, including robberies, assaults, rapes, and murders.

· Public psychiatric treatment services, housing, and rehabilitation services for individuals with schizophrenia are often grossly inadequate and in most states getting worse.

· The total direct and indirect costs of schizophrenia in the United States in 2013 were at least $155 billion.

---

selves, and keeps them there so that the patients' families will not be embarrassed; this abuse was so widespread that an international commission investigated it in 1986. Nowhere in the world has the treatment of schizophrenia been without major problems, although the Scandinavian countries and the Netherlands probably come closest to achieving a reasonable level of care.

How Many People Have Schizophrenia in the United States?

Given the fact that the National Institute of Mental Health (NIMH) has been in business for over half a century, one would think that the answer to this fundamental question would be well established. Not so! The number of people who have schizophrenia in the United

States is widely debated, with advocates for mentally ill persons using higher numbers and those who are responsible for delivering services using lower numbers.

Much of the problem arose from the NIMH-funded Epidemiologic Catchment Area (ECA) study carried out between 1980 and 1985. That study employed lay interviewers using a questionnaire to ascertain symptoms of mental illness among a sample population at five sites. The ECA study reported that 1.5 percent of the U.S. population ages eighteen and over, and 1.2 percent of the population ages nine to seventeen, had schizophrenia in a one-year period. Based on the U.S. population of the year 2000, that translates into 3.5 million individuals with schizophrenia in a one-year period, a prevalence rate approximately twice as high as older studies had shown.

The methodology of the ECA study, however, has been seriously criticized for overdiagnosing mental disorders. A study in Baltimore in which psychiatrists interviewed individuals who had been diagnosed as having schizophrenia in the ECA study found remarkably poor agreement with the ECA diagnosis. Data from previous U.S. prevalence studies; data from the Social Security Administration on the number of individuals receiving benefits for all severe mental illnesses (approximately 3.2 million in 2002); and the 1999 Surgeon General's special report on mental health, which claimed that 1.3 percent of all individuals aged eighteen to fifty-four have schizophrenia, all suggest that 3.5 million individuals with schizophrenia is too high an estimate. In view of the criticisms, NIMH revised its estimate and claimed that schizophrenia affects approximately 1.1 percent of the adult (age eighteen and over) population during any given year. Based on the 2010 census data, that translates into 2.6 million Americans having schizophrenia at any given time.

However, 2.6 million people is a lot of people. It is approximately the same number of people who live in the metropolitan areas of Baltimore, Denver, Pittsburgh, or Tampa. Imagine every person in one of those cities having schizophrenia, and you will begin to appreciate the dimensions of the problem. Another way to express prevalence is the number of cases per 1,000 total population. At any given time, there are 8.4 cases of schizophrenia per 1,000 population. A town of 5,000 people would have about 42 cases; a city of 500,000 would have

4,200 cases; and a city or state of 5 million would have 42,000 cases. These numbers only include individuals with schizophrenia and do not include those with bipolar disorder, which, according to NIMH estimates, affects an additional 2.2 percent of the adult population.

Where are the 2.6 million people with schizophrenia in the United States? A large number of them are living in nursing homes, board-and-care homes, and similar facilities with varying names in different states. Another large group is in jails and prisons, the majority charged with misdemeanor crimes associated with our failure to treat them. Still another large group is living with their families or independently. A smaller but significant group of people with schizophrenia is homeless, living in public shelters, on streets, or under bridges. The smallest group is hospitalized in state hospitals, VA hospitals, or private hospitals, or in the psychiatric units of general hospitals.

Do Some Groups Have More Schizophrenia Than Others?

The distribution of schizophrenia among different geographical areas or ethnic groups, both in the United States and elsewhere, has intrigued researchers for almost two centuries. Although most textbooks assert that schizophrenia has approximately the same incidence (number of new cases) and prevalence (number of existing cases) everywhere in the world, that is clearly not the case. Studies published in 2005 by John McGrath and his colleagues demonstrate an approximately five-fold difference in both the incidence and prevalence of schizophrenia in different parts of the world.

The best-documented geographical difference is the urban risk factor, as discussed in chapter 5. Individuals who are born or raised in an urban area have approximately twice the risk of later being diagnosed with schizophrenia as individuals who are born or raised in a rural area. Suburban areas and small towns fall between these two extremes risk-wise.

Although not as well documented, there are also strong suggestions in the United States that schizophrenia is more prevalent in northern states and less prevalent in southern states. How much of that difference is attributable to the urban risk factor is not known.

Since a large proportion of the African American population lives in large cities, it is not surprising to find that African Americans as a whole have a higher rate of schizophrenia than whites. Five separate studies have confirmed this in highly urbanized states such as New York, Maryland, and Ohio. The higher rate of schizophrenia among African Americans holds up even when corrections are made for the age distribution of the population; thus, in a very careful study in Rochester, New York, African Americans still had a schizophrenia rate one and one-half times that of whites.

When African Americans who live in rural areas are compared with whites who live in rural areas, however, the results are different. Studies were done in Texas and in Louisiana, and no differences were found. This argues strongly against race being the cause of the difference. Rather, it suggests that it is because a higher proportion of African Americans live in the inner city that they have a higher schizophrenia rate. Others have claimed that African Americans appear to have a higher rate of schizophrenia because most psychiatrists are white and unconsciously (or consciously) racist and would more readily label an African Americans patient than a white patient as having schizophrenia. This may well be so but is impossible to measure. Even if it were so, however, it would explain only a small portion of the differences, and we are left with the fact that people in inner cities, whatever their race, have a disproportionately high schizophrenia rate.

Hispanic Americans, on the other hand, appear to have a lower schizophrenia prevalence rate than the general population. In the ECA study discussed above, the prevalence of schizophrenia among Hispanic residents of Los Angeles was less than half that of non-Hispanic residents, confirming the comparatively low prevalence of schizophrenia found in a previous study of Mexican-American residents of Texas.

There are other groups in America that also appear to have a low prevalence of schizophrenia. An extensive study of the rural, communal-living Hutterites published in 1955 reported a schizophrenia prevalence of only 1.1 per 1,000; more recent follow-up studies have confirmed that the Hutterites have continued to have a very low rate of schizophrenia. Studies of the rural Amish have also reported few cases of schizophrenia but a higher rate of bipolar disorder. There have also been impressions reported for over a hundred years that Native Americans have a comparatively low prevalence of schizophrenia, but this has yet to be verified by a careful study.

Studies comparing the prevalence of schizophrenia elsewhere in the world have, until recently, provoked lively controversy among researchers. On one side were those who believed that most reported differences were methodological artifacts or of minor consequence; on the other side were those (including myself) who believed that the differences were real and might provide important clues regarding the causes of the disease. This controversy was settled by the studies of McGrath and his colleagues, who analyzed prevalence and incidence studies from all over the world and concluded that there is indeed at least a *fivefold difference* in the prevalence and incidence of schizophrenia in different areas of the world. It should be pointed out that all major diseases in which both genetic and nongenetic factors are thought to play a role show significant differences in geographic distribution. Heart disease varies approximately sixfold, rheumatoid arthritis tenfold, insulin-dependent diabetes thirtyfold, and multiple sclerosis fiftyfold; some cancers show even greater differences. Schizophrenia would be a unique disease if its prevalence were approximately the same everywhere in the world. The surprising finding, then, would be not that such differences exist, but rather that they do not exist.

By world standards the United States' schizophrenia prevalence rate of 8 per 1,000 is comparatively high. At the lower end of the spectrum are studies from countries such as Ghana, Botswana, Papua New Guinea, and Taiwan with prevalence rates of less than 2 per 1,000. Studies from Canada and from most European and Asian nations fall into the 3 to 6 per 1,000 prevalence range. In addition to the United States, countries that have reported schizophrenia prevalence rates higher than 7 per 1,000 are Ireland, Finland, and Sweden, with a study from northern Sweden reporting the highest rate (17 per 1,000).

Several studies of schizophrenia's prevalence have yielded especially interesting results. Careful studies in Croatia, for example, have shown that villages on the Istrian peninsula have a schizophrenia prevalence rate of 7.3 per 1,000 compared with villages a hundred miles away that have a rate of only 2.9 per 1,000. In Micronesia two surveys found a fourfold difference among various islands, from a low of 4.2 per 1,000 in the Marshall Islands to a high of 16.7 per 1,000 on Palau.

In India nine separate studies have reported that the prevalence of schizophrenia is significantly higher among higher castes than among lower castes.

Ireland is another nation in which schizophrenia has been extensively studied because of reports dating to the last century of a high prevalence both among people who emigrated to other countries and among those who remained in Ireland. As early as 1808, it was claimed that in Ireland "insanity is a disease of as frequent occurrence as in any other country in Europe." Studies in the 1960s and 1970s established that Ireland had more hospitalized patients with schizophrenia per capita than any country in the world, and a three-country community case register reported a schizophrenia prevalence rate of 7.1 per 1,000 in one of the western counties. In 1982 I spent six months in western Ireland studying a small region thought to have an especially high prevalence of schizophrenia; its rate of 12.6 per 1,000 was more than twice that of the surrounding area. This 1982 study also indicated that the high schizophrenia rate in Ireland existed only in older people and not among younger people; subsequent studies have since confirmed that the Irish schizophrenia prevalence rate is lower for individuals born after 1940, suggesting that a change in prevalence, for some unknown reason, took place at approximately that time.

In recent years much interest has been generated by studies of schizophrenia among Caribbean immigrants to England. Such immigrants have been found to have a high schizophrenia prevalence rate that exists not only in the immigrants themselves but also in their offspring born in England. A study in south London, in an area in which many of the Caribbean immigrants live, reported what is perhaps the highest incidence of schizophrenia reported anywhere in the world; the Afro-Caribbean immigrants had a schizophrenia prevalence rate nine times higher than the rate for British whites. Studies in Jamaica, the country of origin of the largest number of Caribbean immigrants, indicate that the schizophrenia rate there is not especially high. Studies in the Netherlands and in Sweden have also reported unusually high rates of schizophrenia among some, but not all, immigrant groups. A summary of these studies suggested that the immigrants themselves have a more than twofold risk of developing schizophrenia and that their first-generation offspring have a more than fourfold risk. The high prevalence among immigrants does not appear to be due to stress.

These are intriguing observations and, in my opinion, may offer important clues to the causes of schizophrenia. If we can understand why the Caribbean immigrants or the western Irish or the Croatian villagers have more than their share of schizophrenia, or why the Hutterites have less than their share, then we may better understand its causes. Sadly, however, this research area has been relatively neglected, especially in the United States.

Is Schizophrenia Increasing or Decreasing?

As noted above, there is evidence in Ireland that the prevalence rate of schizophrenia decreased in recent decades. Since 1985 similar results have been published from studies in Scotland, England, Denmark, Australia, and New Zealand. The average decrease in schizophrenia in these studies is 35 percent over a ten- to twenty-year period. Such studies have been criticized, however, because changing definitions and diagnostic standards make comparisons problematic. Therefore, at this time it can only be said that there is a *suggestion* of a decreasing prevalence of schizophrenia in these countries but that it remains to be confirmed by methodologically careful studies.

Studies in the United States suggest the possibility of a different story. Although no study comparable to the 1980–1984 five-site ECA study was done in the past, independent studies were done at two of the same sites. In Baltimore, a study in 1936 reported a one-year schizophrenia prevalence rate of 2.9 per 1,000. The ECA study, carried out in the same part of Baltimore in 1980–1984, found a six-month rate more than three times as high. Similarly, in New Haven the 1958 study by Hollingshead and Redlich found a six-month schizophrenia prevalence rate of 3.6 per 1,000, whereas the six-month rate for the ECA study was more than twice as high. Case-finding was more complete in the ECA study because a random sampling technique was used, and this would tend to elevate the ECA prevalence rates. However, a narrower definition of schizophrenia was used in the ECA study, which would tend to lower its prevalence rates compared to the two earlier studies. These differences should at least partially cancel each other out.

Despite the numerous methodological problems of the above studies, one is left with an impression that the prevalence of schizophrenia may have increased in the United States in recent decades. This impression is further strengthened by the very high incidence of *new* cases of schizophrenia reported from the ECA study sites. In summary, in the United States schizophrenia may have recently increased, and may still be increasing, in prevalence; this would stand in contrast to several other countries in which schizophrenia may possibly be decreasing in prevalence.

Is Schizophrenia of Recent Origin?

The history of schizophrenia is a curious one that has provoked a lively debate among scholars. On one side are those who claim that "schizophrenia has existed throughout history. . . . There is definite evidence in support of the view that schizophrenia is an ancient illness." Advocates of this view cite early Sanskrit, Babylonian, and biblical figures such as Nebuchadnezzar (who ate "grass as oxen" for seven years) and Ezekiel (who had visual and auditory hallucinations) to support their claims. They also argue that individuals with schizophrenia were kept at home or were considered to be divinely inspired and so were not defined as sick. The other side (which includes myself) acknowledges that there were indeed some people who had brain damage (e.g., from birth injuries or traumas) or brain diseases (e.g., epilepsy, syphilis, or viral encephalitis) that may have produced psychotic symptoms, but that schizophrenia with its hallmark auditory hallucinations and onset in early adulthood was practically never described.

A stronger argument can be made for the existence of occasional cases of schizophrenia beginning in the late Middle Ages. A few small psychiatric hospitals were opened such as Bethlem Hospital (which gave birth to the term "bedlam") in London. King Henry VI, who lived from 1421 to 1471, appears to have had a schizophrenia-like disorder. William Shakespeare selected Henry VI as the subject for his first play in 1591. In *Hamlet* (1601) Shakespeare had Hamlet feign lunacy and Ophelia become insane when she discovered that her father had been killed by the man she loved. Nigel Bark makes a strong case that Poor Mad Tom in *King Lear* (1605) had schizophrenia but also concedes it is possible that he was merely feigning madness. One schizophrenia expert claims that the autobiography of George Trosse, an English minister who, as a young man in 1656, developed delusions, auditory hallucinations, and catatonic behavior, is a description of schizophrenia, but another asserts that alcoholic psychosis was the more likely cause for Trosse's symptoms.

Sporadic cases of what may have been schizophrenia continued to appear in the early 1700s but were remarkably few in number. They increased in the latter 1700s and then, suddenly, at the turn of the century, schizophrenia appeared in unmistakable form. Simultaneously (and apparently independently) John Haslam in England and Philippe Pinel in France in the early 1800s both described cases that were certainly schizophrenia. These cases were followed by a veritable outpouring of descriptions continuing throughout the nineteenth century and also by evidence that schizophrenia was increasing in frequency. It was a dramatic entrance for a disease. Haslam's publication in 1809 was an enlarged second edition of his 1798 book *Observations on Insanity*. It is a remarkable book, with descriptions of delusions, hallucinations, disorders of thinking, and even autopsy accounts of abnormalities in the brains of some of the patients. His descriptions of patients leave no doubt that he was describing what we now call schizophrenia. In 1810 Haslam published an extended description of one patient with schizophrenia, titling it "Illustrations of Madness: Exhibiting a Singular Case of Insanity," which suggested that such cases were very unusual at that time.

From the observations of John Haslam and Philippe Pinel until the end of the nineteenth century there were continuing arguments in Europe about whether insanity was increasing and, if so, why. As early as 1829 Sir Andrew Halliday warned that "the numbers of the afflicted have more than tripled during the last twenty years," and in 1835 J. C. Prichard added that "the apparent increase is everywhere so striking . . . cases of insanity are far more numerous than formerly." In 1856 in France, E. Renaudin published extensive data demonstrating an increase in insanity, especially among young adults and in urban areas, and the following year in England, John Hawkes wrote: "I doubt if ever the history of the world, or the experience of past ages, could show a larger amount of insanity than that of the present day." By 1873 Harrington Tuke warned that "a great wave of insanity is slowly advancing," and three years later Robert Jamieson added that "the most remarkable phenomenon of our time has been the alarming increase of insanity."

Those who believed that the increase in insanity was real offered a variety of possible explanations, ranging from genetics (e.g., increasing consanguineous marriages) and the increasing complexity of civilization to increased masturbation, use of alcohol, or train travel. Those who argued that the increase was not real claimed that it was a statistical artifact due to increased life expectancy of individuals with mental illnesses, part of a social movement to confine troublesome persons to institutions, or the product of increasing industrialization whereby families left home to work and so could no longer maintain their sick relative at home. Dr. Edward Hare in England analyzed these arguments in detail and concluded that the nineteenth century increase in insanity was most probably real. More recently, I coauthored a book, *The Invisible Plague*, on this subject and also concluded that insanity really did increase.

In the United States an awareness of a possible increase in insanity appears to have taken place somewhat later than in Europe. The first American hospital exclusively for mentally ill individuals opened in Williamsburg, Virginia, in 1773 with twenty-four beds, but it was not full for over thirty years. Not a single hospital was opened in the forty-three-year period between 1773 and 1816, but twenty-two hospitals were added between 1816 and 1846.

The accompanying graph illustrates the per capita increase in patients in public mental hospitals in the United States from 1830 to 1950. The initial alarm about increasing insanity in America was sounded in 1852 by Pliny Earle, one of the founders of the American Psychiatric Association, who warned that "insanity is an increasing disease." In 1854 Edward Jarvis undertook an extensive census of insane persons in Massachusetts and became convinced that their numbers were increasing; in 1871 Jarvis wrote that "the successive reports, upon whatever source or means of information procured, all tend to show an increasing number of the insane." In 1894 the superintendent of one Massachusetts state psychiatric hospital added that "the insane have increased twice as fast as the whole people. . . . We find this insane accumulation going on as fast as 50 years ago."

Deinstitutionalization: A Cradle for Catastrophe

During the first half of the twentieth century the number of patients in public psychiatric hospitals in the United States increased three-and-one-half-fold, from 144,653 in 1903 to 512,501 in 1950. The per capita increase based on population was almost twofold. The largest single diagnostic group was patients with schizophrenia. The problem of increasing numbers of persons with schizophrenia received remarkably little public attention, however, until World War II, when two events conspired to bring mental illness to center stage.

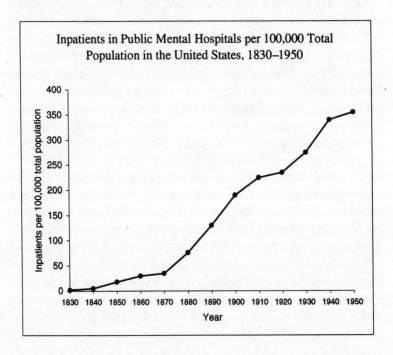

The first event was the extraordinarily high number of young men who were rejected for induction into military service because of mental illness. General Lewis B. Hershey, testifying before House and Senate hearings after the war, asserted that 856,000 men, representing 18 percent of all possible draftees, had been rejected because of mental illness. The second event was the assignment of approximately 3,000 conscientious objectors, who refused to take up arms, to alternate duty in state psychiatric hospitals. These "conchies," as they were popularly called, included many idealistic young Quakers, Mennonites, and Methodists who were appalled by the inhumane conditions they found in the hospitals. They went to the press, organized reports, and testified before Congress regarding these conditions. Kentucky, for example, was said to be spending only $146.11 per hospitalized psychiatric patient *per year*. And during a twelve-year period at St. Elizabeths Hospital in Washington, D.C., twenty patients were said to have been killed by hospital staff members but "no convictions were had in respect of any such cases."

On May 6, 1946, *Life* magazine published a thirteen-page exposé of conditions in state psychiatric hospitals titled "Bedlam 1946: Most U.S. Mental Hospitals Are a Shame and a Disgrace." It was based on the reports of the conscientious objectors and included pictures of naked patients living in filthy conditions. That same month *Reader's Digest* included a condensation of a new novel by Mary Jane Ward titled *The Snake Pit*, which detailed the terrifying experiences of a woman confined to a psychiatric hospital. In September 1946, Mike Gorman, a young reporter with the *Daily Oklahoman*, published a scathing series of articles about Oklahoma's state psychiatric hospitals (e.g., "the dining room made Dante's *Inferno* seem like a country club"), which was published as a book the following year. In 1948 Albert Deutsch published *The Shame of the States*, based on visits to psychiatric hospitals in twelve states. Deutsch claimed that "in some of the wards there were scenes that rivaled the horrors of the Nazi concentration camps—hundreds of naked mental patients herded into huge, barn-like, filth-infested wards," and he included pictures to prove his point. The problem of the mentally ill in America had been etched into the nation's consciousness and conscience as nothing had previously done.

The stage was set for deinstitutionalization, and the introduc-

The Magnitude of Deinstitutionalization: Number of
Patients in Public Mental Hospitals, 1950–2005

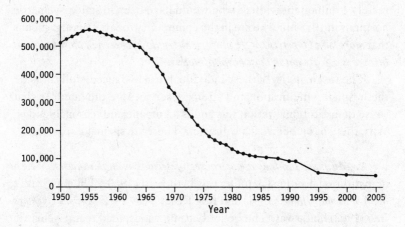

tion in the 1950s of chlorpromazine and reserpine, the first effective
antipsychotic drugs, made it more feasible. The election of John F.
Kennedy as president in 1960 provided the impetus and funds for
emptying the hospitals. Kennedy's younger sister had been publicly
identified as mentally retarded but, as discussed in chapter 3, had also
developed schizophrenia and undergone a lobotomy. Kennedy therefore championed the mentally retarded and the mentally ill and proposed a series of federally funded Community Mental Health Centers
(CMHCs) that, it was said, would function as alternatives to state psychiatric hospitals. In his introduction of the CMHC proposal, Kennedy
specifically noted that "it has been demonstrated that two out of three
schizophrenics—our largest category of mentally ill—can be treated
and released within six months." It was to be the launching of a psychiatric *Titanic*, the largest failed social experiment of twentieth-century
America.

The magnitude of deinstitutionalization is difficult to compre-
hend. In 1955 there were 559,000 seriously mentally ill individuals in
state psychiatric hospitals. In 2015 there were approximately 35,000.
Based on the nation's population increase between 1955 and 2010

from 166 million to 309 million, if there were the same number of patients per capita in the hospitals today as there were in 1955, their total number today would be 1,040,000. This means that there are approximately 1 million individuals who would have been in state psychiatric hospitals in 1955 but who are in the community today. This also means that *more than 96 percent of the people who would have been in those hospitals fifty years ago are not in those hospitals today.*

The vast majority of these individuals can live successfully outside the hospital *if* medication and aftercare services are provided. In that sense deinstitutionalization was and is a humane and reasonable idea. Why, then, has it been such a disaster? There are six major reasons:

1. *Misunderstanding about causes of serious mental illnesses.* When deinstitutionalization got under way in the early 1960s, Thomas Szasz's *Myth of Mental Illness* (1961) and Ken Kesey's *One Flew Over the Cuckoo's Nest* (1962) held sway. The belief became widespread that psychiatric hospitalization *caused* mental illness; that as soon as you released the patients, they would live happily ever after. It was a romantic view but in retrospect incorrect and remarkably naive.

2. *Failure to shift resources from hospitals to community programs.* Despite the massive shift of patients from hospitals to the community, personnel and fiscal resources did not follow them. In New York State, for example, the state hospital patients population was reduced from 93,000 to 24,000 over twenty-five years, yet during the same period not a single hospital was closed and the total number of state hospital employees *increased* from 23,800 to 37,000. The main impediments to shifting resources were unions and powerful members of state legislatures from rural districts in which the state hospital was the largest employer.

3. *Failure of Community Mental Health Centers (CMHCs).* The $3 billion federal CMHC program was a failure from the start. The National Institute of Mental Health provided vague guidelines and almost no oversight and bypassed state departments of mental health, thereby ensuring that there would be no cooperation between state hospitals and the CMHCs. Approximately 5 percent of the 789 federally funded CMHCs took responsibility for the patients being discharged

from the hospitals, whereas the remainder evolved into being counseling and psychotherapy centers for family and personal problems. Some CMHCs built swimming pools and tennis courts with the federal funds, and one Florida CMHC, using a federal staffing grant, even hired swimming instructors.

4. *Lawyers as destructive forces.* Between 1965 and 1990, when deinstitutionalization was taking place, the number of lawyers in America increased from 296,000 to 800,000 more than four times faster than the general population. Some of the lawyers read Szasz's *Myth of Mental Illness* and dedicated their careers to bringing lawsuits against states to get mental patients released from state hospitals, making it more difficult to involuntarily hospitalize or treat them, and passing state legislation to effectively hasten deinstitutionalization. Through organizations such as the American Civil Liberties Union and the Bazelon Center for Mental Health Law (previously known as the Mental Health Law Project), these lawyers accomplished their goals. The numbers of mentally ill homeless persons, with freedom to be perpetually psychotic, are a living testimony to their success.

5. *Mental health professionals as unavailable.* Federal subsidies for the training of psychiatrists, psychologists, and psychiatric social workers began in 1948 and twenty years later had reached $119 million per year. State subsidies were even more generous. The professionals, however, were trained to be mental *health*, not mental *illness*, professionals. No service payback was required in exchange for their publicly subsidized training, so the vast majority of them went immediately to the private practice of psychotherapy. A 1980 survey of private practitioners found that only 6 percent of patients seen by psychiatrists and 3 percent of patients seen by psychologists had ever been hospitalized for mental illness. For most deinstitutionalized individuals with schizophrenia and other serious mental illnesses, the professionals were unavailable.

6. *Federal incentives to empty the hospitals and the IMD exclusion.* Following passage of the federal CMHC legislation, seriously mentally ill individuals being discharged from the hospitals were made eligible

for federal Medicaid, Medicare, Supplemental Security Income (SSI), Social Security Disability Insurance (SSDI), food stamps, special housing, and other programs. In effect, this meant that as long as such individuals were in state mental hospitals, they were the fiscal responsibility of the states; once discharged, however, the majority of the fiscal responsibility for their care was shifted to the federal government. The largest federal incentive to empty state hospitals, as noted above, was the Institutions for Mental Disease (IMD) exclusion, whereby federal Medicaid does not reimburse states for patients in state hospitals but does pay for the patients' care once they are transferred to "semihospitals" not run by the state.

Here is how the IMD exclusion works. In 2000 an individual with schizophrenia in Portland, Oregon, might have been hospitalized in the Oregon State Hospital. The cost was $315 per day, or $114,975 per year. The federal government would have reimbursed Oregon for *none* of the costs because of the IMD exclusion, so the state would have paid the entire cost. However, if the state denied that person with schizophrenia admission to the state hospital and insisted instead on admitting him/her to a "semihosptal" that cost $229 per day, the federal government would have reimbursed Oregon $93 per day, thereby saving the state $65,335 per year compared to the state hospital. And if the state instead admitted the person to a residential facility that cost $126 per day, the federal government would have reimbursed Oregon $76 per day, thereby saving the state $96,725 per year compared to the state hospital. States had, and continue to have, a huge fiscal incentive to shut down state hospitals and hospitalize individuals with schizophrenia anywhere else, regardless of the clinical needs of the patient. The fiscal incentives come entirely from denying intensive hospitalization and emptying the state hospitals; there is no fiscal incentive whatever to provide aftercare. It did not take the states long to learn how to game the system, and this has been a major contributor to the failure of deinstitutionalization.

Given these mistakes, it is no wonder that deinstitutionalization has been a massive failure. Homelessness, jails, violence, victimization, abysmal housing, revolving doors, few professionals, minimal treatment—these consequences were entirely predictable. I could ask the most thought-disordered individual with schizophrenia to set up a scheme for deinstitutionalization and the product would be better than what we have.

Who should be blamed? Blaming conservative politicians, especially former President Reagan, has become the politically correct but factually incorrect answer frequently given by mental health professionals. In fact, the debacle of deinstitutionalization has taken place under five Democratic (Kennedy, Johnson, Carter, Clinton, and Obama) and six Republican (Nixon, Ford, Reagan, Bush, Bush, and Trump) presidents. The *real* blame for the failure of deinstitutionalization rests squarely on the shoulders of the psychiatrists, psychologists, psychiatric social workers, lawyers, and federal and state officials who were, and continue to be, responsible for it.

What Is the Cost of Schizophrenia?

To ask a question about the cost of schizophrenia is, in one sense, meaningless. Anyone who is familiar with schizophrenia knows that its magnitude and tragedy are light-years beyond calculation in dollars and cents. At the same time we live in a society with finite resources, and whether we like it or not, cost-benefit thinking is part of the allocation of those resources. The decision-making process is a political one in which—either explicitly or implicitly—questions are asked such as the following: How much does the disease cost? How much money can be saved by finding better treatments? What is the cost-benefit ratio of spending more research funds on this disease? Because such questions arise, it is important to ascertain the cost of schizophrenia.

The cost of schizophrenia, like any disease, can be calculated in a variety of ways. The economic cost for treating a single case of the disease can be assessed. Or the cost of treating all known cases can be added together. Lost wages because of the disease can be added, as well as the cost of social support (e.g., room and board, rehabilitation programs) needed to keep the person functioning over many years. The cost for treating schizophrenia can also be compared with the cost for treating other diseases, such as heart disease. Finally, but most difficult, the noneconomic cost of schizophrenia can be considered.

The cost for treating schizophrenia in cases in which the person recovers completely is not unreasonable compared with other serious diseases. The person usually requires hospitalization for a few weeks and then medication for several months. However, if the person is not among the fortunate one-quarter of patients who recover completely (see chapter 4), then the costs multiply rapidly.

Estimates have been made of the cost of direct care for treating a single case, for example Sylvia Frumkin, the woman described in Susan Sheehan's *Is There No Place On Earth for Me?* Over eighteen years, she had twenty-seven different admissions to hospitals for schizophrenia. The total cost of her care in 1984 was estimated to be $636,000, which included only hospitalizations, halfway houses, and foster homes. It did not include outpatient medication costs, emergency room services, general health care, social services, law enforcement services needed to return her to the hospital, legal services, court costs, lost wages, or even the direct care costs incurred by Ms. Frumkin's family. I have made a similar approximation of direct care costs for my sister, who had schizophrenia for more than fifty-three years and required hospitalization for long periods; the direct care costs for her hospitalization alone in New York State mental hospitals during that time total over $3 million. Such costs, I would submit, are not unusual for persons with severe schizophrenia.

Two older studies were carried out to calculate the direct costs (e.g., hospitalization costs, medication) as well as the indirect costs (e.g., lost wages) for everyone in the United States who had schizophrenia. One study, done by Drs. Dorothy Rice and Leonard Miller at the University of California, calculated the total cost of schizophrenia for 1990 at $32.5 billion. The other study, done by Dr. Richard Wyatt and colleagues at the National Institute of Mental Health, calculated the cost for 1991 at $65 billion. The two studies were similar in their estimates of direct costs ($19.5 and $18.6 billion, respectively) but differed substantially in estimates of indirect costs such as family caregiving, lost wages, and the losses due to suicides. Remarkably little hard data are available on which to base estimates of indirect costs.

A more recent estimate of the cost of schizophrenia in the United States used data from 2002. Direct health care costs, including inpatient and outpatient services, were estimated to be $22.7 billion. Direct non–health care costs, including the costs of law enforcement and public shelters, were estimated to be $9.3 billion. Indirect costs, including lost wages, were estimated to be $32.4 billion. The total cost, therefore, was said to be $64.4 billion per year, remarkably close to the estimate by Wyatt et al. for 1991. The 2002 study is almost certainly a serious underestimate, however, since it was based on a schizophrenia prevalence estimate of 0.5 percent of the population, less than half the 1.1 percent prevalence now widely used.

The most recent estimate of the economic burden of schizophrenia was based on 2013 data by Cloutier et al. (see "Recommended Further Reading"). They estimated the total annual cost to be $155.7 billion, more than twice the estimated cost in 2002. The excess direct health care costs (e.g., hospitalization, outpatient services) were estimated to be $37.7 billion, compared to $22.7 billion in 2002. The direct non–health care costs (e.g., jails and homeless shelters) in 2013 were estimated to be $9.3 billion, exactly the same as the estimate for 2002. The main difference in 2013 compared to 2002 was the $117.3 billion estimate for indirect costs (e.g., reduced work productivity, caregiving, premature mortality), compared to $32.4 billion in 2002.

A major reason why schizophrenia is such an expensive disease is that it usually begins in early adulthood and often lasts until death fifty or more years later. People who get the disease have been raised and educated through childhood and adolescence, with all the costs associated, only to become disabled at precisely the time they are supposed to become economically contributing members of society. Most of the 2.6 million persons with this disease continue to require services such as occasional hospitalization, foster homes, subsidized income, court costs, social services, outpatient psychiatric services, etc. People with schizophrenia are not beyond their economically most productive years when they become sick, as are patients with Alzheimer's disease. Nor do they die relatively quickly, such as happens to many patients with cancer. If a fiendish economist from another planet were trying to devise a disease that would force our society to incur the maximum costs, then he (or she) could not do better than schizophrenia. Schizophrenia is economically a three-time loser: society must raise and educate the person destined to become afflicted, most people with the disease are unable to contribute economically to society, and at the same time many of them require costly services from society for the rest of their lives.

The cost of schizophrenia has also been compared with other diseases. In Australia the direct and indirect costs for schizophrenia were compared with heart attacks. Despite the fact that heart attacks affect twelve times more people than schizophrenia does in Australia, the overall direct and indirect costs per case of schizophrenia are six times greater than those for heart attacks. These costs did not include pension or Social Security costs that, since persons with schizophrenia live much longer than persons with heart attacks, would make the disparity even greater.

The huge economic cost of schizophrenia leads directly to the question of economic benefits of research on this disease. Schizophrenia is one of the most under-researched diseases in the Western world. In the Australian study referred to above, for example, it was found that research on schizophrenia received only one-fourteenth the funds spent on research on heart attacks. In terms of the relative cost of these diseases to society, this is a foolish allocation of research funds on economic grounds alone. In the United States a calculation was made in 1984 that if research discoveries could have reduced the cost of schizophrenia by only 10 percent by 1998, the savings that would have accrued over the following decade would have totaled $180 billion.

From a public policy viewpoint, therefore, it would be wise to spend more research money on the causes and treatment of schizophrenia. The burden of schizophrenia to taxpayers is substantial; this was noted as early as 1855 by the Massachusetts Commission on Lunacy, which said:

> In whatever way we look at them, these lunatics are a burden upon the Commonwealth. The curable during their limited period of disease, and the incurable during the remainder of their lives, not only cease to produce, but they must eat the bread they do not earn, and consume the substance they do not create, receiving their sustenance from the treasury of the Commonwealth.

The greatest cost of schizophrenia, however, is the noneconomic costs to those who have the disease and to their families. These costs are incalculable. They include the effects of growing up normally until early adulthood, then being diagnosed with a brain disease that may last for the rest of your life. Hopes, plans, expectations, and dreams are abruptly put on hold. Cerebral palsy and Down's syndrome are tragedies for families of newborns; cancer and Alzheimer's disease are tragedies for families of the elderly. There is no known disease, however, with noneconomic costs so great as for schizophrenia. It is the costliest disease of all.

Recommended Further Reading

Cloutier, M., M. S. Aigbogun, A. Guerin, et al. "The Economic Burden of Schizophrenia in the United States in 2013." *Journal of Clinical Psychiatry* 77 (2016): 764–71.

Geller, J. L. "Excluding Institutions for Mental Diseases from Federal Reimbursement for Services: Strategy or Tragedy?" *Psychiatric Services* 51 (2000): 1397–1403.

Hare, E. "Was Insanity on the Increase?" *British Journal of Psychiatry* 142 (1983): 439–55.

Isaac, R. J., and V. C. Armat. *Madness in the Streets.* New York: Free Press, 1990.

James, D. J., and L. E. Glaze. *Mental Health Problems of Prison and Jail Inmates.* Washington, D.C.: U.S. Department of Justice, 2006.

McGrath, J. J. "Myths and Plain Truths about Schizophrenia Epidemiology—the NAPE Lecture 2004." *Acta Psychiatrica Scandinavica* 111 (2005): 4–11.

Saha, S., D. Chant, J. Welham, et al. "A Systematic Review of the Prevalence of Schizophrenia." *PLoS Medicine* 2 (2005): e141.

Torrey, E. F. *Nowhere to Go: The Tragic Odyssey of the Homeless Mentally Ill.* New York: Harper and Row, 1988.

Torrey, E. F. *Out of the Shadows: Confronting America's Mental Illness Crisis.* New York: John Wiley and Sons, 1997.

Torrey, E. F. *Schizophrenia and Civilization.* New York: Jason Aronson, 1980.

Torrey, E. F., and J. Miller. *The Invisible Plague: Rising Insanity from 1750 to the Present.* New Brunswick, N.J.: Rutgers University Press, 2001.

Torrey, E. F. *The Insanity Offense: How America's Failure to Treat the Seriously Mentally Ill Endangers Its Citizens.* New York: W. W. Norton, revised paperback edition, 2012.

Torrey, E.F. *American Psychosis: How the Federal Government Destroyed the Mental Illness Treatment System.* New York: Oxford University Press, 2014.

Wu, E. Q., H. G. Birnbaum, L. Shi, et al. "The Economic Burden of Schizophrenia in the United States in 2002." *Journal of Clinical Psychiatry* 66 (2005): 1122–29.

15

Issues for Advocates

And, once more, we may say, that we have reason to plead for this class, because they cannot plead for themselves. It is one of the evils of insanity, that it cannot gain a fair hearing, or make known its wants. It laughs in horrid mirth, while coals of fire are on its head. It shrinks and shudders before the phantoms of its own creation. It sits in morbid silence while disease is gnawing upon its life. The insane plead not for themselves, but will not every generous heart feel yet more for them, in remembrance of their forlorn condition?
Robert Waterston, 1843

They say, "Nothing can be done here!"
I reply, "I know no such word in the vocabulary I adopt!"
Dorothea Dix, 1848

Dorothea Dix was an extremely effective advocate for persons with serious mental illnesses. She went into the poorhouses and jails to witness the atrocious conditions. She emphasized that mentally ill persons are not hopeless cases but rather can function much better if given adequate care and humane living conditions. She testified before innumerable state legislatures and investigatory commissions, always emphasizing the consequences of poor psychiatric care for individuals. She confronted and embarrassed officials, from local clerks to governors, publicly accusing them of not doing their jobs. Most important, she never took "no" for an answer.

Dorothea Dix has much to teach us today. Although not every patient and family member can achieve her stature as an advocate, we all can do some work to improve the lives of people with schizophrenia. If we would do so, it is useful to keep in mind the following four general principles.

THE FOUR PRINCIPLES OF ADVOCACY

1. Master the facts of the situation. Credibility comes from facts, not merely from emotions.

2. Many people with schizophrenia make excellent advocates for trying to improve services. There is no substitute for the credibility that comes from having had schizophrenia or another serious mental disorder.

3. Put everything in writing, including your summary of meetings with officials. Send copies to everyone concerned. Officials can deny ever hearing you say something, but it is much more difficult for them to deny having received your letter when you have a copy of it.

4. Be careful of being co-opted. Politicians are experts at verbally agreeing with people and then doing nothing. Judge public officials by what they do, not by what they say. Don't accept crumbs when what is needed is a seven-course meal.

Advocacy Organizations

Improving services and research for people with schizophrenia necessitates understanding how the system works. Until the 1960s, almost all decisions for public services for mentally ill individuals rested at the state level. Since then, the decision making has become much more complex. As noted in chapter 14, the federal government has become the major player in funding services, mostly through Medicaid reimbursement. Many states, meanwhile, have attempted to shift their remaining responsibility for services to the counties or cities, although the state government is still ultimately responsible. Thus, advocacy efforts, to be effective, must often be carried out at all three levels—federal, state, and local.

Effective advocacy for individuals with schizophrenia did not begin until the 1980s. Prior to that time, the organizations that might have been expected to provide leadership for individuals with schizophrenia neglected this patient population.

Present advocacy organizations include the following:

Treatment Advocacy Center (TAC): By way of full disclosure, I founded TAC in 1998 and continue to be an active member. In addition, all royalties from the sale of this book go to TAC. Based in Arlington, Virginia, TAC advocates exclusively for individuals with severe psychiatric disorders, mostly with diagnoses of schizophrenia, bipolar disorder, and severe depression with psychotic features. It has focused on such problems as mentally ill people in jails and prisons, those who are homeless, those being victimized, and those who have committed suicide or violent acts because of a lack of treatment. TAC attempts to change state laws to make it easier to treat affected individuals before they suffer the consequences of nontreatment. TAC was instrumental in passing Kendra's Law in New York State and Laura's Law in California and has improved laws for the treatment of mentally ill people in thirty-five other states. TAC also played a significant role in the passage in 2016 of the 21st Century Cures Act, including the establishment of the position of Assistant Secretary for Mental Health in the Department of Health and Human Services. Assisted outpatient treatment (AOT) (see chapter 10) has been a central focus of TAC's advocacy efforts and has been shown to significantly reduce hospitalizations, incarcerations, homelessness, and violent behavior of mentally ill individuals and to save money. Recently it has also focused advocacy efforts on increasing the supply of public psychiatric beds, the reform of HIPAA, and the abolition of the IMD exclusion. TAC is completely funded by foundations and private donations and does not accept contributions from pharmaceutical companies. Its website is www.treatmentadvocacycenter.org.

MentalIllnessPolicyORG (MIPO): This organization was started in 2011 by D.J. Jaffe, who had also been one of the founders of TAC. MIPO works on many of the same issues as TAC and also played a significant role in the passage of the 21st Century Cures Act. Based in New York City, MIPO has also focused its advocacy efforts at improving mental illness treatment services in New York City and state. Of special note is the book published by Mr. Jaffe in 2017 which is essentially a handbook for would-be mental illness advocates: *Insane Consequences: How the Mental Health Industry Fails the Mentally Ill*. MIPO is completely funded by private donations. Its website is www.mentalillnesspolicy.org.

NAMI: NAMI, in Arlington, Virginia, was previously known as the National Alliance for the Mentally Ill. It was founded in 1979, an outgrowth of efforts by families in San Mateo County, California, and Madison, Wisconsin, to advocate for improved services for their seriously mentally ill relatives. Although it originally focused its efforts on the most severe psychiatric disorders, it subsequently broadened its agenda to include post-traumatic stress disorder (PTSD), anxiety disorders, and some personality disorders. NAMI's strength lies in its hundreds of local chapters, which provide education and support to individuals with mental illnesses and their families. Its Family-to-Family education programs (see chapter 11) have made a major contribution to improving public understanding of mental illnesses. At the national level, it has produced some important studies, such as ratings of the states, reports on state mental health budgets, and promotion of PACT programs (see chapter 9). Unfortunately, NAMI's effectiveness and credibility as an advocacy organization has been increasingly compromised at the national level by its heavy reliance on pharmaceutical company funding and at the state level by reliance on funding from state mental health agencies. NAMI's website is www.nami.org.

Mental Health America (MHA): Previously known as the National Mental Health Association, MHA is located in Alexandria, Virginia. It was founded in 1909 by Clifford Beers, who had manic-depressive illness (bipolar disorder), as an attempt to reform state psychiatric hospitals. Sadly, the organization was kidnapped first by psychoanalysts and later by mental health advocates, and its mission became as nebulous as it is all-inclusive. MHA posters ask: "Have you hugged your kid today?", which is nice for children but offers nothing for individuals with serious psychiatric disorders. At the local level, some MHA affiliates have contributed significantly to advocating for individuals with schizophrenia, including in Pittsburgh, Philadelphia, Dallas, Los Angeles, and Honolulu. However, at the national level it does virtually no schizophrenia-related advocacy. The MHA website is www.mentalhealthamerica.net.

Schizophrenia and Related Disorders Alliance of America (SARDAA): SARDAA is a continuation and expansion of Schizophrenics Anonymous, founded by the late Joanne Verbanic in Michigan. It focuses on providing support for individuals with this disorder, doing public education and advocacy. It's exclusive focus is schizophrenia and related psychoses. The website is www.sardaa.org.

NIMH and SAMHSA

Several federal agencies run programs that directly impact people with schizophrenia. For example, the Social Security Administration administers the SSDI and SSI programs (see chapter 8), and the Centers for Medicaid and Medicare Services (CMS) administers Medicaid and Medicare. The two federal government programs that should theoretically be advocates for people with schizophrenia are the National Institute of Mental Health (NIMH) and the Substance Abuse and Mental Health Services Administration (SAMHSA).

National Institute of Mental Health (NIMH): NIMH was created by Congress in 1946 in response to the increasing number of individuals with serious mental illnesses, as recognized during the drafting of soldiers to serve in World War II, and the deteriorating conditions in state psychiatric hospitals. Its original name was the National Neuropsychiatric Institute, but at the last minute mental health advocates got its name changed. Its original mission was to support research on serious psychiatric disorders and support the training of mental health professionals. Except for service demonstration projects, services for mentally ill people explicitly remained the responsibility of state and local governments, as it had been for more than a century.

Like many government agencies, NIMH's original mission got lost over time. Research-wise, it assumed responsibility for all behavioral science issues. Services-wise, it developed a program of federally funded Community Mental Health Centers, thereby shifting the fiscal responsibility for mentally ill people from the states to the federal government. A 2003 report found that less than 29 percent of NIMH's research grants had *any* relationship to serious mental illnesses, and only 6 percent of the grants were "reasonably likely to improve the treatment and quality of life for individuals presently affected" by serious mental illnesses. At the time, NIMH was supporting eighteen research grants to study how pigeons think but only one research grant on postpartum psychosis. In 2002, when Dr. Thomas Insel was appointed director of NIMH, the institute substantially increased its focus on schizophrenia and other severe mental illnesses, including the funding of a program to encourage the early treatment of schizophrenia (Recovery After an Initial Schizophrenia Episode or RAISE). In 2016, Dr. Joshua Gordon became the director of NIMH; his commitment to schizophrenia research and treatment has been minimal to date.

Substance Abuse and Mental Health Services Administration (SAMHSA): SAMHSA was formed in 1991 with an official mission to reduce "the impact of substance abuse and mental illness on America's communities." It has virtually ignored the "mental illness" part of its mandate. For example, in its plan *SAMHSA's Roles and Actions 2011–2014*, neither schizophrenia nor manic-depressive illness (bipolar disorder) is even mentioned in the 41,804-word document. Among its hundreds of publications, there are 194 on alcohol abuse, 5 on peer pressure, and 1 on "Hurricane Recovery Guides" and "Oil Spill Response," but not a single one on schizophrenia. Thus SAMHSA was a classic failed federal agency until 2016. Under the leadership of Congressman Tim Murphy from Pennsylvania, the 21st Century Cures Act was passed by Congress which, among other things, created an Assistant Secretary for Mental Health in the Department of Health and Human Services to oversee SAMHSA. Reform of the agency, long needed, is under way.

Educating the Public

One of the major reasons why services and research for schizophrenia have been so neglected is that most people do not understand this disease. The number of people who still believe that schizophrenia is a "split personality," for example, is shockingly high. We should not expect legislators or the public at large to support improved services or research unless we are willing to help educate them. Education, therefore, is one of the most important tasks for us all, and there are many different groups that need to be educated.

What you can do as an advocate:

• Develop a speakers' bureau and offer to talk to community service organizations (e.g., Kiwanis, Lions, Rotary), school assemblies, and local companies. Mr. and Ms. Ron Norris in Wilmington, Delaware, persuaded the Du Pont Corporation to fund the making of a film that can be used for such presentations. It is called "When the Music Stops" and is twenty minutes long.

• Organize an education campaign. For example, one group of families created "Nothing to Hide: Mental Illness in the Family," an exhibit of photographs and interviews with twenty families affected by severe mental illnesses.

• Schools are an especially fertile ground for education. Several NAMI state affiliates have developed working groups that target the schools. For example, in 1993 NAMI New York State developed a lesson plan on mental illness for grades 4–6, 7–8, and 9–12, then sent it to the health coordinators in every school district in the state and urged local NAMI members to encourage the health coordinator to use it.

• There are 344,000 churches, synagogues, and mosques in the United States. The clergy are often the first people consulted by individuals with schizophrenia and their families, so the clergy are natural allies. Offer to give a talk on schizophrenia to the congregation; Mental Illness Awareness Week is a good time to do so. NAMI Maine developed a Religious Outreach Committee to educate all clergy in the state. Pathways to Promise, which started as part of NAMI St. Louis, has attempted to educate clergy on a national level. Religious groups are the main providers of care for the homeless mentally ill, since these groups operate most public shelters; they are therefore aware of the vast numbers of untreated individuals with schizophrenia and are potentially strong allies in advocacy efforts.

• Establish contact with officials of local newspapers and radio and television stations. Encourage them to consider more coverage of the problems of the seriously mentally ill (e.g., an exposé of a rundown boardinghouse). Educate them about schizophrenia and bipolar disorder. Ask them to speak at a meeting of your support group.

• Educate mental health professionals-in-training by offering to make presentations to local nursing schools, schools of social work, university departments of psychology, schools of medicine, and psychiatric residency training programs.

• Initiate a dialogue between your group and the local psychiatric society. Ask them to make a presentation to your group and ask to make one to their group. Both sides will emerge with a better understanding of each other's problems and with ideas on how to be helpful to each other. The Northeast Ohio Alliance for the Mentally Ill in Cleveland has done this very effectively. Offer to write articles for the local or state APA newsletter, presenting your point of view on an issue for which you need their support.

• Educate lawyers and judges about schizophrenia. Request time to make a presentation to the monthly meeting of the local bar association and offer to teach a class at the law school.

• Offer to give a lecture to police trainees. Police officers come into frequent contact with individuals with schizophrenia on the street; the more education they have, the more humane will be the services they render.

• For all educational efforts, utilize informed patients whenever possible. They have much more credibility with laypersons than do either family members or professionals. They should—they have been there.

Decreasing Stigma

Decreasing the stigma associated with schizophrenia and other mental illnesses is a task for Sisyphus—every time you start to make some progress, the stone rolls back downhill and you must begin all over again. What repeatedly pushes the stone downhill are episodes of violence committed by individuals with schizophrenia or other severe psychiatric disorders.

As noted in chapter 13, research studies in both the United States and Europe have demonstrated that episodes of violence are the largest single cause of stigma against individuals with mental illness. Such studies suggest that it will be extremely difficult to decrease stigma against individuals with mental illnesses until the episodes of violence are decreased. This has not been widely recognized by some advocacy groups who prefer instead to deny that episodes of violence exist, or to suggest that the media not report them. This is the traditional stance of the ostrich, which does, indeed, keep the problem out of sight but simultaneously leaves important bodily areas exposed.

The single most important thing advocates can do to decrease stigma, therefore, is to support attempts to decrease violence. An important part of these attempts is the use of assisted treatment for individuals with severe mental illnesses who have limited awareness of their illness and who have demonstrated a propensity for violence. Dr. Richard Lamb made this point in an editorial when he said: "We can reduce stigma by doing what needs to be done to ensure that persons with severe mental illness who resist treatment receive the treatment they so clearly need." To claim that you are working to decrease stigma but that you oppose all assisted treatment is simply to identify yourself as an admirer of Sisyphus.

One other strategy to decrease the stigma against schizophrenia was carried out in Japan. The Japanese Society of Psychiatry and Neurology officially changed the term for schizophrenia from *Seishin-Bunretsu-Byo* (literally "mind-split-disease") to *Togo-Shitcho-Sho* ("integration disorder"). A study in 2009 reported that the old term was associated in the minds of the Japanese with being "criminal," but the new term was significantly less so. However, follow-up studies on the effect of the name change in 2015 and 2016 reported that it had had a very modest effect on the association of schizophrenia with dangerousness and overall little effect on newspaper coverage. There have also been proposals in the United States to change the term *schizophrenia* to something like *Haslam's disease* or *Pinel's disease*, Haslam and Pinel being the first to clearly describe schizophrenia at the beginning of the nineteenth century (see chapter 14). So far, nothing has come of such efforts.

How to Organize for Advocacy

Your advocacy efforts will be more effective if you have a well-organized and strong group. Numbers of members help, but in fact effective advocacy in most organizations is usually accomplished by a small number of its members. Individuals with schizophrenia, siblings, children of mentally ill individuals, spouses, parents, grandparents, friends, and mental illness professionals who are interested can all play important roles. Considering the fact that there are 2.6 million persons with schizophrenia today in the United States, a coalition of them, their families, and friends should theoretically be able to accomplish almost anything. To do so, however, it is necessary to get more of them out of the closets and into the streets. Some suggestions for doing so are the following:

• Increase membership in your local support group. Leave brochures for your group with all local mental illness professionals. Give brochures to drug salesmen who visit physicians. Leave leaflets on the windows of cars parked in the visitors lot of the state hospital. Put notices on community bulletin boards, in church bulletins, and in company and local newspapers. One NAMI group persuaded a grocery chain to print its name and telephone number on milk cartons. Another persuaded the telephone company to include information on their group with telephone bills.

• Organize special support groups for siblings, children of mentally ill individuals, wives and husbands, the parents of seriously mentally ill children, and individuals being treated in the VA system. These special support groups have been started by some state and local NAMI chapters.

• Enlist the help of the individuals who run the local homeless shelter and your local law enforcement officials, including the police, sheriffs, jail officials, and parole officers. These people are acutely aware of the failure of public services for individuals with serious mental illnesses. They are potentially excellent allies.

• Enlist the assistance of local civic groups that are also concerned about problems of individuals with severe mental illnesses. For example, some Kiwanis Clubs have been helpful, and the League of Women Voters in Illinois undertook a major survey of services for mentally ill individuals.

• Utilize the advocacy ideas on the websites listed in appendix B.

• Utilize the many advocacy suggestions in D.J. Jaffe's excellent book *Insane Consequences: How the Mental Health Industry Fails the Mentally Ill.*

• If *none* of the above suits your aptitudes or abilities and you still want to help, there is one thing left that you can do. As advocated in the movie *Network*, when fed up with existing conditions, you should lean out your window and yell loudly: "I'm mad as hell and I'm not going to take it anymore!" After doing this you will be forced to explain to your neighbors what is going on, and several more families will thereby become educated about schizophrenia.

Services for individuals with schizophrenia and other serious mental illnesses are not likely to improve until enough individuals become angry and get organized. Persons with schizophrenia will continue to be fourth-class citizens, leading twilight lives, often shunned, ignored, and neglected. They will continue to be, in the words of President Carter's Commission on Mental Health, "a minority within minorities. They are the most stigmatized of the mentally ill. They are politically and economically powerless and rarely speak for themselves. . . . They are the totally disenfranchised among us." The mad will become truly liberated only when those of us fortunate enough to have escaped the illness show how mad we really are.

In closing, I can do no better than to quote the closing lines of R. Walter Heinrichs' engaging book, *In Search of Madness: Schizophrenia and Neuroscience.* Heinrichs bravely wrestles with the entire corpus of recent schizophrenia research data, then concludes that, until we have

solved the problem, we are obligated to provide the best care possible
for those individuals who suffer from this disease:

> Schizophrenia is the flaw that is woven into the fabric of a child's life.
> It is the sudden wound in the mind's secret body, the hemorrhage of
> meaning disguised as wisdom. It is the clever voice, singing lies. It is
> the illness of the imagination, beyond imagination; beyond the com-
> fort of memory, beyond the reach of human tenderness and the hope
> of safety. It is the illness that conspires against love. It is the illness
> that forces what is intimate and what is alien into strange unions.
> It is the illness that comes and goes on a tide of chemistry and in
> its wake leaves a violent sorrow and a longing for the pleasures of
> darkness. Tomorrow may bring the answers that escaped in the past,
> the answers that lead to cause and cure. In the meantime, madness
> is among us and diminishes to the extent that we care for those who
> endure it.

Recommended Further Reading

Jaffe, D. J. *Insane Consequences: How the Mental Health Industry Fails the Mentally Ill.* Amherst, New York: Prometheus Books, 2017.

Torrey, E. F. *Out of the Shadows: Confronting America's Mental Illness Crisis.* New York: John Wiley and Sons, 1997.

Torrey, E. F. "Stigma and Violence: Isn't It Time to Connect the Dots?" *Schizophrenia Bulletin* 37 (2011): 892–96.

Torrey, E. F. *The Insanity Offense: How America's Failure to Treat the Seriously Mentally Ill Endangers Its Citizens.* New York: W. W. Norton, paperback edition, 2012.

Torrey, E. F., M. T. Zdanowicz, S. M. Wolfe, et al. *A Federal Failure in Psychiatric Research: Continuing NIMH Negligence in Funding Sufficient Research on Serious Mental Illnesses.* Arlington, Va.: The Treatment Advocacy Center, 2003.

Torrey, E. F. *American Psychosis: How the Federal Government Destroyed the Mental Illness Treatment System.* New York: Oxford University Press, 2014.

APPENDIX A

An Annotated List of the Best and the Worst Books on Schizophrenia

The Best

The following books, listed alphabetically by author, are useful for becoming familiar with all phases of schizophrenia. Some of them are out of print, but used copies are available over the Internet or at your local library. Those that I have found to be especially useful I have marked with an asterisk. With rare exceptions, I did not include fictional accounts. In addition to these books, there are also several good professional textbooks for individuals who wish to do advanced reading. These include J. Lieberman and R. Murray, eds., *Comprehensive Care of Schizophrenia* (London: Martin Dunitz, 2000); P. F. Buckley and J. L. Waddington, eds., *Schizophrenia and Mind Disorders* (Boston: Butterworth Heinmann, 2000); S. R. Hirsch and D. R. Weinberger, *Schizophrenia* (Oxford: Blackwell Science, 2001); P. B. Jones and P. F. Buckley, *Schizophrenia* (London: Mosby, 2003); M. F. Green, *Schizophrenia Revealed: From Neurons to Social Interaction* (New York, Norton, 2003); J. A. Lieberman, T. S. Stroup, and D. O. Perkins, eds., *Essentials of Schizophrenia* (Washington, D.C.: American Psychiatric Press, 2012); R. Reddy and M. Keshavan, *Schizophrenia: A Practical Primer* (Abingdon, England: Informa Healthcare, 2006); K. Mueser and D. V. Jeste, *Clinical Handbook of Schizophrenia* (New York: Guilford Press, 2008);

R. Freedman, *The Madness Within Us: Schizophrenia as a Neuronal Process* (New York: Oxford University Press, 2010).

Adamec, Christine. *How to Live with a Mentally Ill Person: A Handbook of Day-to-Day Strategies.* New York: John Wiley, 1996. This is a solid and practical how-to book by a professional writer whose daughter developed schizophrenia. It utilizes a positive, "cheerleading" approach "to energize you and give you the hope you need." Included are a multitude of practical suggestions, such as a model "Crisis Information Form" to be prepared ahead of time for emergency admissions or if you have to call the police. The author emphasizes the importance of accepting the illness and moving on, of not being bogged down by the "myth of the 'before' person" or the "ghost of patient past."

Alexandra, Christina. *Five Lost Years: A Personal Exploration of Schizophrenia.* Roseville, Calif.: Day Bones Press, 2000. This is a first-person account by a young woman who experienced several psychotic episodes and subsequent hospitalizations, one for eighteen months. It is well written as a series of staccato vignettes that provide the reader with a sense of the author's internal experiences. In the end, she recovers and becomes a born-again Christian.

*Amador, Xavier. *I Am Not Sick, I Don't Need Help.* Peconic, N.Y.: Vida Press, 2011. This is a very important book, the first that attempts to address the elephantine question running roughshod over families of individuals with schizophrenia: Why won't the sick person take his/her medicine? Amador, a psychologist who had a brother with schizophrenia, has pioneered research on anosognosia, also known as insight, or awareness of illness. He blends clinical vignettes skillfully with his erudition, and the resulting mix is edifying. Most important, Amador provides families and mental illness professionals with a concrete, step-by-step plan to improve awareness of illness in the person who has schizophrenia. It will not work all the time but is well worth trying before having to utilize involuntary hospitalization and various forms of assisted treatment.

Backlar, Patricia. *The Family Face of Schizophrenia: Practical Counsel from America's Leading Experts.* Los Angeles: Tarcher, 1994. "Being a family member of someone with schizophrenia is a difficult job. No one ever applies for these jobs and there is no standard job description." This quite nicely summarizes this book, which includes seven true stories of schizophrenia, each followed by a commentary by a professional (two psychiatrists, two psychologists, a psychiatric nurse, a social worker, and a lawyer). It is an unusual format, but it works surprisingly well.

*Bartók, Mira. *The Memory Palace: A Memoir.* New York: Free Press, 2011. The author is a writer of children's books and has written a memoir of being raised by a mother with schizophrenia. It is at once terrifying and deeply affecting, a reminder of both how difficult it can be for such children and how little we do to protect them. Mira ultimately has to change her name and cut off all contact with her mother for seventeen years, reconciling with her only when her homeless mother is dying. Even then, the author admits that "in my mind she was still the madwoman on the street . . . who follows you down alleyways, lighting matches in your hair."

Bernheim, Kayla F., Richard R. J. Lewine, and C. T. Beale. *The Caring Family: Living with Chronic Mental Illness*. New York: Random House, 1982. Although this was one of the first books written for family members of someone with a severe mental illness, its message is as useful today as when it was published. The authors discuss such common reactions as guilt, shame, fear, anger, and despair, and offer suggestions for resolving them. The book discusses "chronic mental illness" as a whole and does not focus specifically on schizophrenia, but its discussion of individual and family dynamics as a consequence of the illness is certainly applicable.

Button, Margo. *The Unhinging of Wings*. Lantzville, British Columbia, Canada: Oolichan Books, 1996. This is a remarkable collection of sixty-six poems written by Margo Button about her son, afflicted with schizophrenia, who committed suicide at age twenty-seven. Many of the poems had been previously published in literary journals, and the collection is a poignant and moving memorial.

> Now I know there is no one to blame,
> but that impassive god
> who shoots stray bullets
> through the brain.

The preface for the book is by Dr. Michael Smith, who won the 1993 Nobel Prize for Chemistry and donated his prize money to schizophrenia research.

Cockburn, Patrick, and Henry Cockburn. *Henry's Demons: Living with Schizophrenia, a Father and Son's Story*. New York: Scribner's, 2011. Patrick Cockburn is a British newspaper writer and has written an account of his son's schizophrenia. Alternate chapters were contributed by the son. It is a well-written account of how both father and son attempt to come to terms with the disease that has profoundly affected them both.

Cutting, John, and Anne Charlish. *Schizophrenia: Understanding and Coping with the Illness*. London: Thorsons, 1995. Written by a respected schizophrenia researcher and a journalist, this has been a popular book in England for families of schizophrenia sufferers. The descriptions of symptoms by patients themselves are especially noteworthy (e.g., "I seem to be empty inside. Nothing touches me anymore. It's as if I am an object without feelings, without the urge to do anything."). The sections on the diagnosis of schizophrenia are also strong.

DeLisi, Lynn E. *100 Questions and Answers about Schizophrenia: Painful Minds*. Sudbury, Mass.: Jones and Bartlett, 2016. Written by a veteran schizophrenia researcher, this is a useful primer on schizophrenia framed around one hundred questions and answers. As such, it is easy for the reader to go directly to the information he or she is seeking.

*Deveson, Anne. *Tell Me I'm Here*. New York: Penguin Books, 1992. This is a powerfully written account of a son's schizophrenia as seen through his mother's eyes. Deveson is a broadcaster and filmmaker, well known to the Australian public, and her account of her son's illness enabled many Australian families with a seriously mentally ill family member to come out of the closet. Because it is real, her story is more terrifying than the worst fictional horror story. Deveson skillfully captures the various shades and nuances of the tragedy we call schizophrenia. This is one of the best books.

Dobbins, Carolyn. *What a Life Can Be: One Therapist's Take on Schizo-Affective Disorder*. Dundas, Ontario: Bridgeross Communications, 2011. This is a nicely written memoir by a therapist with schizoaffective disorder. She notes that functioning well is very difficult, "a full-time job, 24/7, for most of my life." She also emphasizes that "not every fibre of our being is crazy when we're mentally ill. Part of the spirit remains untouched and free." It is a hopeful book about someone who has put her life together despite her illness.

*Earley, Pete. *Crazy: A Father's Search Through America's Mental Health Madness*. New York: G. P. Putnam's Sons, 2006. Pete Earley's son was diagnosed with schizoaffective disorder, then he broke into a house and was charged with a felony crime. Earley, a reporter by profession, has written an excellent and appropriately grim account of how seriously mentally ill individuals end up in the criminal justice system. He mixes experiences of his son with accounts of mentally ill individuals in Miami's Dade County Jail. This is the best account to date of this increasingly common phenomenon, one of the most serious, yet relatively invisible, consequences of our failed mental illness treatment system. Parents who have watched their mentally ill offspring become part of the criminal justice system will easily empathize with Pete Earley's frustration and calls for reform.

Hatfield, Agnes B., and Harriet P. Lefley. *Surviving Mental Illness: Stress, Coping and Adaptation*. New York: Guilford Press, 1993. Eminently practical and well written, this book will be useful for families trying to sort out the myriad problems confronting them when a family member becomes seriously mentally ill. Emphasis is put on the importance of understanding what the sick person is experiencing, so the book includes some useful personal accounts by Dr. Frederick Frese, Esso Leete, and Daniel Link.

Holman, Virginia. *Rescuing Patty Hearst*. New York: Simon & Schuster, 2003. When Virginia Holman was eight years old, her mother, then age thirty-two, developed paranoid schizophrenia. This is Ms. Holman's recollection of growing up with an intermittently psychotic mother who would not allow her to read many books because of "secret messages" therein and who makes Virginia's younger sister "eat a bowl of cereal crawling with ants." Written as a series of flashbacks with shifting time frames, the book would have been stronger if the author had allocated more space to discussing her mother and less to the details of playing games with her cousins.

Inman, Susan. *After Her Brain Broke: Helping My Daughter Recover Her Sanity.* Dundas, Ontario: Bridgeross Communications, 2010. This is a very nicely written account by a mother whose daughter has been diagnosed with schizoaffective disorder. She describes the occasional highlights and more common lowlights of the Canadian psychiatric care system as experienced by her daughter. The author's attempt to educate herself as she wends her way through the treatment maze is a model for others.

*Isaac, Rael Jean, and Virginia C. Armat. *Madness in the Streets.* New York: Free Press, 1990; paperback published by the Treatment Advocacy Center, 2000. This is an important history of the "mental health" movement and how so many individuals with serious mental illnesses ended up homeless and on the streets. There is enough blame to go around for just about everyone involved in the "mental health" scene, but the lawyers with the American Civil Liberties Union and the Bazelon Center for Mental Health Law collect (and deserve) the largest share. It is a well-written and depressing history and essential to understand if we expect to improve things.

*Jaffe, D. J. *Insane Consequences: How the Mental Health Industry Fails the Mentally Ill.* Amherst, New York: Prometheus Books, 2017. For anyone who wants to be an advocate and improve the mental illness treatment system, this is the only book you need. D. J. Jaffe, who worked in advertising before becoming an advocate, understands the levers of change and lays it out in clear prose for the reader. He is especially lucid in describing how government programs that were originally implemented to help the mentally ill can become corrupted; what was supposed to be part of the solution merely becomes another part of the problem. The author also contributed Appendix B to this book.

Karp, David. *Burden of Sympathy: How Families Cope with Mental Illness.* New York: Oxford University Press, 2000. Karp, a professor of sociology at Boston College, himself suffered from severe depression. Based on sixty intensive interviews he did with family members of individuals with schizophrenia, bipolar disorder, and severe depression, he has written an excellent book "about the social tango between emotionally ill people and those who try to help them." In examining the lives of the family members, he demonstrates that "sustaining an appropriate level of involvement with a mentally ill child, parent, sibling, or spouse is extraordinarily difficult." Karp writes well and, perhaps because of his own experience with depression, captures the essence of caring and caregivers.

Kleier, Maxene. *Possessed Mentalities.* New York: iUniverse, 2005. Two of Ms. Kleier's daughters developed schizophrenia, and then one killed the other. This is an honest, if somewhat rambling, narrative of the tragedy and reminds us what a cruel disease schizophrenia can be. The account by the surviving daughter at the end of the book provides interesting insight into the mind of those who kill because of their psychotic thinking.

Lachenmeyer, Nathaniel. *The Outsider: A Journey into My Father's Struggle with Madness*. New York: Broadway Books, 2000. Charles Lachenmeyer had a Ph.D. in sociology before he developed paranoid schizophrenia and ultimately became homeless. This story is his son's reconstruction of his father's life. It is painful and poignant, and all the more so because the father responded to medications when he took them for brief periods. The story also abounds in ironies, including the fact that the father had worked as an attendant in a state hospital while in college and had written his thesis on the double-bind theory of schizophrenia.

Lefley, Harriet P. *Family Psychoeducation for Serious Mental Illness*. New York: Oxford University Press, 2009. This is the most recent book by a psychologist who is also a professor at the University of Miami. In this book she focuses on family psychoeducation but also incorporates much helpful material from her previous books, especially *Families as Allies in Treatment of the Mentally Ill*, coedited with Dale Johnson (1990); *Helping Families Cope with Mental Illness* (1994); and *Family Caregiving in Mental Illness* (1996). These books are especially useful for trainees in the mental health and illness professions.

Levine, Jerome, and Irene Levine. *Schizophrenia for Dummies*. New York: Wiley, 2009. Written by a psychiatrist-psychologist husband and wife with extensive experience with and expertise on schizophrenia, this book is reliable and readable. Like most *Dummies* books, it is short on details but includes abundant coping tips, which makes it especially useful.

*Lieberman, Jeffrey A. *Shrinks: The Untold Story of Psychiatry*. New York: Little, Brown and Co., 2015. For anyone trying to understand the American psychiatric profession—and this is no easy task—this is by far the best book. Individuals with schizophrenia and their families will especially like the historical development of modern treatments. The author is one of America's leading psychiatrists and knows his subject well.

Marsh, Diane T. *Serious Mental Illness and the Family: The Practitioner's Guide*. New York: John Wiley, 1998. This is the best book available for mental illness professionals providing care for individuals with severe mental illnesses. The author, a psychologist who specializes in treating individuals with these illnesses and their families, also authored the useful *Families and Mental Illness: New Directions in Professional Practice*, published in 1992. As the author notes, *Serious Mental Illness and the Family* "is designed to assist practitioners in developing the competencies necessary for working with families." Although aimed at mental health professionals, families will find the sections on siblings, spouses, and offspring of seriously mentally ill individuals especially useful.

Marsh, Diane T., and Rex Dickens. *How to Cope with Mental Illness in Your*

Family: A Self-Care Guide for Siblings, Offspring, and Parents. New York: Putnam, 1997. This is an excellent book on how severe psychiatric disorders affect other members of the family and, more important, what to do about it. The authors, a psychologist specializing in severe psychiatric disorders and a man whose mother and three siblings have been affected, have been active members of NAMI for many years. Their book is a synthesis of what they have been told by hundreds of families, including extended personal accounts that they published in an earlier book, *Anguished Voices.* The emphasis in this book is on self-help and coping skills. Most important, the authors emphasize the tremendous variability of the effect of having a family member with a severe psychiatric disorder. On one end is devastation, divorce, and what has been called "a funeral that never ends." On the other end is the young woman described by Marsh and Dickens who remembers "standing up in second grade and sharing the mental condition of my brother as my contribution to Show and Tell. I thought it was the most unique thing about my life and certainly better than any hamster!"

McLean, Richard. *Recovered, Not Cured: A Journey through Schizophrenia.* Crows Nest, Australia: Allen and Unwin, 2003. This is one of the best in describing the symptoms of schizophrenia. The author, a young drug-using Aussie, lives with his gradually increasing symptoms for several years before seeking treatment. He bases his brutally honest recollections on diary entries and intersperses these with drawings and accounts of symptoms from those he is talking to on the Internet. The book is especially good in describing his denial of his illness.

Moorman, Margaret. *My Sister's Keeper.* New York: Norton, 1992. The effect on siblings of having a seriously mentally ill brother or sister has been little studied or written about. Moorman's account of her older sister's schizophrenia goes a long way toward filling that gap. She is especially articulate about the problems of role reversal as a younger sister who had to, in effect, become an older sister to her older sister. Part of the book was originally published in the *New York Times,* and Moorman also appeared on the *Oprah Winfrey Show* to discuss her experiences.

Mueser, Kim T., and Susan Gingerich. *The Complete Family Guide to Schizophrenia.* New York: Guilford Press, 2006. Written by a psychologist and a social worker, this book updates their earlier collaborative effort, *Coping with Schizophrenia: A Guide for Families* (1994). Although its thirty chapters and 480 pages appear somewhat daunting, it is well written and very useful, with abundant worksheets and resources.

Nasar, Sylvia. *A Beautiful Mind: A Biography of John Forbes Nash, Jr., Winner of the Nobel Prize in Economics, 1994.* New York: Simon & Schuster, 1998. Paperback published by Touchstone Books, 1999. This is a nicely written account of John Nash. A brilliant mathematician in his twenties, he then developed schizophrenia but partially recovered in his late fifties and was awarded the

Nobel Prize for Economics in 1994 for his earlier work. The book describes clearly the early premorbid asociality and other symptoms of illness that precede the illness in approximately one-third of cases. It also provides a poignant account of the devastating effects of the illness on Nash's wife, sons, mother, and friends, as well as a good description of the confused etiological ambience of the early 1960s.

North, Carol. *Welcome, Silence: My Triumph over Schizophrenia.* New York: Simon & Schuster, 1987. This is the personal account of a young woman's fight against the symptoms of schizophrenia. Although her case is quite atypical in many ways, the book includes excellent descriptions of what it is like to experience auditory hallucinations and to fight the symptoms of the disease. North was one of the few patients who responded dramatically to renal dialysis as an experimental treatment, and she is today a fully trained psychiatrist who specializes in serious mental illness.

Pfeiffer, Mary Beth. *Crazy in America: The Hidden Tragedy of Our Criminalized Mentally Ill.* New York: Carroll and Graf, 2007. In title and content, this book is similar to Pete Earley's *Crazy*, since both focus on the tragic plight of mentally ill persons in jails. The author is an investigative reporter and spares the reader none of the tragic details. One mentally ill man is shot by the police, another hangs himself in jail, and still another tears out her eyes while in solitary confinement. This is grim stuff, but it accurately reflects today's grim reality.

*Powers, Ron. *No One Cares About Crazy People.* New York: Hachette, 2017. The author, a Pulitzer Prize–winning author, recounts what happens when both his sons develop schizophrenia. One suicides shortly before his twenty-first birthday and the second undergoes the usual cycle of hospitalization and medication refusal before finally becoming stable. Powers has a writer's eye for detail and the absurdities of the mental illness care non-system. If you were not angry when you started the book, you will be when you finish.

Riley, Jocelyn. *Crazy Quilt.* New York: Morrow, 1984. An unusual children's book, this is the fictional account of a thirteen-year-old girl whose mother has schizophrenia. It is a poignant reminder of the effects of this disease on other family members and the fact that children need education and support just as siblings and parents need them. We need many more such books so that children, too, may understand. An earlier book by the same author, *Only My Mouth Is Smiling* (1982), is also good. Other worthy children's books are Betty Hyland, *The Girl with the Crazy Brother* (New York: Watts, 1987), in which a sixteen-year-old girl has to cope with the onset of schizophrenia in her brother; Gayle Glass, *Catch a Falling Star* (iristhedragon@hotmail.com); Regina Hanson, *The Face at the Window* (New York: Clarion Books, 1997); and Marie Day, *Edward the Crazy Man* (SANE Australia, admin@sane.org).

Ross, Marvin. *Schizophrenia: Medicine's Mystery, Society's Shame.* Dundas, Ontario: Bridgeross Communications, 2008. Written by a journalist who is one of the leading Canadian advocates for individuals with serious psychiatric disorders, this short book summarizes the neurobiology and treatment of this disease. Chapter 6, "Treatment Strategies," is especially good.

Russell, L. Mark, and Arnold E. Grant. *Planning for the Future: Providing a Meaningful Life for a Child with a Disability After Your Death,* 5th Palatine, Ill: Planning for the Future Inc., 2005. For anyone who is trying to plan for the future for a mentally disabled family member, this is essential reading. The authors cover everything from SSI, SSDI, Medicaid, Medicare, and other government benefits to wills, trusts, estate planning, power of attorney, and nursing home expenses. The book is replete with detailed examples and includes sample letters of intent. It has been especially popular with parents who worry about what will happen to their mentally ill child after they are gone.

*Sanghera, Sathnam. *The Boy with the Topknot.* New York: Penguin, 2009. Originally published in 2008 as *If You Don't Know Me by Now.* Written by a writer for the *London Times,* this is the account of schizophrenia in a family of Indian immigrants in England. Sanghera slowly comes to realize that his father has schizophrenia and details the effect of that fact on his family, especially himself. It is masterfully written, with an unusual combination of pathos, humor, and honesty.

Schiller, Lori, and Amanda Bennett. *The Quiet Room: A Journey Out of the Torment of Madness.* New York: Warner Books, 1994. This is a brave book by a woman whose schizoaffective disorder began at age seventeen with auditory hallucinations as the only symptom. The hallucinations remained her only symptom for several years, allowing her to complete college and start working; in this respect, her atypical course is similar to that described by Carol North in *Welcome, Silence.* Lori Schiller tells her story from the perspective of several other people (mother, father, brother) as well as from her own.

Sellers, Heather. *You Don't Look Like Anyone I Know.* New York: Riverhead Books, 2010. So you think you had a rough childhood? Heather Sellers describes being woken in the middle of the night by her mother, who had paranoid schizophrenia, to drive around and write down the license plate numbers of trucks that her mother believed were following them. When Heather tired of that she would go crosstown to live with her father who was an alcoholic who cross-dressed. Heather also has face-blindness but that is the least of her problems and the book is mistitled. The author teaches literature in college and is an excellent writer with a wild story to tell.

*Sheehan, Susan. *Is There No Place on Earth for Me?* Boston: Houghton, Mifflin, 1982. Paperback published by Random House, 1983. Susan Sheehan's superb study originally appeared in *The New Yorker* magazine. It provides the best available description of the course of a chronic schizophrenic illness, the difficulties encountered by a person with the disease, the frustrations for the family, and the mediocre care available at the state hospital. It is searingly accurate and mandatory reading for anyone who wants to understand the tragedy of this disease. The patient described has the schizoaffective subtype.

Sherman, Michelle D., and DeAnne M. Sherman, *I'm Not Alone: A Teen's Guide to Living with a Parent Who Has a Mental Illness*. Edina, Minn.: Beaver Pond Press, 2006. This is a useful, simple book for children whose parent has a serious psychiatric disorder. It mixes anecdotes with advice in a practical manner, focusing on such questions as "Are all of my feelings normal?," "How can I cope with all this?," and "What do I tell other people?" The book fills an important gap, since there has been little written for such children.

*Simon, Clea. *Mad House: Growing Up in the Shadow of Mentally Ill Siblings*. New York: Doubleday, 1997. What is it like, as an eight-year-old girl, to have your older brother and sister both develop schizophrenia? Clea Simon lived it and eloquently describes it. She is especially articulate in describing being caught between fear and guilt, the traditional Scylla and Charybdis of relatives of those afflicted. Simon, who writes for the *Boston Globe*, is an excellent writer and has created a lovely book about a very cruel disease.

*Swados, Elizabeth. *The Four of Us: A Family Memoir*. New York: Farrar, Straus and Giroux, 1991. Paperback published by Penguin Books, 1993. This is an extraordinary account of how severe mental illness can devastate an entire family. The son is officially diagnosed with schizophrenia but appears to have the schizoaffective type or even bipolar disorder. The effects of the disease's malignant ripples are stunning, as the young man spirals downward to a failed suicide attempt, throwing himself beneath a subway train, then to homelessness. It is beautifully written, brutally honest, and profoundly depressing. Recommended for reading on sunny days in pleasant gardens.

Taylor, Robert. *Distinguishing Psychological from Organic Disorders: Screening for Psychological Masquerade*. 2nd ed. New York: Springer, 2000. This is an updated, second edition of an excellent book. The author lays out a method for mental illness professionals and others to use to distinguish organic brain diseases (e.g., brain tumors) from schizophrenia, manic-depressive illness, and other psychiatric conditions. Taylor's method is lucid, eminently practical, and remarkably easy to implement, and any professional who reads this book will be a better clinician.

Torrey, E. Fuller. *American Psychosis: How the Federal Government Destroyed the Mental Illness Treatment System*. New York: Oxford, 2014. It seems like bad manners to recommend one's own books, but in fact the book has been well received. It is a sequel to *The Insanity Offense* (2012), *Nowhere to Go* (1988), and *Out of the Shadows* (1997). Together, they describe how the American mental illness treatment system went down the drain and the consequences of this for seriously mentally ill individuals: incarceration, victimization, homelessness, and homicides. These books tell a sad and tragic tale but one we must understand if we are to have any hope of improving things.

Torrey, E. Fuller, Ann E. Bowler, Edward H. Taylor, and Irving I. Gottesman. *Schizophrenia and Manic-Depressive Disorder: The Biological Roots of Mental Illness as Revealed by a Landmark Study of Identical Twins.* New York: Basic Books, 1994. Paperback edition, 1996. This is the report of a study of sixty-six pairs of identical twins; in twenty-seven pairs, one had schizophrenia and the other was well, and in thirteen pairs, both had schizophrenia. As one twin researcher wrote, identical twins are " 'experiments' which nature has conducted for us, starting in each case with identical sets of genes and varying environmental factors." And as "experiments," they indeed are both interesting and useful.

Tracey, Patrick. *Stalking Irish Madness: Searching for the Roots of My Family's Schizophrenia.* New York: Bantam, 2008. The author is a former journalist whose grandmother, uncle, and two sisters were all diagnosed with schizophrenia. He recounts his journey, both literal and spiritual, to discover the history of his family and causes of the illness. The journey takes him to a part of Ireland where schizophrenia appeared to be especially prevalent in the past. It is a story well told.

*Wagner, Pamela Spiro, and Carolyn S. Spiro. *Divided Minds: Twin Sisters and Their Journey through Schizophrenia.* New York: St. Martin's Press, 2005. For most of us, it is almost impossible to imagine what it would be like to be an identical twin, to say nothing of being one of a pair in which one gets schizophrenia. *Divided Minds* describes this situation. Pam, initially the more accomplished of the twins, begins hearing vague voices in sixth grade and is hospitalized for the first of many times during her freshman year of college. Carolyn becomes a physician and psychiatrist, largely in reaction to her sister's illness. This is an excellent book, written in alternate sections by the women, who are both accomplished writers. Pam's description of her symptoms and Carolyn's ambivalence about her role as caring sibling are related with brutal honesty. Of special note is the depiction of the medieval psychiatric treatment offered by the Medical Center at Yale and other psychiatric hospitals in the 1970s, just before biological psychiatry took hold. The sisters' story also reminds us how devastating schizophrenia can be for the whole family. There is no sugarcoating this story, just as there is no sugarcoating this disease.

*Wasow, Mona. *The Skipping Stone: Ripple Effects of Mental Illness on the Family.* Palo Alto, Calif.: Science and Behavioral Books, 1995. This is a lyrical summary of one hundred interviews done with family members of individuals with a serious mental illness. Mona Wasow is a social worker and the mother of a son with schizophrenia. "The ripple effect of mental illness on the entire family is enormous," she states, and she proceeds to document this effect on the siblings, spouses, grandparents, and children of affected individuals. Her chapters on grief, coping, and hope are excellent (e.g., "trying to capture the essence of grief in writing is like trying to capture the wind in a box or the ocean in a glass"). Her understanding of these illnesses is beautifully and brutally frank: "But let us be honest with ourselves: the tortures of hallucinations, the failure to connect with people, and the anxieties, desperate isolation, and loneliness of people with serious mental illness take a staggering toll." This is one of the best books.

Williamson, Wendell J. *Nightmare: A Schizophrenia Narrative.* Durham, N.C.: The Mental Health Communication Network, 2001. On January 26, 1995, Wendell Williamson, in a high-profile case, shot two strangers to death in Chapel Hill, North Carolina. He was heavily armed and had planned to kill many more, before he was himself shot and subdued. Williamson had been an Eagle Scout, student council president in high school, and an honors graduate from UNC; he was a law student at the time of the shooting. This book is very useful for telling three stories. First, it clearly describes Williamson's descent into paranoid schizophrenia and his feelings of being telepathic and being able to exchange thoughts with everyone from the president in the White House to strangers in bars. The second story is of the utter failure of the local mental health system to treat Williamson prior to his crimes. The third story, and the most important aspect of the book, is Williamson's recollections of his ongoing internal dialogue about whether he was truly telepathic or just psychiatrically ill. This is a unique account of the nuances of anosognosia as told by the person affected. Amy Martin, who edited the book and got it published, deserves credit for her contribution.

Winerip, Michael. *9 Highland Road.* New York: Pantheon Books, 1994. Michael Winerip, a respected reporter for the *New York Times*, spent two years hanging around a group home on Long Island. The result is an engaging, lively, and very well-written narrative that captures the home's ambience, including the struggles and joys of its residents diagnosed with schizophrenia and other severe psychiatric disorders. "Schizophrenia," writes Winerip, "is the most monstrous of the mental illnesses." Perhaps the book's greatest contribution is to illustrate that individuals with schizophrenia need more than medication to reclaim their lives. They also need friends, guidance, support, and people who believe in them.

Woolis, Rebecca. *When Someone You Love Has a Mental Illness: A Handbook for Family, Friends, and Caregivers.* New York: Perigee Books, 1992. This is a handy book to have around because of its numerous "Quick Reference Guides" for such subjects as "Handling Your Relative's Anger," "Dealing with Bizarre Behavior," "Preventing Suicide," and "Rules for Living at Home or Visiting." It does not provide long discourses on the various subjects but instead tells you what to *do*. It is a practical book par excellence.

Wyden, Peter. *Conquering Schizophrenia: A Father, His Son, and a Medical Break-*

through. New York: Knopf, 1998. This is the story of a dedicated father, who died shortly after publication of the book, and his search for an effective treatment for the schizophrenia suffered by one of his sons. It provides a good history of antipsychotic drug development and focuses especially on olanzapine (Zyprexa), to which his son responded. The author was a professional writer, so the book is well written. The author's other son is the current U.S. senator from Oregon.

The Worst

The following are some of the worst books on schizophrenia. If you own any of them, don't throw them away; someday they may be worth money as intellectual curiosities. Your grandchild will ask, incredulously, "Did they *really* believe that then?"

Barnes, Mary, and Joseph Berke. *Mary Barnes: Two Accounts of a Journey through Madness*. New York: Ballantine Books, 1973. This is the book that made Ronald Laing's approach to schizophrenia widely known. Schizophrenia, it says, is a "career" that is "launched with the aid and encouragement of one's immediate family." The family member with schizophrenia is often "the least disturbed member of the entire group." This assertion is preposterous in any context, but it is also sad when one realizes that Laing's own daughter was diagnosed with schizophrenia. Moreover, the authors claim that suffering from schizophrenia can be a growth experience—"psychosis may be a state of reality, cyclic in nature, by which the self renews itself." There is no end to such absurd drivel in this book.

Boyle, Mary. *Schizophrenia: A Scientific Delusion?* New York: Routledge, 1990. The author is the head of a training program for clinical psychologists in London and doubts that schizophrenia exists. Like Thomas Szasz, she acknowledges that auditory hallucinations, disconnected thought processes, and bizarre behavior exist but believes that they should be viewed within their "social context." Although the book was published in 1990, most of it appears to have been written a decade earlier, since it fails to consider most of the existing biological evidence for schizophrenia as a brain disease. If you are having trouble getting to sleep at night, this book should do it!

Breggin, Peter R. *The Psychology of Freedom*. Buffalo, N.Y.: Prometheus Books, 1980. It is difficult to select the worst books about schizophrenia from the many Dr. Breggin has written, but this is one of my favorites. "Craziness," as Breggin refers to schizophrenia, "is a failure of nerve. . . . Insanity is cowardice; utter insanity is utter cowardice." Individuals who develop schizophrenia, says Breggin, are responsible for making themselves that way. "The individual makes himself or herself helpless" because he does not have the courage to face his own shortcomings. "People who are grossly deluded and hallucinating are grossly cowardly and have forfeited responsibility for the control of their own inner life. . . . It is the self-imposed crippling of the individual by himself or herself." This extraordinary drivel continues page after page; it is a wonder that people with schizophrenia haven't yet chased Breggin up a tree for his vitriolic attacks on them.

Breggin, Peter R. *Toxic Psychiatry*. New York: St. Martin's Press, 1991. It would have been difficult to imagine that Dr. Breggin could have written a worse book on psychiatric medications than his previous one, *Psychiatric Drugs: Hazards to the Brain*, but he has accomplished this considerable feat. Schizophrenia, Breggin tells us, is "a psychospiritual overwhelm" caused by child abuse and/or the drugs used to treat it. His style is a disjointed hysteria in which he grossly exaggerates the negatives and ignores the positives.

Colbert, Ty C. *Broken Brains or Wounded Hearts: What Causes Mental Illness*. Santa Ana, Calif.: Kevco, 1996. There seems to be no end to the repackaging of traditional psychoanalytic theory and attempts to sell it as something new. Colbert, a California psychologist in private practice, would have us believe that "schizophrenia is not a brain disease" but rather merely the product of "an overload of emotional pain." He claims that "the mind *purposely* creates the defenses necessary to deal with that pain. Thus, the disorders of schizophrenia, depression, and other so-called mental illnesses are seen as the person's own strategy for adapting to the pain." The person *chooses* to have schizophrenia.

Cooper, David. *Psychiatry and Anti-Psychiatry*. New York: Ballantine Books, 1967. Another confused protégé of R. D. Laing, Cooper in this book romanticized the individual with schizophrenia as merely expressing the pathology of the family. Specifically he speculated that "in the 'psychotic' families the identified schizophrenic patient member by his psychotic episode is trying to break free of an alienated system and is, therefore, in some sense less 'ill' or at least less alienated than the 'normal' offspring of the 'normal' families." This is pure bunkum.

Dorman, Daniel. *Dante's Cure: A Journey Out of Madness*. New York: Other Press, 2003. Yet another book in the mode of *I Never Promised You a Rose Garden*, this one features a presumably kind and caring psychoanalyst who treats a young woman with severe depression, auditory hallucinations, and anorexia. The treatment consists of eight years of traditional psychoanalysis, including four years of psychiatric hospitalization. During many of the sessions, the psychoanalyst and patient sit completely silent. The patient occasionally requests medication, but the psychiatrist insists that she must instead understand her lack of ego strength and close relationship with her mother. The most heartening thing about the book, in fact, is that after twenty-eight years of teaching psychoanalytic psychotherapy to residents in training, UCLA finally told Dr. Dorman he was no longer needed.

Goffman, Erving. *Asylums: Essays on the Social Situation of Mental Patients and Other Inmates.* Garden City, N.Y.: Anchor Books, 1961. Supported by funds from the National Institute of Mental Health, sociologist Erving Goffman spent a year at St. Elizabeths Hospital in Washington, D.C., observing the patients. He concluded that most of the patients' behavior was a reaction to being hospitalized, not a result of their illnesses. The logical corollary was that one needed only to open the gates of the hospital and let the patients go free, no strings (or medication) attached, and they would live happily ever after.

Green, Hannah. *I Never Promised You a Rose Garden.* New York: Holt, Rinehart and Winston, 1964. If a prize were to be given to the book that has produced the most confusion about schizophrenia over the past half century, this book would win going away. The young woman with "schizophrenia" is helped to become well by psychoanalytic psychotherapy. In fact, the woman almost certainly never had schizophrenia; her symptoms were much more consistent with hysteria, and she went on to marry, have a family, write fifteen books, and lecture all over the country—not exactly a typical course of schizophrenia. Furthermore, psychoanalytic therapy is about as likely to cure schizophrenia as it is likely to cure multiple sclerosis. The book belongs in the Kingdom of Ur with the young woman's fantasies.

Kesey, Ken. *One Flew Over the Cuckoo's Nest.* New York: Signet Books, 1962. Made into a popular movie, this is a fictional version of the idea promoted by Erving Goffman in *Asylums* and by the movie *King of Hearts.* Randle McMurphy tries to mobilize the patients in the state hospital to challenge Big Nurse Ratched and the evil psychiatrists who work there. The patients are depicted as oppressed, not sick, and in the end Chief Broom escapes from the hospital to live happily ever after. In reality, Chief Broom probably joined the legion of homeless mentally ill individuals living under some bridge, ended up in jail, was beaten up, or all of the above. Kesey was a guru of psychedelic drugs at the time, and his story also has a hallucinatory ring to it.

Lidz, Theodore. *The Relevance of the Family to Psychoanalytic Theory.* Madison, Conn.: International Universities Press, 1992. This book completes forty-five years of pumpkin-headed publications by the late Dr. Lidz, who was a professor of psychiatry at Yale University. His career started in 1949 with "Psychiatric Problems in the Thyroid Clinic," which asserted that individuals with hyperthyroidism "had in childhood felt less wanted than a sibling." He then moved on to his study of sixteen families in which one member had schizophrenia: "In each family at least one parent suffered from serious and crippling psychopathology, and in many both were markedly disturbed . . . the father appeared to be seriously disturbed just as often as the mother." It is doubtful if ever in the history of medicine so many papers and books have been published on so few patients in studies of such doubtful scientific merit.

Mahoney, J. Michael. *Schizophrenia: The Bearded Lady Disease.* Authorhouse, 2002. Self-published and heavily advertised by the author, this book illustrates that anyone who has enough money can promote a nutty idea. The author contends that schizophrenia is caused by "severe bisexual conflict" and can only be successfully treated by long-term psychoanalysis. The author uses as his model Freud's theory that repressed homosexuality is the cause of paranoid schizophrenia, based on Freud's analysis of the case of Daniel Paul Schreber, whom Freud never actually met. The author's method of proving his "severe bisexual conflict" thesis was to collect 639 quotations and editorialize on each. The book's text is as strange as its title.

Modrow, John. *How to Become a Schizophrenic: The Case Against Biological Psychiatry.* Everett, Wash.: Apollylon Press, 1992. This is a pathetic book by a man who was once diagnosed with schizophrenia. "My fate had been sealed not by my genes, but by the attitudes, beliefs, and expectations of my parents [who] had serious psychological problems of their own." His symptoms, says Modrow, were merely the consequence of the stress his mother and father subjected him to. In one chapter he claims that "schizophrenia is largely caused by feelings of intense self-loathing." Elsewhere he reassures us that "there is no vast difference between schizophrenia and normalcy."

Penney, Darby, and Peter Stasney. *The Lives They Left Behind.* New York: Bellevue Literary Press, 2008. The authors started out with a worthy idea and then proceeded to butcher it. They examined suitcases and personal effects of patients who had died at New York's Willard State Hospital in an effort to give a human face to the patients who died there, and in this they were successful. However, the authors use the suitcases as a pretext to promote their own radical agenda: "So-called schizophrenia," as they call it, is a response to stress, not a biological disease. The patients described were not in the hospital for treatment of their disease but rather as "prisoners of the mental health system." A review in the *New York Times* (March 25, 2008) got it exactly right: "The authors' strident prose . . . proves to be almost unreadable."

Read, John, Loren R. Mosher, and Richard P. Bentall, eds. *Models of Madness: Psychological, Social and Biological Approaches to Schizophrenia.* New York: Brunner-Routledge, 2004. This is a multi-authored book and valuable insofar as it collects together in a single volume almost everyone who knows nothing about schizophrenia. It is thus an opus of ignorance. John Read, the lead editor and a clinical psychologist in New Zealand, wrote all or part of twelve of the twenty-four chapters and thus has ample opportunity to promote his theories about child abuse and parental deviance as the causes of schizophrenia. Predictably, the consensus treatment promoted by most of the authors is psychoanalytic psychotherapy. The book's title is grossly misleading insofar as the only "biological" aspect of the book is a chapter titled "Biological Psychiatry's Lost Cause."

Robbins, Michael. *Experiences of Schizophrenia*. New York: Guilford Press, 1993. This book may well become a collector's item as one of the last books written in which psychoanalysis and other forms of insight-oriented psychotherapy are recommended as the treatment of choice for schizophrenia. As such, it follows in the tradition of Boyer and Giovacchini's *Psychoanalytic Treatment of Schizophrenic, Borderline and Characterological Disorders* (1980) and Karon and Van den Bos's *Psychotherapy of Schizophrenia: Treatment of Choice* (1981). Robbins describes selected cases of schizophrenia that he treated with psychoanalysis for up to seven years. Like most psychoanalysts, Robbins blames families for causing schizophrenia, describing them as "quietly totalitarian and controlling, suppressive of the autonomy and potential for separation of individual members."

Rubin, Theodore I. *Lisa and David*. New York: Macmillan, 1961. This book is included because it became a movie (*David and Lisa*) and thus influenced a generation of thinking about schizophrenia. Lisa, a thirteen-year-old girl with "hebephrenic schizophrenia," and David, a fifteen-year-old boy with "pseudoneurotic schizophrenia," are eloquently described in their daily activities in a residential treatment center in 1959 and 1960. Unfortunately, the author is a psychoanalyst whose only plan for treatment for the two is continued psychotherapy until they can "become involved in problems of . . . neurotic defenses, sexuality, and family relations." The two case histories cry out for antipsychotic drug therapy, which was available in 1959 and 1960 but is nowhere to be seen. One only hopes that in the intervening years the families of Lisa and David have taken them out of such an anachronistic treatment facility and found them more up-to-date treatment.

Szasz, Thomas. *Schizophrenia: The Sacred Symbol of Psychiatry*. New York: Basic Books, 1976. Starting with *The Myth of Mental Illness* in 1961 and continuing with *The Manufacture of Madness* (1970), *Schizophrenia: The Sacred Symbol of Psychiatry* (1976), and *Psychiatric Slavery* (1977), Szasz produced more erudite nonsense on the subject of schizophrenia than any writer. As a historian, Szasz was first class, but as a psychiatrist he never moved beyond a strictly psychoanalytic approach to treating schizophrenia. He argued, for example, that schizophrenia is merely a creation of psychiatry and "if there is no psychiatry there can be no schizophrenics." What wonderful simplicity! One wonders whether he ever saw a patient with this disease.

Whitaker, Robert. *Anatomy of an Epidemic: Magic Bullets, Psychiatric Drugs, and the Astonishing Rise of Mental Illness in America*. New York: Crown, 2010. The author, formerly a respected journalist, has many important criticisms of American psychiatry (e.g., broadening of diagnostic classification) and the pharmaceutical industry (e.g., promoting the use of medications in children). On the subjects of schizophrenia and antipsychotic drugs, however, he is wrong on almost every count. Whitaker seems unsure whether schizophrenia is even a disease and claims that most of its symptoms are caused by the antipsychotic drugs used to treat it. He relies on discredited studies, such as those claiming that the outcome of schizophrenia is more benign in developing countries where antipsychotics are less common. Most remarkably, he believes that patients would do better if not treated with drugs. In promoting this idea, he seems to be remarkably unaware of history: between 1800 and 1950, this approach was (of necessity) tried for literally hundreds of thousands of patients. The results of this "experiment" were abysmal.

APPENDIX B

Useful Online Resources on Schizophrenia
(This review was done by D. J. Jaffe, Executive Director of Mental Illness
Policy Org., and author of *Insane Consequences: How the Mental Health Industry
Fails the Mentally Ill.*)

The virtual world gives individuals and families facing schizophrenia ready
access to information and connections to others without leaving home. Some
websites, social media platforms, blogs, podcasts, and apps offer the best of
information, while others can be dangerous. Anyone with Facebook, Twitter,
Pinterest, Instagram, Linked-in, a blog, podcast, or website now has a bull-
horn. Pop psychology ("5 ways to cure mental illness!") regularly mixes with
pseudo-science ("Hiking better than medication for depression") to create a
wealth of misinformation. Snake-oil salesmen abound, and phone apps promise to wash your schizophrenia problems away. For-profit companies often disguise their ads to look like they are from news outlets or satisfied customers.
Stories that start off legitimate are broadcast and rebroadcast with each broadcaster putting his or her own spin on it, much like the game of telephone,
where one person whispers a story to the next person who whispers to the
next, until finally the last person has to repeat what they heard, and what they
repeat has no relation to the original story. So a research report that finds say,
toxoplasmosis generated by cats may be associated with some incidence of

schizophrenia, in the final telling becomes "Schizophrenia researchers urge you to kill your cats."

Be Wary of these Online Resources

Avoid Citizens Commission on Human Rights (CCHR), Scientology, Mad in America, National Empowerment Center (NEC), Excellence in Mental Health, mindfreedom, Bazelon, National Coalition for Mental Health Recovery (NCMHR), and sites that extol Thomas Szasz, Peter Breggin, or Robert Whitaker. Avoid sites and blogs that only list the side-effects of medications without discussing potential benefits, or promote eCPR, Open Dialogue, Hearing Voices, Mental Health First Aid (MHFA), or claim that it has discovered the cause, the cure or way to predict or prevent schizophrenia. While it is getting better under Assistant Secretary of Mental Health, Dr. Elinore McCance-Katz, I would still avoid information from the Substance Abuse and Mental Health Services Administration (SAMHSA) as it tends to be supportive of interventions that are politically correct but lack a scientific foundation. NAMI National used to provide reputable information on serious mental illness but has moved far from that.

Rely on these Reputable Resources

The schizophrenia page of the National Institute of Mental Health (https://www.nimh.nih.gov/health/topics/schizophrenia/index.shtml) contains basic reliable information on schizophrenia and links to studies that are looking for participants. Because NIMH materials are in the public domain, pamphlets from other organizations are often an outdated version of NIMH materials. Other sites with robust information include the Schizophrenia Society of Canada (http://www.schizophrenia.ca), the British Columbia Schizophrenia Society (http://www.bcss.org, Facebook: https://www.facebook.com/BCSchizophreniaSociety, @BCSchizophrenia), and Pathways (http://pathwayssmi.org, @PathwaysSMI), formerly known as North Shore Schizophrenia Society.

Individuals seeking other information on schizophrenia are usually looking for one of four discrete types: information on new treatments and research; financial entitlements and government protections; local services and coping tips; and advocacy. Here's where to look.

1. Information on New Treatments and Research

Most of the reputable information about new treatments and new research emanates from studies published in science journals, including Schizophrenia Research (https://www.journals.elsevier.com/schizophrenia-research), Schizophrenia Bulletin (https://academic.oup.com/schizophreniabulletin), Psychiatric News (https://psychnews.psychiatryonline.org), and Psychiatric Times (http://www.psychiatrictimes.com). By relying on them, you can keep up-to-date while monitoring fewer sites.

When a new study is published in one of these journals, it usually includes a summary (abstract). Unfortunately, reporters, bloggers, and site administrators often take information from the study's abstract, or even just the press release, combine it with an interview with the author of the study, and rebroadcast it without reading the underlying study. This is problematic because the abstract and the press release, as well as the resultant story, will likely highlight only the positive findings, and not any negative results or weaknesses in the study. Likewise, the number of people who dropped out of a study is not always reported, making it hard to determine if those who were still in the study at the end were typical or atypical.

Read the actual study, rather than the abstract. If you can only find the abstract online, it often gives the email address of the lead author. If you send a fawning appreciative email, they will usually send you the full study. If not, your library may be able to get it for you.

Look closely to determine who conducted the study. Studies that lack independence or are paid for by pharmaceutical companies or inventors of new psychosocial approaches with a financial interest in the result deserve an extra grain of skepticism. Just as important as reading the full study: don't spread information you haven't verified.

Here are free sources of science-based research and treatment information. Some link to the abstracts and some to the actual studies.

PubMed Central and PubMed

https://www.ncbi.nlm.nih.gov/pmc
https://www.ncbi.nlm.nih.gov/pubmeds
The National Institutes of Health's National Library of Medicine's PubMed Central provides free access to the full text of studies that were supported by the National Institutes of Health and published in scientific journals. However, the information is only available twelve months after its publication. It's a good resource if you want to look up the actual studies on a particular medication, treatment, or side-effects. Studies can also be sorted by date. The Library of Medicine's PubMed offers a search of all published abstracts regardless of their funding source. Some abstracts link to the full study.

The Mental Elf

https://www.nationalelfservice.net/mental-health/schizophrenia
The Mental Elf is based in the United Kingdom and run by Dr. Andre Tomlin, an information scientist and blogger who has worked in mental health. He keeps readers up-to-date on the latest mental health research and while highlighting the limitations of the studies. His Facebook page and Twitter feed (@Mental_Elf) cover a wider range of mental illnesses.

Science Daily
https://www.sciencedaily.com/news/mind_brain/schizophrenia
The Science Daily schizophrenia section publishes summaries of studies as they come in, but they don't objectively analyze the studies to see if the summaries reflect the most important points.

Schizophrenia Warriors Smart Academy
https://www.facebook.com/SchizophreniaWarriors
This Facebook page contains a robust feed of the often overstated press releases, news articles and abstracts. It's a good place to find out what is being published, but do read and critique the actual studies yourself.

Clozapine
Individuals interested in learning more about clozapine may be interested in Dr. Robert Laitman's Running for Daniel site (https://www.teamdanielrun ningforrecovery.org/talks) and the CURESZ Foundation site (https://curesz .org run by Bethany Yeiser and Dr. Henry Nasrallah. Both have a lot of info on clozapine and how to deal with side-effects.

Neuro-critics
To understand the limitations of highly publicized research, follow the Twitter feeds and blogs of some "neuro-critics." Unlike anti-psychiatrists, neuro-critics acknowledge serious mental illness exists, but they are appalled by the shoddy research that passes as science and the overstated claims that are often made by study authors.

James Coyne blogs at PLOS (blogs.plos.org/mindthebrain/author/jcyone/) and has a Twitter Feed (@CoyneoftheRealm) and Facebook page (https:// www.facebook.com/james.c.coyne) that expose the faulty math, modeling, and conclusions that work their way into both the mass media and peer-reviewed press. Neuroskeptic blogs at Discover Magazine (http://blogs.discovermaga zine.com/neuroskeptic), @Neuro_Skeptic) and covers a broad swath of psychiatry with a skeptical eye that exposes the sham science behind putting the prefix 'neuro' in front of everything ("Neuro Golf Clubs" anyone?).

Keith Laws (@Keith_Laws), a professor of Cognitive Neuropsychology, covers the overstated claims for many of the cognitive treatments. The Neurocritic (@neurocritic) looks at some of the most sensationalistic findings concerning neuroscience and brain imaging. Dr. Sidney Wolfe at Public Citizen Health Research Group, publishes Best Pills/Worst Pills (www.worstpills.org) which is useful for looking up efficacy and side effects of specific drugs. Public Citizen does not accept any support from the pharmaceutical industry, but the site does require registering.

2. Information on Financial Entitlements and Government Protections

The best, most accurate information on financial benefits for people with schizophrenia is found on the websites of the government agencies that administer the benefits. Use these sites rather than the reprints of the information found elsewhere, because the reprints may not be up-to-date, while the agency website likely will be.

- Medicaid information is at medicaid.gov and Medicare information is at medicare.gov. Both programs are administered by the Centers for Medicaid and Medicare Services (cms.gov), but there are important state-by-state bells and whistles, so look for state-specific websites as well.
- The Supplemental Security Income (SSI) and Social Security Disability Income (SSDI) programs are administered by the Social Security Administration (ssa.gov).
- Section 8 housing falls under the Department of Housing and Urban Development (hud.gov), but each state offers state-specific information.
- Benefits for U.S. veterans can be found at the Department of Veterans Affairs (va.gov).
- Benefits for federal employees are found at https://www.usa.gov /benefits-for-federal-employees.
- Information on educational, transportation, and other services you are entitled to under the Americans with Disability Act can be found at ada.gov.
- Information on the emergency room services you are entitled to under the Emergency Medical Treatment and Labor Act (EMTALA) can be found on the Center for Medicare and Medicaid Services (CMS) site at https://www.cms.gov/Regulations-and-Guidance/Legislation /EMTALA.
- Information on patient privacy protections embedded in HIPAA are available at https://www.hhs.gov/hipaa/index.html.
- The Department of Justice publishes information on privacy protections for students that are part of FERPA at https://www2.ed.gov/policy /gen/guid/fpco/ferpa/index.html.
- Parity regulations can be found at https://www.cms.gov/cciio/programs -and-initiatives/other-insurance-protections/mhpaea_factsheet.html

3. Information on Local Services and Coping Tips

Finding doctors, housing, clinics, rehabilitation, therapy, clubhouses, and other services online is difficult because nationwide sites are less useful for geo-specific needs. The *state or local* Mental Health Association, NAMI, or mental health agency may provide an online resource or app that purports to list local services, but the majority of listed programs likely do not accept people with schizophrenia, and those that do are likely full. However, their Facebook pages may be useful because you can ask a question and get answers from locals. There are also many Facebook groups and pages dedicated to helping caregivers of people with serious mental illness and people with serious mental illness cope better. Some are public, so you can only use them to ask a question if you don't mind others seeing it. Others are private.

For caregivers, two good non-public Facebook groups are Amy Welty Peterson's Parents of Kids with Schizophrenia (https://www.facebook.com /groups/461789313858387) and Deborah Fabos's Circle of Comfort and Assistance Community (CCA). To join CCA, email Deborah at CCA Community@outlook.com explaining why you want to join. Parents in both groups offer a wealth of practical knowledge and emotional support to others.

There are many "peer" or "consumer" groups on Facebook where you can ask questions. But peers should be extra cautious because there are people in these groups who espouse policies and "solutions" that are flat-out wrong. On Facebook, people with schizophrenia trade information and concerns at Schizophrenia Haven (https://www.facebook.com/groups/Schizophre niaHaven) and Schizophrenia Support Group (https://www.facebook.com /groups/schizophreniasupportgroup.) Brian Chiko's schizophrenia.com has not been updated in a while, but still has the most vibrant schizophrenia forums.

While many websites have information on coping skills like managing symptoms, handling violence and substance abuse, estate planning, or fighting recalcitrant health care officials, no one has aggregated the information in a single, easy-to-access site. Try the coping section of Mental Illness Policy Org. (https://mentalillnesspolicy.org/coping) described below.

4. Information on Advocacy

It's important for people with schizophrenia and their families to advocate for improvement of the treatment system. If we don't, who will? If your primary goal is to "eliminate stigma," any site can help, as "eliminating stigma" is the meat and potatoes of most mental "health" websites. But for those into more hardcore advocacy designed to improve how services are delivered, increase access and decrease suffering, you need to take two steps: monitor policies and politics, and organize to change them.

Monitoring Policies and Politics

Mental health department policies originate in the political sphere, so monitoring policies and politics is key. Bookmark your state and county mental health departments, the mental health committees of your state assembly and senate, and Protection and Advocacy groups. Explore the sites frequently and sign up for their blogs, alerts, and Twitter feeds. Set a Google email alert for "mental illness," "mentally ill," "mental health," "schizophrenia," "psychiatric," and other terms, so that you get daily updates on what is going on.

To get leads about new legislation or policies, follow national, state, and local "peer," "consumer," and "survivor" groups, because they do a better job of monitoring and alerting members than pro-psychiatry groups do, even though they are often on the wrong side of the issue. You can find a useful state list here: http://power2u.org/consumerrun-statewide.html. Also follow Bazelon (bazelon.org), National Disabilities Rights Network (http://www .ndrn.org), and Mental Health America (nmha.org). However, understand that these groups often publicize and support legislation that is the exact opposite of what would help people with serious mental illnesses like schizophrenia.

Also follow the websites of trade associations representing those involved in the provisioning of mental health services. Their websites all have policy sections, and many publish useful data you can use in your advocacy. Here are just a few: the National Association of State Mental Health Program Directors (https://nasmhpd.org); the National Council for Community Behavioral Health (https://www.thenationalcouncil.org); the National Association for Behavioral Healthcare, primarily representing hospital systems (nabh.org); and the American Psychiatric Association (psychiatry.org).

Government agencies that provide benefits create annual and subject matter reports that are a rich source of data to inform your advocacy. Likewise with reports from the Treatment Advocacy Center discussed below.

Organizing for Change
By far the two best sources of online information for those organizing for change are those provided by the Treatment Advocacy Center and Mental Illness Policy Org.*

Treatment Advocacy Center
http://treatmentadvocacycenter.org
Facebook: https://www.facebook.com/TreatmentAdvocacyCtr
Twitter: @TreatmentAdvCtr
Blog: http://tac2.nonprofitsoapbox.com/stay-informed
The Treatment Advocacy Center provides a wealth of information on the consequences of failing to treat people with serious mental illness and what changes in the mental health system are needed to remedy those failures. Highlights include three informative blogs; state-by-state information about emergency hospitalization, civil commitment laws, and other issues (http:// tac2.nonprofitsoapbox.com/browse-by-state); and original research on violence, the hospital bed shortage, criminalization, and other critical issues that are ignored by most advocacy organizations.

---

*Disclosure: Dr. Torrey is associated with the Treatment Advocacy Center, and D. J. Jaffe is Executive Director of Mental Illness Policy Org.

Mental Illness Policy Org

http://mentalillnesspolicy.org
Facebook: https://www.facebook.com/mentalillnesspolicyorg/
Twitter: @MentalIllPolicy
Blog: https://mentalillnesspolicy.org/blog.html

The Mental Illness Policy Org website attempts to make the best information easily accessible in order to empower advocates. Entrée to the site is through a massive table of contents that provides access to documents in a single click. The site focuses almost exclusively on five issues: involuntary commitment, assisted outpatient treatment, preserving psychiatric inpatient capacity, not guilty by reason of insanity, and reorienting mental health expenditures towards the 4% with serious mental illness, rather than improving mental wellness in the masses. Subsites exist for New York (kendras-law.org) and California (lauras-law.org).

If you are focused on helping the most seriously ill, and want to facilitate change at the state level, you will probably have to start your own group, as there are few state groups focused on the seriously ill in the United States. Start your own community by using Facebook, Linked-in, Twitter, email lists, and blogs. They allow you to create a core group of people who share your passion for whatever change you want.

Blogs and Apps

Blogs: My favorite blogs are written by Pete Earley and Natasha Tracy. Pete Earley, author of *Crazy*, and a former *Washington Post* reporter writes a very popular blog (http://www.peteearley.com/blog, @peteearley) that deliciously covers the more difficult issues surrounding severe mental illness and often uncovers important and disturbing trends before others. Natasha Tracy (technically bipolar, author of *Lost Marbles*) writes a hip and often-contrarian blog from the peer perspective (natashatracy.com, @natasha_tracy) that is consistently original and thoughtful. They're both active on Facebook too. Many people enjoy The Mighty, which publishes inspirational stories by people with various mental health issues, sometimes including schizophrenia (https://themighty.com/topic/schizophrenia).

Apps: Apps for the phone are getting a lot of attention but are in their infancy. Most are merely standard social media type things (connect with others, access information) wrapped in a mental health narrative. Further, it appears that the information shared on them is not HIPAA protected, and may be sold to third-parties. Some apps connect you to unknown therapists for a monthly or per-use fee, but it is not likely reimbursable. Some apps may include a not-ready-for-prime-time biometric twist that the vendor promises is useful. PsyberGuide (https://psyberguide.org), run by Dr. Stephen Schueller and backed by several reputable organizations, is a new site that is trying to independently evaluate apps and would be a good place to start for those interested in exploring them.

NOTES

Epigraph

Van Gogh letter, quoted by J. Rewald, *Post-Impressionism: From van Gogh to Gauguin* (New York: Museum of Modern Art, 1962), p. 321.

Chapter 1

"What then does": H. R. Rollin, *Coping with Schizophrenia* (London: Burnett Books, 1980), p. 162. **"Sympathy"**: R. W. Emerson, *Journals* (1836). *"strangeness has"*: R. Porter, *A Social History of Madness* (New York: Weidenfeld and Nicolson, 1987), p. 9. **"My greatest"**: P. J. Ruocchio, "First person account: the schizophrenic inside," *Schizophrenia Bulletin* 17 (1991): 357–60. *I Never Promised You a Rose Garden:* See C. North and R. Cadoret, "Diagnostic Discrepancy in Personal Accounts of Patients with 'Schizophrenia,'" *Archives of General Psychiatry* 38 (1981): 133–37. **"Perceptual dysfunction"**: J. Cutting and F. Dunne, "Subjective Experience of Schizophrenia," *Schizophrenia Bulletin* 15 (1989): 217–31. **"either entirely"**: N. Dain, *Concepts of Insanity in the United States, 1789–1865* (New Brunswick: Rutgers University Press, 1964), p. 226, quoting the 1861–62 *Reports of the Illinois State Hospital for the Insane*. **"During the last"**: A. McGhie and J. Chapman, "Disorders of Attention and Perception in Early Schizophrenia," *British Journal of Medical Psychology*, 34

(1961): 103–16. **"Colours seem"**: Ibid. **"Everything looked vibrant"**: Cutting and Dunne. **"Lots of things"**: Ibid. **"People looked deformed"**: Ibid. **"I saw everything"**: G. Burns, "An Account of My Madness," mimeo, 1983. **"These crises"**: M. Sechehaye, *Autobiography of a Schizophrenic Girl* (New York: Grune and Stratton, 1951), p. 22. **"Everything seems"**: McGhie and Chapman. **"Occasionally during"**: Anonymous, "An Autobiography of a Schizophrenic Experience," *Journal of Abnormal and Social Psychology* 51 (1955): 677–89. **"My focus"**: M. Vonnegut, *The Eden Express* (New York: Praeger, 1975), p. 107. **"An outsider"**: E. Leete, "Mental Illness: An Insider's View," presented at annual meeting of National Alliance for the Mentally Ill, New Orleans, 1985. **In one study**: Cutting and Dunne. **"Sometimes when people"**: McGhie and Chapman. **"Social situations"**: R. McLean, *Recovered, Not Cured* (Crows Nest, Australia: Allen and Unwin, 2003), p. 35. **"it was terrible"**: M. Barnes and J. Berke, *Mary Barnes: Two Accounts of a Journey through Madness* (New York: Ballantine, 1973), p. 44. **"touching any patient"**: P. S. Wagner, "Life in the Closet," *Hartford Courant*, August 26, 1993. **"decay in my"**: Rollin, p. 150. **"a genital sexual"**: Ibid. **One psychiatrist**: See M. B. Bowers, *Retreat from Sanity: The Structure of Emerging Psychosis* (Baltimore: Penguin, 1974). **"My trouble is"** and **"My concentration is"**: McGhie and Chapman. **"Childhood feelings"**: Bowers, p. 152. **"All sorts of"**: W. Mayer-Gross, E. Slater, and M. Roth, *Clinical Psychiatry* (Baltimore: Williams and Wilkins, 1969), p. 268. **"In college"**: Wagner. **"I was invited"**: A. Boisen, *Out of the Depths*, 1960. Quoted in B. Kaplan, ed., *The Inner World of Mental Illness* (New York: Harper and Row, 1964), p. 118. **"It was evening"**: E. Leete, "The Interpersonal Environment," in A. B. Hatfield and H. P. Lefley, *Surviving Mental Illness* (New York: Guilford Press, 1993), p. 117. **"Suddenly my whole"**: M. Coate, *Beyond All Reason* (Philadelphia: Lippincott, 1965), p. 21. **"I was in"**: Bowers, p. 27. **"nearly all patients"**: J. Parnas and P. Handset, "Phenomenology of Anomalous Self-Expression in Early Schizophrenia," *Comprehensive Psychiatry* 44 (2003): 121–34. **"as if a heavy"**: B. J. Freedman, "The Subjective Experience of Perceptual and Cognitive Disturbances in Schizophrenia," *Archives of General Psychiatry* 30 (1974): 333–40. **"However hard"**: Rollin, p. 150. **One sensation**: See E. F. Torrey, "Headaches After Lumbar Puncture and Insensitivity to Pain in Psychiatric Patients," *New England Journal of Medicine* 301 (1979): 110; G. D. Watson, P. C. Chandarana, and H. Merskey, "Relationship between Pain and Schizophrenia," *British Journal of Psychiatry* 138 (1981): 33–36; and L. K. Bickerstaff, S. C. Harris, R. S. Leggett, et al., "Pain Insensitivity in Schizophrenic Patients," *Archives of Surgery* 123 (1988): 49–51. **"The walk of"**: N. McDonald, "Living with Schizophrenia," *Canadian Medical Association Journal* 82 (1960): 218–21, 678–81. **"When people are"**: McGhie and Chapman. **"I can concentrate"**: Ibid. **"I used to get"**: Cutting and Dunne. **"I have to"**: J. Chapman, "The Early Symptoms of Schizophrenia," *British Journal of Psychiatry* 112 (1966): 225–51. **"the teeth, then"**: Sechehaye, foreword. "This morning": S. Sheehan, *Is There No Place on Earth for Me?* (Boston: Houghton Mifflin, 1982), p. 69. "I can't concentrate": McGhie and Chapman. "I tried sitting": B. O'Brien, *Operators and Things: The Inner Life of a Schizophrenic* (New York: Signet, 1976), pp. 97–98. "During the visit": Sechehaye, p. 28. "If I do": Chapman. "My thoughts get": McGhie and Chapman. "How could a": O'Brien, p. 100. "It seemed": McLean, p. 20. "Big magnified": Chapman. "I feel that": Mayer-Gross, Slater, and Roth, pp. 281, 267. "For instance, I": G. Bateson, ed., *Perceval's Narrative: A Patient's Account of His Psychosis 1830–1832* (1838, 1840) (New York: Morrow, 1974), p. 269. "I may be": McGhie and Chapman. Chapman claims: See Chapman. "I am so": Anonymous, "I Feel Like I Am Trapped Inside My Head, Banging Desperately against Its Walls," *New York Times*, March 18, 1986, p. C–3. "How could": S. Nasar, *A Beautiful Mind* (New York: Simon & Schuster, 1998), p. 11. "A policeman walking": A. Chekhov, "Ward No. 6," quoted in A. A. Stone and S. S. Stone, eds., *The Abnormal Personality through Literature* (Englewood Cliffs, N.J.: Prentice-Hall, 1966), p. 5. "During the paranoid": Anonymous, "Schizophrenic Experience." "I felt that": Ibid. de Clerembault: G. Remington and H. Book, "Case Report of de Clerembault Syndrome, Bipolar Affective Disorder and Response to Lithium," *American Journal of Psychiatry* 141 (1984): 1285–88. "telepathic force": Rollin, p. 132. "I believed": C. Hubert, "Woman Defies Her Demons to Excel," *Sacramento Bee*, February 1, 2002, p. A-1. "I was really upset": McLean, p. 76. A 1999 study: E. F. Torrey, et al., *Threats to Radio and Television Station Personnel in the United States by Individuals with Severe Mental Illnesses* (Washington, D.C.: Public Citizen's Health Research Group and the Treatment Advocacy Center, 1999). "millions and billions": P. Earle, "Popular Fallacies in Regard to Insanity and the Insane," *Journal of Social Science* 26: 107–17, 1890. "This phenomenon can": J. Lang, "The Other Side of Hallucinations," *American Journal of Psychiatry* 94 (1938): 1090–97. "No doubt I": Poe, "The Tell-Tale Heart." "Thus for years": D. P. Schreber, *Memoirs of My Nervous Illness* (1903), translated and with introduction by I. Macalpine and R. A. Hunter (London: William Dawson, 1955), p. 172. "There was music": Boisen, quoted in Kaplan, p. 119. "For about almost": Schreber, p. 225. "a constant state": E. Goode, "Experts See Mind's Voices in New Light," *New York Times*, May 6, 2003, p. F-1. "I don't just sit": D. Terry and D. Terry, "My Private Chorus of Chaos," *Chicago Tribune*, February 23, 2003, p. 8. recent studies: P. K. McGuire, G. M. S. Shah, and R. M. Murray, "Increased Blood Flow in Broca's Area during Auditory Hallucinations in Schizophrenia," *Lancet* 342 (1993): 703–6. temporoparietal junction: M. Plaze, M.-L. Paillère-Martinot, J. Penttilä, et al., "'Where Do Auditory Hallucinations Come From?'—A Brain Morphometry Study of Schizophrenia Patients with Inner or Outer Space Hallucinations," *Schizophrenia Bulletin* 37 (2011): 212–21. born deaf: E. M. R. Critchley, "Auditory Experiences of Deaf Schizophrenics," *Journal of the Royal Society of Medicine* 76 (1983): 542–44. "At an early": Lang.

Silvano Arieti: *Creativity: The Magic Synthesis* (New York: Basic Books 1976), p. 251. **"On a few":** Ibid. **"To the person":** Lang. **"I have no contact":** Parnas and Handset. **"A young man":** Ibid. **In extreme cases:** H. Faure, "L'Investissement Delirant de L'Image de Soi," *Evolution Psychiatrique* 3 (1956): 545–77. **"I get shaky":** Chapman. **"This was equally":** Sechehaye, p. 87. **"My breast gives":** Schreber, p. 207. **"81 percent":** S. Bustamante, K. Maurer, W. Loffler, et al., "Depressive Symptoms in the Early Course of Schizophrenia," abstract, *Schizophrenia Research* 11 (1994): 187. **"During the first":** Lang. **"Later, considering them":** Sechehaye, p. 35. **"I sat":** M. Stakes, "First Person Account: Becoming Seaworthy," *Schizophrenia Bulletin* 11 (1985): 629. **"there has been":** P. Cramer, J. Bowen, and M. O'Neill, "Schizophrenics and Social Judgment," *British Journal of Psychiatry* 160 (1992): 481–87. **"patients performed":** C. G. Kohler, T. H. Turner, W. B. Bilker, et al., "Facial Emotion Recognition in Schizophrenia: Intensity Effects and Error Pattern," *American Journal of Psychiatry* 160 (2003): 1768–74. **"Half the time":** McGhie and Chapman. **"one of the earliest":** Chapman. **"During my first":** Anonymous, "Schizophrenic Experience." **"Instead of wishing":** E. Meyer and L. Covi, "The Experience of Depersonalization: A Written Report by a Patient," *Psychiatry* 23 (1960): 215–17. **"I wish I":** J. A. Wechsler, *In a Darkness* (New York: Norton, 1972), p. 17. **"reported experiencing":** A. M. Kring, S. L. Kerr, D. A. Smith, et al., "Flat Affect in Schizophrenia Does Not Reflect Diminished Subjective Experience of Emotion," *Journal of Abnormal Psychology* 102 (1993): 507–17. **"Loneliness needs":** J. K. Bouricius, "Negative Symptoms and Emotions in Schizophrenia," *Schizophrenia Bulletin* 15 (1989): 201–7. **"I still have":** I. Chovil, "First Person Account: I and I, Dancing Fool, Challenge You the World to a Duel," *Schizophrenia Bulletin* 26 (2000): 745–47. **One study of changes:** T. C. Manschreck, et al., "Disturbed Voluntary Motor Activity in Schizophrenic Disorder," *Psychological Medicine* 12 (1982): 73–84; see also M. Jones and R. Hunter, "Abnormal Movements in Patients with Chronic Psychotic Illness," in G. E. Crane and R. Gardner, *Psychotropic Drugs and Dysfunctions of the Basal Ganglia*, publication no. 1938 (Washington, D.C.: U.S. Public Health Service, 1969). **In another study:** Cutting and Dunne. **"I became":** Ibid. **eye blinking:** See J. R. Stevens, "Eye Blink and Schizophrenia: Psychosis or Tardive Dyskinesia," *American Journal of Psychiatry* 135 (1978): 223–26. **"[He] stood":** H. de Balzac, "Louis Lambert" (1832), in A. A. Stone and S. S. Stone, eds., *The Abnormal Personality through Literature* (Englewood Cliffs, N.J.: Prentice-Hall, 1966), pp. 63–64. **"When I am":** McGhie and Chapman. **"I don't like":** Ibid. **"I am not":** Ibid. **"As the work":** Kindwall and Kinder (1940), quoted in C. Landis and F. A. Mettler, *Varieties of Psychopathological Experience* (New York: Holt, Rinehart, and Winston, 1964), p. 530. **"to help to":** Chapman. **Chapman believes:** Chapman. **"the only way":** Wagner. **the Abominable Snowman:** B. Hoffman, "Weird But True," *New York Post,*

May 28, 2002, p. 19. **body temperature:** T. W. H. Chong and D. J. Castle, "Layer upon Layer: Thermoregulation in Schizophrenia," *Schizophrenia Research 69* (2004): 149–57. **One young lady:** E. Herrig, "First Person Account: A Personal Experience," *Schizophrenia Bulletin* 21 (1995): 339–42. **John Hinckley:** "Hinckley Sr. Seeks Support in Fight against Mental Illness," *Psychiatric News*, November 16, 1984. **"Generally, insane":** "Confinement of the Insane," *American Law Review* (1869): 215. **"an enchanted loom":** Quoted by O. Sacks, *The Man Who Mistook His Wife for a Hat* (New York: Summit Books, 1985), p. 140. **"self-measuring ruler":** Burns. **"You will realize":** *The Complete Letters of Vincent Van Gogh*, vol. 3 (Boston: New York Graphic Society, 1978), p. 524. **cited by one woman:** A. Sobin and M. N. Ozer, "Mental Disorders in Acute Encephalitis," *Journal of Mount Sinai Hospital* 33 (1966): 73–82. **"Something inside":** B. Bick, "Love and Resentment," *New York Times*, March 25, 1990. **"No doubt Louis":** Balzac.

Chapter 2

"To one": M. Coate, *Beyond All Reason* (Philadelphia: Lippincott, 1965), pp. 1–2. **Studies have shown:** C. S. Mellor, "First Rank Symptoms of Schizophrenia," *British Journal of Psychiatry* 117 (1970): 15–23, **patients with bipolar disorder:** W. T. Carpenter, J. S. Strauss, and S. Muleh, "Are There Pathognomonic Symptoms in Schizophrenia?" *Archives of General Psychiatry* 28 (1973): 847–52. **DSM-IV:** *Diagnostic and Statistical Manual of Mental Disorders* (Washington, D.C.: American Psychiatric Association, 1994). **Rosenhan study:** D. L. Rosenhan, "On Being Sane in Insane Places," *Science* 179 (1973): 250–58; see also R. L. Spitzer, "More on Pseudoscience in Science and the Case for Psychiatric Diagnosis," *Archives of General Psychiatry* 33 (1976): 459–70. **"If I were":** S. S. Kety, "From Rationalization to Reason," *American Journal of Psychiatry* 131 (1974): 957–63. **deficit schizophrenia:** W. T. Carpenter Jr., D. W. Heinrichs, and A.M.I. Wagman, "Deficit and Nondeficit Forms of Schizophrenia: The Concept," *American Journal of Psychiatry* 145 (1988): 578–83. **endophenotypes:** I. I. Goffman and T. D. Gould, "The Endophenotype Concept in Psychiatry: Etymology and Strategic Intentions," *American Journal of Psychiatry* 160 (2003): 636–45. **5 percent:** J. van Os, R. J. Linscott, I. Myin-Germeys, et al., "A Systematic Review and Meta-Analysis of the Psychosis Continuum: Evidence for a Psychosis Proneness-Persistence-Impairment Model of Psychotic Disorder," *Psychological Medicine* 39 (2008): 1–17. **cross-national survey:** R. Nuevo, S. Chatterji, E. Verdes, et al., "The Continuum of Psychotic Symptoms in the General Population: A Cross-National Study," *Schizophrenia Bulletin* 38 (2012): 475–85. **"should not be":** D. B. Smith, "Can You Live with the Voices in Your Head?" *New York Times Magazine*, March 25, 2007, pp. 49–53.

Chapter 3

"What consoles me": J. Rewald, *Post-Impressionism: From van Gogh to Gauguin* (New York: Museum of Modern Art, 1962), p. 320. **marijuana:** J. McGrath, J. Welham, J. Scott, et al., "Association between Cannabis Use and Psychosis-Related Outcomes Using Sibling Pair Analysis in a Cohort of Young Adults," *Archives of General Psychiatry* 67 (2010): 440–47; M. De Hert, M. Wampers, T. Jendricko, et al., "Effects of Cannabis Use on Age at Onset in Schizophrenia and Bipolar Disorder," *Schizophrenia Research* 126 (2011): 270–76. **The best study:** M. Harbrecht and H. Häfner, "Substance Abuse and the Onset of Schizophrenia," *Biological Psychiatry* 40 (1996): 1155–63. **widely quoted study:** R. C. W. Hall, E. R. Gardner, S. K. Stickney, et al., "Physical Illness Manifesting as Psychiatric Disease," *Archives of General Psychiatry* 37 (1980): 989–95. **Koran and his colleagues:** L. M. Koran, H. C. Sox, K. I. Marton, et al., "Medical Evaluation of Psychiatric Patients," *Archives of General Psychiatry* 46 (1989): 733–40. **One English study:** K. Davison, "Schizophrenia-like Psychoses Associated with Organic Cerebral Disorders: A Review," *Psychiatric Developments* 1 (1983): 1–34. **Another English study:** E. C. Johnstone, J. F. Macmillan, and T. J. Crow, "The Occurrence of Organic Disease of Possible or Probable Aetiological Significance in a Population of 268 Cases of First Episode Schizophrenia," *Psychological Medicine* 17 (1987): 371–79. **A postmortem study:** Davison. **Viral Encephalitis:** E. F. Torrey, "Functional Psychoses and Viral Encephalitis," *Integrative Psychiatry* 4 (1986): 224–36. **One study:** Davison. **In 2004:** S. Saik, J. E. Kraus, A. McDonald, et al., "Neurosyphilis in Newly Admitted Psychiatric Patients: Three Case Reports," *Journal of Clinical Psychiatry* 65 (2004): 919–21. **one report:** A. G. Awad, "Schizophrenia and Multiple Sclerosis," *Journal of Nervous and Mental Disease* 171 (1983): 323–24. **"a common":** Davison. **AIDS:** N. Buhrich, D. A. Cooper, and E. Freed, "HIV Infection Associated with Symptoms Indistinguishable from Functional Psychosis," *British Journal of Psychiatry* 152 (1988): 649–53. **There is some:** A. S. Nielsen, P. B. Mortensen, E. O'Callaghan, et al., "Is Head Injury a Risk Factor for Schizophrenia?" *Schizophrenia Research* 55 (2002): 93–98; G. E. Jaskiw and J. F. Kenny, "Limbic Cortical Injury Sustained during Adulthood Leads to Schizophrenia-like Syndrome," *Schizophrenia Research* 58 (2002): 205–12. **An MRI study:** P. Buckley, J. P. Stack, C. Madigan, et al., "Magnetic Resonance Imaging of Schizophrenia-like Psychoses Associated with Cerebral Trauma: Clinicopathological Correlates." *American Journal of Psychiatry* 150 (1993): 146–48. **Rosemary Kennedy:** E. F. Torrey, *Nowhere to Go* (New York: Harper and Row, 1988), pp. 102–6. **study reported:** J. Rimmer and B. Jacobsen, "Antisocial Personality in the Biological Relatives of Schizophrenics." *Comprehensive Psychiatry* 21 (1980): 258–62.

Chapter 4

"Such a disease": Quoted in V. Norris, *Mental Illness in London* (London: Oxford University Press, 1959), p. 15. "it is only": J. Hawkes, "On the Increase of Insanity," *Journal of Psychological Medicine and Mental Pathology* 10 (1857): 508–21. "in a considerable": E. Kraepelin, *Dementia Praecox and Paraphrenia* (Huntington, N.Y.: Robert E. Krieger, 1971), pp. 236–37. **study in Finland:** M. Isohanni, I. Isohanni, P. Jones, et al., "School Predictors of Schizophrenia in the 1966 Northern Finland Birth Cohort," *Schizophrenia Research* 36 (1999): 44. **Especially interesting:** A. Shaner, G. Miller, and J. Mintz, "Evidence of a Latitudinal Gradient in the Age of Onset of Schizophrenia," *Schizophrenia Research* 94 (2007): 58–63. **Researchers in Germany and Canada:** M. Hambrecht, H. Häfner, and W. Löffler, "Beginning Schizophrenia Observed by Significant Others," *Social Psychiatry and Psychiatric Epidemiology* 29 (1994): 53–60; J. Varsamis and J. D. Adamson, "Somatic Symptoms in Schizophrenia," *Canadian Psychiatric Association Journal* 21 (1976): 1–6. **"monster themes":** A. T. Russell, L. Bett, and C. Sammons, "The Phenomenology of Schizophrenia Occurring in Childhood," *Journal of the American Academy of Child and Adolescent Psychiatry* 28 (1989): 399–407. **Recent MRI studies:** J. L. Rapoport, J. N. Giedd, J. Blumenthal, et al., "Progressive Cortical Change During Adolescence in Childhood-Onset Schizophrenia," *Archives of General Psychiatry* 56 (1999): 649–54; A. L. Sporn, D. K. Greenstein, N. Gogtay, et al., "Progressive Brain Volume Loss during Adolescence in Childhood-Onset Schizophrenia," *American Journal of Psychiatry* 160 (2003): 2181–89. **follow-up of ten:** J. G. Howells and W. R. Guirguis, "Childhood Schizophrenia 20 Years Later," *Archives of General Psychiatry* 41 (1984): 123–28. **Vladimir Nabokov:** V. Nabokov, *The Stories of Vladimir Nabokov* (New York: Vintage, 1995), pp. 598–603. **Louise Wilson:** *This Stranger, My Son* (New York: Putnam, 1968). **study in Denmark:** I. M. Terp, G. Engholm, H. Moller, et al., "A Follow-Up Study of Postpartum Psychoses: Prognosis and Risk Factors for Readmission," *Acta Psychiatrica Scandinavica* 100 (1999): 40–46. **One study:** H. Brodaty, P. Sachdev, A. Koschera, et al., "Long-term Outcome of Late-Onset Schizophrenia: 5-year Follow-up Study," *British Journal of Psychiatry* 183 (2003): 213–19. **recent studies:** A. Aleman, R. S. Kahn, J. P. Selten, "Sex Differences in the Risk of Schizophrenia," *Archives of General Psychiatry* 60 (2003): 565–71. **gender differences:** See M. V. Seeman, "Gender Differences in Schizophrenia," *Canadian Journal of Psychiatry* 27 (1982): 107–11; J. M. Goldstein, "Gender Differences in the Course of Schizophrenia," *American Journal of Psychiatry* 145 (1988): 684–89; and S. Lewis, "Sex and Schizophrenia: Vive la Difference," *British Journal of Psychiatry* 161 (1992): 445–50. **"were considered to be":** J. Lieberman, et al., "Time Course and Biologic Correlates of Treatment Response in First-Episode Schizophrenia," *Archives of General Psychiatry* 50 (1993): 369–76. **best summary:** J. H. Stephens, "Long-term Prognosis and Follow-up in

Schizophrenia," *Schizophrenia Bulletin* 4 (1978): 25–47. **"About three-fifths":** L. Ciompi, "Catamnestic Long-term Study of the Course of Life and Aging of Schizophrenics," *Schizophrenia Bulletin* 6 (1980): 606–16. **"the current picture":** C. M. Harding and J. S. Strauss, "The Course of Schizophrenia: An Evolving Concept" in M. Alpert, ed., *Controversies in Schizophrenia* (New York: Guilford Press, 1985), p. 347. **"The patient":** W. Mayer-Gross, E. Slater, and M. Roth, *Clinical Psychiatry* (Baltimore: Williams and Wilkins, 1969), p. 275. **community survey in Baltimore:** M. Von Korff, G. Nestadt, A. Romanoski, et al., "Prevalence of Treated and Untreated *DSM-III* Schizophrenia," *Journal of Nervous and Mental Disease* 173 (1985): 577–81. **biasing the sample:** J. Thirthalli and S. Jain, "Better Outcome of Schizophrenia in India: A Natural Selection against Severe Forms?," *Schizophrenia Bulletin* 35 (2009): 655–57. **"is not consistent":** R. J. Sullivan, J. S. Allen, and K. L. Nero, "Schizophrenia in Palau," *Current Anthropology* 48 (2007): 189–213. **A 2008 report:** A. Cohen, V. Patel, R. Thara, et al., "Questioning an Axiom: Better Prognosis for Schizophrenia in the Developing World?," *Schizophrenia Bulletin* 34 (2008): 229–44. **A 2009 study:** A. Alem, D. Kebede, A. Fekadu, et al., "Clinical Course and Outcome of Schizophrenia in a Predominantly Treatment Naïve Cohort in Rural Ethiopia," *Schizophrenia Bulletin* 35 (2009): 646–54. **"about twice":** P. Allebeck, "Schizophrenia: A Life-Shortening Disease," *Schizophrenia Bulletin* 15 (1989): 81–89. **"nearly a threefold":** D. W. Black and R. Fisher, "Mortality in *DSM-IIIR* Schizophrenia," *Schizophrenia Research* 7 (1992): 109–16. **"5.05 times":** P. Corten, M. Ribourdouille, and M. Dramaix, "Premature Death among Outpatients at a Community Mental Health Center," *Hospital and Community Psychiatry* 42 (1991): 1248–51. **A 1999 study:** B. P. Dembling, D. T. Chen, and L. Vachon, "Life Expectancy and Causes of Death in a Population Treated for Serious Mental Illness," *Psychiatric Services* 50 (1999): 1036–42. **study from Sweden:** B. Logdberg and L. Nilsson, "Mortality in Schizophrenia over the Last 70 Years in the Township of Malmo," abstract, *Schizophrenia Bulletin* 31 (2005): 229. **double the rate:** M. J. Edlund, C. Conrad, and P. Morris, "Accidents among Schizophrenic Outpatients," *Comprehensive Psychiatry* 30 (1989): 522–26. **12 percent of the excess:** S. Brown, "Excess Mortality of Schizophrenia," *British Journal of Psychiatry* 171 (1997): 502–8. *Diseases:* See A. E. Harris, "Physical Disease and Schizophrenia," *Schizophrenia Bulletin* 14 (1988): 85–96; and S. Mukherjee, D. B. Schnur, and R. Reddy, "Family History of Type 2 Diabetes in Schizophrenic Patients," *Lancet* 1 (1989): 495. **prostate cancer:** P. B. Mortensen, "Neuroleptic Medication and Reduced Risk of Prostate Cancer in Schizophrenic Patients," *Acta Psychiatrica Scandinavica* 85 (1992): 390–93 **102 individuals:** S. Brown, J. Birtwistle, L. Roe, et al., "The Unhealthy Lifestyle of People with Schizophrenia," *Psychological Medicine* 29 (1999): 697–701. **41 percent less:** B. G. Druss, D. W. Bradford, R. A. Rosenheck, et al., "Mental Disorders and Use of Cardiovascular Procedures after Myocardial Infarction," *Journal of the American Medical Association* 283

(2000): 506–11. **study in England:** M. Marshall and D. Gath, "What Happens to Homeless Mentally Ill People? Follow-up of Residents of Oxford Hostels for the Homeless," *British Medical Journal* 304 (1992): 79–80. **in Oklahoma:** J. Cannon, "Remains Identified," *Norman Transcript*, December 21, 1990, p. 2. **In Houston:** S. K. Bardwell, "Services Saturday for Homeless Woman, Son Killed in Traffic Accident," *Houston Chronicle*, April 29, 1999, p. A-32. **In Santa Ana:** R. Hinch, "Woman Killed by Train Has Final Resting Place," *Orange County Register,* February 23, 2000, p. A-1.

Chapter 5

"Insanity in": J. F. Duncan, "President's Address," *Journal of Mental Science* 21 (1875): 316. **"If the brain":** Lyall Watson, quoted in J. Hooper and D. Teresi, *The 3-Pound Universe* (New York: MacMillan, 1986), p. 21. **A 1933 study:** M.T. Moore, D. Nathan, A.E. Elliot et al., "Encepalographic Studies in Schizophrenia," *American Journal of Psychiatry* 89 (1933): 801–10. **A 2015 review:** K. Bakhshi and D.A. Chance, "The Neuropathology of Schizophrenia: A Selective Review of Past Studies and Emerging Themes in Brain Structure and Cytoarchitecture," *Neuroscience* 303 (2015): 82–102. A 2013 Review: S.V. Haijma, N.V. Haren, W. Cahn, et al., "Brain Volume in Schizophrenia: A Meta-analysis of Over 18,000 Subjects," *Schizophrenia Bulletin* 29 (2013): 1129–38. **"three-quarters of the schizophrenic":** M. A. Taylor and R. Abrams, "Cognitive Impairment in Schizophrenia," *American Journal of Psychiatry* 141 (1984): 196–201. **A 1988 review:** D. W. Heinrichs and R. W. Buchanan, "Significance and Meaning of Neurological Signs of Schizophrenia," *American Journal of Psychiatry* 145 (1988): 11–18. **more than twenty:** Torrey, "Studies of Individuals." **"a broad":** J. A. Grebb, D. R. Weinberger, and J. M. Morihisa, "Electroencephalogram and Evoked Potentials Studies of Schizophrenia," in H. A. Nasrallah and D. R. Weinberger, eds., *The Neurology of Schizophrenia* (Amsterdam: Elsevier, 1986), pp. 121–40. **Known risk factors:** E. F. Torrey, J. J. Bartko, and R. H. Yolken, "*Toxoplasma gondii* and Other Risk Factors for Schizophrenia: An Update," *Schizophrenia Bulletin* 38 (2012): 642–47. **Known risk factors:** Ibid. **"Psychiatry and neuropathology":** H. Griesinger, cited by G. Zilboorg and G. W. Henry, *A History of Medical Psychology* (New York: Norton, 1941), p. 436. **"I was looked":** "Britain's Offbeat Psychoanalyst," *Newsweek*, November 1, 1982, p. 16. **Hubbard taught:** "Hubbard's Teachings Guide Treatment of Mental Illness," *St. Petersburg Times*, November 14, 1998. **"a feeling of":** S. Arzy, M. Seeck, S. Ortigue, et al., "Induction of an Illusory Shadow Person," *Nature* 443 (2006): 287. **feelings that your actions:** C. Farrar and C. D. Frith, "Experiencing Oneself vs Another Person as Being the Cause of an Action: The Neural Correlates of the Experience of Agency," *NeuroImage* 15 (2002): 596–603. **"insanity, then, is":** W.A.F. Browne, *What Asylums Were, Are, and*

Ought to Be (Edinburgh: Black, 1837), p. 6. **"important molecular"**: H. Maudsley, *Physiology and Pathology of the Mind* (London: Macmillan, 1867), p. 367. **"a meteoric shower"**: from Sonnet 137, in her 1934 collection *Huntsman, What Quarry?* Excerpted in *Poems by Edna St. Vincent Millay* (New York: Harper and Brothers, 1939). **"a hereditary"**: D. R. Weinberger, "Implications of Normal Brain Development for the Pathogenesis of Schizophrenia," *Archives of General Psychiatry* 44 (1987): 660–69. **A 1992 study**: E. S. Susser and S. P. Lin, "Schizophrenia after Prenatal Exposure to the Dutch Hunger Winter of 1944–1945," *Archives of General Psychiatry* 49 (1992): 983–88; E. Susser, R. Neugebauer, H. W. Hoek, et al., "Schizophrenia after Prenatal Famine," *Archives of General Psychiatry* 53 (1996): 25–31. **A 2005 study**: D. St Clair, M. Xu, P. Wang, et al., "Rates of Adult Schizophrenia following Prenatal Exposure to the Chinese Famine of 1959–1961," *Journal of the American Medical Association* 294 (2005): 557–62. **a 2010 study**: J. J. McGrath, T. H. Burne, F. Féron, et al., "Developmental Vitamin D Deficiency and Risk of Schizophrenia: A 10-Year Update," *Schizophrenia Bulletin* 36 (2010): 1073–78. **"there is no good"**: C. C. Tennant, "Stress and Schizophrenia: A Review," *Integrative Psychiatry* 3 (1985): 248–61. **46 such studies**: E. Susser, C.S. Widom, "Still Searching for Lost Truths About the Bitter Sorrows of Childhood," *Schizophrenia Bulletin* 38 (2012): 672–5. **"An extensive literature"**: S. Bendall, H. J. Jackson, C.A. Hulbert et al., "Childhood Trauma and Psychotic Disorders: A Systematic, Critical Review of the Evidence," *Schizophrenia Bulletin* 34 (2008): 568–79. **"In cases"**: E. Bleuler, *Dementia Praecox or the Group of Schizophrenias* (New York: International Universities Press, 1950), p. 345; first published in 1911. **"I seldom see"**: Letter from Sigmund Freud to Karl Abraham in E. Jones, *The Life and Work of Sigmund Freud*, vol. 2 (New York: Basic Books, 1955), p. 437. **"I do not like"**: Quoted in M. Shur, *The Id and the Regulatory Principle of Mental Functioning* (London: Hogarth, 1967), p. 21. **"in some sense"**: C. Lasch, *The Culture of Narcissism* (New York: Norton, 1979), p. 76. **"psychosis is the final"**: Ibid. **"we share"**: R. C. Lewontin, S. Rose, and L. J. Kamin, *Not in Our Genes* (New York: Pantheon Books, 1984), p. ix. **"An adequate"**: Ibid, p. 231.

Chapter 6

"To lighten": Charles Dickens, "A Curious Dance around a Curious Tree," in *Household Words*, January 17, 1852. **"as a suffering"**: W. J. Annitto, "Schizophrenia and Ego Psychology," *Schizophrenia Bulletin* 7 (1981): 199–200. **A 1996 survey**: C. Blanco, C. Carvalho, M. Olfson, et al., "Practice Patterns of International and U.S. Medical Graduate Psychiatrists," *American Journal of Psychiatry* 156 (1999): 445–50. **"What does mean"**: B. J. Ennis, *Prisoners of Psychiatry* (New York: Harcourt Brace Jovanovich, 1972); for a more complete discussion of this problem, see R. L. Taylor and E. F. Torrey, "The Pseudo-regulation of

American Psychiatry," *American Journal of Psychiatry* 129 (1972): 658–62. **diagnostic algorithm:** H. C. Sox, L. M. Koran, C. H. Sox, et al., "A Medical Algorithm for Detecting Physical Disease in Psychiatric Patients," *Hospital and Community Psychiatry* 40 (1989): 1270–76. **German study:** B. von der Stein, W. Wittgens, W. Lemmer, et al., "Schizophrenia Mimicked by Neurological Diseases," presented at the International Conference on Schizophrenia, Vancouver, July 1992. **"The hospital becomes":** B. Silcock, "Three Experiences of Madness," *Sane Talk*, summer 1994, p. 5. **A 2002 study:** P. V. Rosenau and S. H. Linder, "A Comparison of the Performance of For-Profit and Nonprofit U.S. Psychiatric Inpatient Care Providers since 1980," *Psychiatric Services* 54 (2003): 183–87. **"cozy relationship":** "JCAHO Responds to Concern over Psychiatric Hospital Oversight," *Mental Health Weekly*, vol. 9, October 4, 1999, p. 1. **"a man barricaded":** C. Holden, "Broader Commitment Laws Sought," *Science* 230 (1985): 1253–55. **"Public defender":** D. A. Treffert, "The Obviously Ill Patient in Need of Treatment: A Fourth Standard for Civil Commitment," *Hospital and Community Psychiatry* 36 (1985): 259–64. **"significant changes":** J. M. Kane, F. Quitkin, A. Rifkin, et al., "Attitudinal Changes in Involuntarily Committed Patients Following Treatment," *Archives of General Psychiatry* 40 (1983): 374–77. **"the combination of drug":** B. Pasamanick, F. R. Scarpitti, and S. Dinitz, *Schizophrenics in the Community: An Experimental Study in the Prevention of Hospitalization* (New York: Appleton-Century-Crofts, 1967), p. ix. **A 1998 study:** J. Rabinowitz, E. Bromet, J. Lavelle, et al., "Relationship between Type of Insurance and Care during the Early Course of Psychosis," *American Journal of Psychiatry* 155 (1998): 1392–97. **A 1985 study:** G. Geis, P. Jaslow, H. Pontell, et al., "Fraud and Abuse of Government Medical Benefit Programs by Psychiatrists," *American Journal of Psychiatry* 142 (1985): 231–34. **"The reason":** Editorial, "Mind and Money," *Wall Street Journal*, December 17, 1999, p. A-14.

Chapter 7

"Lunacy, like the rain": *The Philosophy of Insanity*, by an inmate of the Glasgow Royal Asylum for Lunatics at Gartnavel, 1860; used as an epigraph by Albert Deutsch, *The Shame of the States* (New York: Harcourt, Brace, 1948). **John Davis:** J. M. Davis, "Overview: Maintenance Therapy in Psychiatry: 1. Schizophrenia," *American Journal of Psychiatry* 132 (1975): 1237–45. **Stefan Leucht:** S. Leucht, M. Tardy, K. Komossa, et al., "Antipsychotic Drugs Versus Placebo for Relapse Prevention in Schizophrenia: A Systematic Review and Meta-Analysis," *Lancet* 379 (2012): 2063–71. **neurological symptoms:** G. Goldstein, R. D. Sanders, S. D. Forman, et al., "The Effects of Antipsychotic Medication on Factor and Cluster Structure of Neurologic Examination Abnormalities in Schizophrenia," *Schizophrenia Research* 75 (2005): 55–64. Approximately 40%: R. Mojtabai, L. Fochtmann, S-W. Chang, et al., "Unmet Need For Mental Health Care in Schizophrenia: An Overview of Literature and New Data From a First-Admission Study," *Schizophrenia Bulletin* 35 (2009): 678–95. **Two large studies:** M. Torniainen, E. Mittendorfor-Rutz, A. Tanksanen, et al., "Antipsychotic Treatment and Mortality in Schizophrenia," *Schizophrenia Bulletin* 41 (2015): 656–63. J. Vermeulen, G. van Rooijen, P. Doedens, et al., "Antipsychotic Medication and Long-Term Mortalitty Risk in Patients with Schizophrenia; A Systemic Review and Meta-Analysis," *Psychological Medicine* 47 (2017): 2217–18. **PORT:** R. W. Buchanan, J. Kreyenbuhl, D. L. Kelly, et al., "The 2009 Schizophrenia PORT Psychopharmacological Treatment Recommendations and Summary Statements," *Schizophrenia Bulletin* 36 (2010): 71–93. **15 drugs in 212 trials:** S. Leucht, A. Cipriani, L. Spineli, et al., "Comparative Efficacy and Tolerability of 15 Antipsychotic Drugs in Schizophrenia: A Multiple-Treatments Meta-Analysis," *Lancet* 382 (2013): 951–62. **"extraordinary prevalence":** T. Turner, "Rich and Mad in Victorian England," *Psychological Medicine* 19 (1989): 29–44. **study of spontaneous:** W. S. Fenton, "Prevalence of Spontaneous Dyskinesia in Schizophrenia," *Journal of Clinical Psychiatry* 61 (2000) (Suppl 4): 10–14. **less than 20 percent:** V. Khot and R. J. Wyatt, "Not All That Moves Is Tardive Dyskinesia," *American Journal of Psychiatry* 148 (1991): 661–66. **ten-year follow-up:** R. Yassa and N.P.V. Nair, "A 10-Year Follow-Up Study of Tardive Dyskinesia," *Acta Psychiatrica Scandinavica* 86 (1992): 262–66. **abused to get high:** O. V. Tcheremissine, "Is Quetiapine a Drug of Abuse? Reexamining the Issue of Addiction," *Expert Opinion on Drug Safety* 7 (2008): 739–48. **A recent review:** S. Gentile, "Antipsychotic Therapy during Early and Late Pregnancy: A Systematic Review," *Schizophrenia Bulletin* 36 (2010): 518–44. **a useful article:** P. E. Deegan and R. E. Drake, "Shared Decision Making and Medication Management in the Recovery Process," *Psychiatric Services* 57 (2006): 1636–39. **the difference between:** "Fluphenazine Levels—Short and Long," *Biological Therapies in Psychiatry* 4 (1981): 33–34. **racial group differences:** P. Ruiz, R. V. Varner, D. R. Small, et al., "Ethnic Differences in the Neuroleptic Treatment of Schizophrenia," *Psychiatric Quarterly* 70 (1999): 163–72. **shown no improvement:** S. Leucht, R. Busch, W. Kissling, et al., "Early Prediction of Antipsychotic Nonresponse among Patients with Schizophrenia," *Journal of Clinical Psychiatry* 68 (2007): 352–60. **"many first-episode":** J. A. Gallego, D. G. Robinson, S. M. Sevy, et al., "Time to Treatment Response in First-Episode Schizophrenia: Should Acute Treatment Trials Last Several Months?" *Journal of Clinical Psychiatry* 72 (2011): 1691–96. **$80 million:** J.L. Goren, A.J. Rose, E.G. Smith, et al., "The Business Case for Expanded Clozapine Utilization," Pscyhiatric Services 67 (2016): 1197–1205. **"reduce relapses by 30 percent":** C. Leucht, S. Heres, J. M. Kane, et al., "Oral versus Depot Antipsychotic Drugs for Schizophrenia—A Critical Systematic Review and Meta-Analysis of Randomised Long-term Trials," *Schizophrenia Research* 127 (2011): 83–92. **epi-**

sodes of violence: C. Arango, I. Bombín, T. González-Salvador, et al., "Randomised Clinical Trial Comparing Oral versus Depot Formulations of Zuclopenthixol in Patients with Schizophrenia and Previous Violence," *European Psychiatry* 21 (2006): 34–40. A 2017 study: H. Taipale, E. Mittendorfer-Rutz, K. Alexanderson, et al., "Antipsychotics and Mortality in a Nationwide Cohort of 29,823 Patients with Schizophrenia," *Schizophrenia Research.* 197 (2018): 274–80. "33 percent of patients": G. Goodwin, W. Fleischhacker, C. Arango, et al., "Advantages and Disadvantages of Combination Treatment with Antipsychotics," *European Neuropsychopharmacology* 19 (2009): 520–32. "Fortune magazine": D. Cauchon, "Americans Pay More; Here's Why," *USA Today*, November 10, 1999. Robert Whitaker: R. Whitaker, *Anatomy of an Epidemic* (New York: Crown, 2010). several recent studies: S. Teferra, T. Shibre, A. Fekadu, et al., "Five-year Clinical Course and Outcome of Schizophrenia in Ethiopia," *Schizophrenia Research* 136 (2012): 137–42; A. Cohen, V. Patel, R. Thara, et al., "Questioning an Axiom: Better Prognosis for Schizophrenia in the Developing World?," *Schizophrenia Bulletin* 34 (2008): 229–44. supersensitivity psychosis: J. Moncrieff, "Does Antipsychotic Withdrawal Provoke Psychosis? Review of the Literature on Rapid Onset Psychosis (Supersensitivity Psychosis) and Withdrawal-related Relapse," *Acta Psychiatrica Scandinavica* 114 (2006): 3–13. In monkeys: G. T. Konopaske, K.-A. Dorph-Petersen, J. N. Pierri, et al., "Effect of Chronic Exposure to Antipsychotic Medication on Cell Numbers in the Parietal Cortex of Macaque Monkeys," *Neuropsychopharmacology* 32 (2007): 1216–23. "when the onset": W. Z. Potter and M. V. Rudorfer, "Electroconvulsive Therapy—A Modern Medical Procedure," *New England Journal of Medicine* 328 (1993): 882–83. TMS: P. B. Fitzgerald and Z. J. Daskalakis, "A Review of Repetitive Transcranial Magnetic Stimulation Use in the Treatment of Schizophrenia," *Canadian Journal of Psychiatry* 53 (2008): 567–76; C. W. Slotema, J. D. Blom, H. W. Hoek, et al., "Should We Expand the Toolbox of Psychiatric Treatment Methods to Include Repetitive Transcranial Magnetic Stimulation (rTMS)? A Meta-Analysis of the Efficacy of rTMS in Psychiatric Disorders," *Journal of Clinical Psychiatry* 71 (2010): 873–84. studies to date: P. McGorry, "At Issue: Cochrane, Early Intervention, and Mental Health Reform: Analysis, Paralysis, or Evidence-Informed Progress?," *Schizophrenia Bulletin* 38 (2012): 221–24; M. Weiser, "Early Intervention for Schizophrenia: The Risk-Benefit Ratio of Antipsychotic Treatment in the Prodromal Phase," editorial, *American Journal of Psychiatry* 168 (2011): 761–63. One survey: J. Unützer, R. Klap, R. Sturm, et al., "Mental Disorders and the Use of Alternative Medicine: Results from a National Survey," *American Journal of Psychiatry* 157 (2000): 1851–57. evening primrose: A.H.C. Wong, M. Smith, and H. S. Boon, "Herbal Remedies in Psychiatric Practice," *Archives of General Psychiatry* 55 (1998): 1033–44. lithium toxicity: D. Pyevich and M. P. Bogenschutz, "Herbal Diuretics and Lithium Toxicity, letter, *American Journal of Psychiatry* 158 (2001): 1329. In one study: G. Hogarty and S. Goldberg, "Drug and

Sociotherapy in the Post-Hospital Maintenance of Schizophrenia," *Archives of General Psychiatry* 24 (1973): 54–64. **"a longer duration"**: M. Clarke, P. Whitty, S. Browne, et al., "Untreated Illness and Outcome of Psychosis," *British Journal of Psychiatry* 189 (2006): 235–40. **"reducing the DUP"**: I. Melle, T. K. Larsen, U. Haahr, et al., "Prevention of Negative Symptom Psychopathologies in First-Episode Schizophrenia," *Archives of General Psychiatry* 65 (2008): 634–40. **"barely better"**: P. B. Jones and J. J. Van Os, "Predicting Schizophrenia in Teenagers: Pessimistic Results from the British 1946 Birth Cohort," abstract, *Schizophrenia Research* 29 (1998): 11. **a study from Scotland**: E. C. Johnstone, K. P. Ebmeier, P. Miller, et al., "Predicting Schizophrenia: Findings from the Edinburgh High-Risk Study, *British Journal of Psychiatry* 186 (2005): 18–25.

Chapter 8

"Expecting the": J. Halpern, P. R. Binner, C. B. Mohr, et al., *The Illusion of Deinstitutionalization* (Denver: Denver Research Institute, 1978). **"If, for example"**: W. M. Mendel, *Treating Schizophrenia* (San Francisco: Jossey-Bass, 1989), p. 128. **"pessimistic outcome"**: H. Hoffman, Z. Kupper, and B. Kunz, "The Impact of 'Resignation' on Rehabilitation Outcome in Schizophrenia," *Schizophrenia Research* 36 (1999): 325–26. **"an inability to engage"**: Social Security Administration, Department of Health and Human Services, *Supplemental Security Income Regulations* (these regulations are available in all Social Security offices). **"graduated independent"**: "Diabetic Lay Dead at Group Home 3 Days," *Washington Post*, April 19, 1986, p. C-3. **"the police found"**: "21 Ex-Mental Patients Taken from 4 Private Homes," *New York Times*, August 5, 1979, p. B-3. **documented in 2002**: C. Levy, "Broken Homes," *New York Times*, April 28–30, 2002. **In one study**: H. R. Lamb, "Board-and-Care Home Wanderers," *Hospital and Community Psychiatry* 32 (1981): 498–500. **Fairweather Lodges**: G. W. Fairweather, ed., *The Fairweather Lodge: A Twenty-Five-Year Retrospective* (San Francisco: Jossey-Bass, 1980). **patient characteristics**: F. B. Dickerson, N. Ringel, and F. Parente, "Predictors of Residential Independence among Outpatients with Schizophrenia," *Psychiatric Services* 50 (1999): 515–19. **"the presence of"**: *There Goes the Neighborhood* (White Plains, N.Y.: Community Residences Information Services Program, 1986). **one recent study**: R. M. Friedrich, B. Hollingsworth, E. Hradek, et al., "Family and Client Perspective on Alternative Residential Settings for Person with Severe Mental Illness," *Psychiatric* Services 50 (1999): 509–14. **6 percent**: R. J. Turner, "Jobs and Schizophrenia," *Social Policy* 8 (1977): 32–40. **"in the morning"**: H. R. Lamb and Associates, *Community Survival for Long-term Patients* (San Francisco: Jossey-Bass, 1976), p. 8. **"I get lost"**: S. E. Estroff, *Making It Crazy: An Ethnography of Psychiatric Clients in an American Community* (Berkeley: University of California Press, 1981), p. 233. **"I just can't"**: C. Smith, "Schizophrenia in the 1980s," presented at the Alberta Schizophrenia Conference, May 1986. **26 to 53 percent:** R. P. Roca, W. R. Breakey, and P. J. Fisher, "Medical Care of Chronic Psychiatric Outpatients," *Hospital and Community Psychiatry* 38 (1987): 741–44. **"the treatment of":** L. E. Adler and J. M. Griffith, "Concurrent Medical Illness in the Schizophrenic Patient," *Schizophrenia Research* 4 (1991): 91–107. **two-day conference:** S. R. Marder, S. M. Essock, A. L. Miller, et al., "Physical Health Monitoring of Patients with Schizophrenia," *American Journal of Psychiatry* 161 (2004): 1334–49. **dental care:** R. G. McCreadie, H. Stevens, J. Henderson, et al., "The Dental Health of People with Schizophrenia," *Acta Psychiatrica Scandinavica* 110 (2004): 306–10. **Hearing Voices is not:** T. Styron, L. Utter, L. Davidson, "The Hearing Voices Network: Initial Lessons and Future Directions for Mental Health Professionals and Systems of Care," *Psychiatric Quarterly* 88 (2017): 769-85. **"I am proud":** A. Woods, "The Voice-Hearer," *Journal of Mental Health* 22 (2013): 263-270. **29 percent:** T. Styron, L. Utter, L. Davidson, op. cit.

Chapter 9

"Madness is": W. L. Perry-Jones, The Trade in Lunacy (London: Routeldge and Kegan Paul, 1972), p. 11. **A 2008 survey:** E. F. Torrey, K. Entsminger, J. Geller, et al. The Shortage of Public Hospital Beds for Mentally Ill Persons, Treatment Advocacy Center, March 17, 2008. **2016 data:** D. A. Fuller, E. Sinclair, J. Geller, et al., Going Going Gone: Trends and Consequences of Eliminating State Psychiatric Beds, 2016, Treatment Advocacy Center, June 2016. **FACT:** See E. F. Torrey, L. Dailey, H. R. Lamb, et al.; Treat or Repeat: A State Survey of Serious Mental Illness, Major Crimes and Community Treatment, Treatment Advocacy Center, September 2017. **PSRB:** See E. F. Torrey, L. Dailey, H. R. Lamb, et al.; Treat or Repeat: A State Survey of Serious Mental Illness, Major Crimes and Community Treatment, Treatment Advocacy Center, September 2017.

Chapter 10

"Although insanity": Anonymous, "Admissions to Hospitals for the Insane," *American Journal of Insanity* 25 (1868): 74. **between 1999 and 2016:** F. Dickerson, J. Schroeder, E. Katsafanas, et al., "Cigarette Smoking by Patients with Serious Mental Illness, 1999–2016: An Increasing Disparity," *Psychiatric Services* 69 (2018): 147–53. **smoking on life expectancy:** C. Cather, G. N. Pachas, K. M. Cieslak, et al., "Achieving Smoking Cessation in Individuals with Schizophrenia," *CNS Drugs* 31 (2017): 471–81. **decreases cognitive**

function: F. Dickerson, M. B. Adamos, E. Katsafanas et al., "The Association Among Smoking, HSV-1 Exposure, and Cognitive Functioning in Schizophrenia, Bipolar Disorder, and Non-Psychiatric Controls," *Schizophrenia Research* 176 (2016): 566–71. **instant coffee:** J. I. Benson and J. J. David, "Coffee Eating in Chronic Schizophrenic Patients," *American Journal of Psychiatry* 143 (1986): 940–41. **adenosine receptors:** P. B. Lucas, D. Pickar, J. Kelsoe, et al., "Effects of the Acute Administration of Caffeine in Patients with Schizophrenia," *Biological Psychiatry* 28 (1990): 35–40. **caffeine may decrease:** S. R. Hirsch, "Precipitation of Antipsychotic Drugs in Interaction with Coffee or Tea," letter, *Lancet* 2 (1979): 1130–31. **worsening of their symptoms:** Lucas, et al., "Effects of the Acute Administration of Caffeine"; M. O. Zaslove, R. L. Russell, and E. Ross, "Effect of Caffeine Intake on Psychotic In-Patients," *British Journal of Psychiatry* 159 (1991): 565–67. **interfere with the absorption:** F. Kulhanek, O. K. Linde, and G. Meisenberg, "Precipitation of Antipsychotic Drugs in Interaction with Coffee or Tea," letter, *Lancet* 2 (1979): 1130. **In one study:** J. A. Cabarillo, A. G. Herraiz, S. I. Ramos, et al., "Effects of Caffeine Withdrawal from the Diet on the Metabolism of Clozapine in Schizophrenic Patients," *Journal of Clinical Psychopharmacology* 18 (1998): 311–16. **47 percent abused:** D. A. Regier, M. E. Farmer, D. S. Rae, et al., "Comorbidity of Mental Disorders with Alcohol and Other Drug Abuse," *Journal of American Medical Association* 264 (1990): 2511–18. **A 2002 national:** Substance Abuse and Mental Health Services Administration, *Results from the 2002 National Survey on Drug Use and Health: Detailed Tables* (U.S. Department of Health and Human Services, 2003). **One study:** C. A. Pristach and C. M. Smith, "Self-Reported Effects of Alcohol Use on Symptoms of Schizophrenia," *Psychiatric Services* 47 (1996): 421–23. **higher relapse rate:** R. E. Drake and M. A. Wallach, "Substance Abuse among the Chronically Ill," *Hospital and Community Psychiatry* 40 (1989): 1041–46. **Hair analysis:** M. S. Swartz, J. W. Swanson, and M. J. Hannon, "Detection of Illicit Substance Use among Persons with Schizophrenia by Radioimmunoassay of Hair," *Psychiatric Services* 54 (2003): 891–95. **Disulfiram can be used:** S. J. Kingsbury and C. Salzman, "Disulfiram in the Treatment of Alcoholic Patients with Schizophrenia," *Hospital and Community Psychiatry* 41 (1990): 133–34. **Marijuana improves:** R. Warner, D. Taylor, J. Wright, et al., "Substance Use among the Mentally Ill: Prevalence, Reasons for Use, and Effects on Illness," *American Journal of Orthopsychiatry* 64 (1994): 30–39; V. Peralta and M. J. Cuesta, "Influence of Cannabis Abuse on Schizophrenic Psychopathology," *Acta Psychiatrica Scandinavica* 85 (1992): 127–30. **73 percent of them:** J. Coverdale, J. Aruffo, and H. Grunebaum, "Developing Family Planning Services for Female Chronic Mentally Ill Outpatients," *Hospital and Community Psychiatry* 43 (1992): 475–77. **62 percent were:** J. A. Kelly, D. A. Murphy, G. R. Bahr, et al., "AIDS/HIV Risk Behavior among the Chronically Mentally Ill," *American Journal of Psychiatry* 149 (1992): 886–89. **66 percent had:** K. McKinnon,

F. Courrios, H.F.L. Meyer-Bahlburg, et al., "Reliability of Sexual Risk Behavior Interviews with Psychiatry Patients," *American Journal of Psychiatry* 150 (1993): 972–74. **"sexual activity was"**: D. Civic, G. Walsh, and D. McBride, "Staff Perspectives on Sexual Behavior of Patients in a State Psychiatric Hospital," *Hospital and Community Psychiatry* 44 (1993): 887–90. **"had never had"**: K. Bhui, A. Puffet, and G. Strathdee, "Sexual and Relationship Problems amongst Patients with Severe Chronic Psychoses," *Social Psychiatry and Psychiatric Epidemiology* 32 (1997): 459–67. **"vividly described"**: M. B. Rosenbaum, "Neuroleptics and Sexual Functioning," *Integrative Psychiatry* 4 (1986): 105–6. **30 to 60 percent:** G. Sullivan and D. Lukoff, "Sexual Side Effects of Antipsychotic Medication: Evaluation and Interventions," *Hospital and Community Psychiatry* 41 (1990): 1238–41. **reported sexual side effects:** S. Smith, P. Mostyn, S. Vearnals, et al., "The Prevalence of Sexual Dysfunction in Schizophrenic Patients Taking Conventional Antipsychotic Medication," *Schizophrenia Research* 41 (2000): 218. **"would routinely engage"**: D. D. Gold and J. D. Justino, "'Bicycle Kickstand' Phenomenon: Prolonged Erections Associated with Antipsychotic Drugs," *Southern Medical Journal* 81 (1988): 792–94. **"the rate of children"**: M. V. Seeman, M. Lang, and N. Rector, "Chronic Schizophrenia: A Risk Factor for HIV?" *Canadian Journal of Psychiatry* 35 (1990): 765–68. **31 percent of the women:** J. H. Coverdale and J. A. Aruffo, "Family Planning Needs of Female Chronic Psychiatric Outpatients," *American Journal of Psychiatry* 146 (1989): 1489–91. **"schizophrenia was associated"**: L. M. Howard, G. Thornicroft, M. Salmon, et al., "Predictors of Parenting Outcome in Women with Psychotic Disorders Discharged from Mother and Baby Units," *Acta Psychiatrica Scandinavica* 110 (2004): 347–55. **"chronic psychiatric outpatients"**: Coverdale and Aruffo, "Family Planning Needs." **better mothers:** M. Mullick, L. J. Miller, and T. Jacobsen, "Insight into Mental Illness and Child Maltreatment Risk among Mothers with Major Psychiatric Disorders," *Psychiatric Services* 52 (2001): 488–92. **guidelines have been proposed:** L. B. McCullough, J. Coverdale, T. Bayer, et al., "Ethically Justified Guidelines for Family Planning Interventions to Prevent Pregnancy in Female Patients with Chronic Mental Illness," *American Journal of Obstetrics and Gynecology* 167 (1992): 19–25. **study from Denmark:** B. E. Bennedsen, P. B. Mortensen, A. V. Olesen, et al., "Preterm Birth and Intra-Uterine Growth Retardation among Children of Women with Schizophrenia," *British Journal of Psychiatry* 175 (1999): 239–45. **report from Australia:** A. Jablensky, S. Zubrick, V. Morgan, et al., "The Offspring of Women with Schizophrenia and Affective Psychoses: A Population Study," *Schizophrenia Research* 41 (2000): 8. **breastfeeding:** A. Buist, T. R. Norman, and L. Dennerstein, "Breastfeeding and the Use of Psychotropic Medication: A Review," *Journal of Affective Disorders* 19 (1990): 197–206. **1.6 percent in Texas:** D. Gamino, "1 in 24 New Austin State Hospital Patients Has HIV," *Austin American-Statesman*, August 22,

1991. **5.5 percent in New York:** F. Cournos, M. Empfield, E. Horwath, et al., "HIV Seroprevalence among Patients Admitted to Two Psychiatric Hospitals," *American Journal of Psychiatry* 148 (1991): 1225–30. **3.4 percent were positive:** M. Sacks, H. Dermatis, S. Looser-Ott, et al., "Seroprevalence of HIV and Risk Factors for AIDS in Psychiatric Inpatients," *Hospital and Community Psychiatry* 43 (1992): 736–37. **6.2 percent:** W. D. Klinkenberg, J. Caslyn, G. A. Morse, et al., "Prevalence of Human Immunodeficiency Virus, Hepatitis B, and Hepatitis C among Homeless Persons with Co-occurring Severe Mental Illness and Substance Use Disorders," *Comprehensive Psychiatry* 44 (2003): 293–302. **AIDS by shaking hands:** J. F. Aruffo, J. H. Coverdale, R. C. Chacko, et al., "Knowledge about AIDS among Women Psychiatric Outpatients," *Hospital and Community Psychiatry* 41 (1990)\: 326–28. **A 1993 study:** F. Cournos, K. McKinnon, H. Meyer-Bahlburg, et al., "HIV Risk Activity among Persons with Severe Mental Illness: Preliminary Findings," *Hospital and Community Psychiatry* 44 (1993): 1104–6. **In another study:** J. A. Kelly, et al., "AIDS/HIV Risk Behavior." **AIDS education programs:** R. M. Goisman, A. B. Kent, E. C. Montgomery, et al., "AIDS Education for Patients with Chronic Mental Illness," *Community Mental Health Journal* 27 (1991): 189–97; J. A. Kelly, T. L. McAuliffe, K. J. Sikkema, et al., "Reduction in Risk Behavior among Adults with Severe Mental Illness Who Learned to Advocate for HIV Prevention," *Psychiatric Services* 48 (1997): 1283–88. **Connecticut study:** D. J. Sells, M. Rowe, D. Fisk, et al., "Violent Victimization of Persons with Co-occurring Psychiatric and Substance Use Disorders," *Psychiatric Services* 54 (2003): 1253–57. **278 residents:** A. F. Lehman and L. S. Linn, "Crimes against Discharged Mental Patients in Board-and-Care Homes," *American Journal of Psychiatry* 141 (1984): 271–74. **185 individuals:** V. A. Hiday, M. S. Swartz, J. W. Swanson, et al., "Criminal Victimization of Persons with Severe Mental Illness," *Psychiatric Services* 50 (1999): 62–68. **"The mentally ill":** C. W. Dugger, "Big Shelters Hold Terrors for the Mentally Ill," *New York Times*, January 12, 1992, pp. 1 and 22. **twenty women:** S. Friedman and G. Harrison, "Sexual Histories, Attitudes, and Behavior of Schizophrenic and 'Normal' Women," *Archives of Sexual Behavior* 13 (1984): 555–67. **In Washington:** L. A. Goodman, M. A. Dutton, and M. Harris, "Episodically Homeless Women with Serious Mental Illness: Prevalence of Physical and Sexual Assault," *American Journal of Orthopsychiatry* 65 (1995): 468–78. **In France:** J. M. Darvez-Bornoz, T. Lemperiere, A. Degiovanni, and P. Grillard, "Sexual Victimization in Women with Schizophrenia and Bipolar Disorder," *Social Psychiatry and Psychiatric Epidemiology* 30 (1995): 78–84. **"I know one":** C. J. Cooper, "Brutal Lives of Homeless S. F. Women," *San Francisco Examiner*, December 18, 1988, p. A-1. **half the time:** J. A. Marley and S. Buila, "When Violence Happens to People with Mental Illness: Disclosing Victimization," *American Journal of Orthopsychiatry* 69 (1999): 398–402. **"were confused":** T. Marshall and P. Solomon, "Professionals' Responsibilities in Releasing Information to Families of Adults with Mental Illness," *Psychiatric Services* 54 (2003): 1622–28. **"I was never":** N. Dearth, B. J. Labenski, M. E. Mott, et al., *Families Helping Families* (New York: Norton, 1986), p. 61. **Riverside County:** T. Bogart and P. Solomon, "Procedures to Share Treatment Information among Mental Health Providers, Consumers, and Families," *Psychiatric Services* 50 (1999): 1321–25. **70 percent of patients:** P. J. Weiden, L. Dixon, A. Frances, et al., "Neuroleptic Noncompliance in Schizophrenia," in C. A. Tamminga and S. C. Schulz, eds., *Advances in Neuropsychiatry and Psychopharmacology. Vol. 1: Schizophrenia Research* (New York: Raven Press, 1991), pp. 285–96. **$136 million per year:** P. J. Weiden and M. Olfson, "Measuring Costs of Rehospitalization in Schizophrenia," presented at the annual meeting of the American Psychiatric Association, San Francisco, California, May 1993. Costs averaged for first two years. **twice as high:** I. E. Lin, R. Spiga, and W. Fortsch, "Insight and Adherence to Medication in Chronic Schizophrenics," *Journal of Clinical Psychiatry* 40 (1979): 430–32. **"I did not want":** D. Minor, quoted in A. B. Hatfield and H. P. Lefley, *Surviving Mental Illness* (New York: Guilford Press, 1993), p. 134. **"Unfortunately the side":** E. Leete, "The Treatment of Schizophrenia: A Patient's Perspective," *Hospital and Community Psychiatry* 38 (1987): 486–91. **recent studies:** M. Vanelli, P. Burstein, and J. Cramer, "Refill Patterns of Atypical and Conventional Antipsychotic Medications at a National Retail Pharmacy Chain," *Psychiatric Services* 52 (2001): 1248–50; M. Valenstein, F. C. Blow, L. A. Copeland, et al., "Poor Antipsychotic Adherence among Patients with Schizophrenia: Medication and Patient Factors," *Schizophrenia Bulletin* 30 (2004): 255–64. **"the major finding":** P. J. Weiden, J. J. Mann, G. Haas, et al., "Clinical Nonrecognition of Neuroleptic-Induced Movement Disorders: A Cautionary Study," *American Journal of Psychiatry* 144 (1987): 1148–53. **"psychiatrists misjudged":** S. E. Finn, J. M. Bailey, R. T. Schultz, et al., "Subjective Utility Ratings of Neuroleptics in Treating Schizophrenia," *Psychological Medicine* 20 (1990): 843–48. **"the reluctance":** T. Van Putten, "Why Do Schizophrenic Patients Refuse to Take Their Drugs?" *Archives of General Psychiatry* 31 (1974): 67–72. **"it is still":** R. Diamond, "Drugs and the Quality of Life: The Patient's Point of View," *Journal of Clinical Psychiatry* 46 (1985): 29–35. **"Many of the mistakes":** B. Blaska, "The Myriad Medication Mistakes in Psychiatry: A Consumer's View," *Hospital and Community Psychiatry* 41 (1990): 993–98. **"A few months":** R. McLean, *Recovered, Not Cured* (Crow's Nest, Australia: Allen and Unwin, 2003), pp. 160–61. **found that 37 percent:** C. Clary, A. Dever, and E. Schweizer, "Psychiatric Inpatients' Knowledge of Medication at Hospital Discharge," *Hospital and Community Psychiatry* 43 (1992): 140–44. **In a Baltimore study:** A. F. Lehman, L. B. Dixon, E. Kernan, et al., "A Randomized Trial of Assertive Community Treatment for Homeless Persons with Severe Mental Illness," *Archives of General Psychiatry* 54 (1997): 1038–43. **"approximately one-third":** L. Dixon, P. Weiden, M.

Torres, et al., "Assertive Community Treatment and Medication Compliance in the Homeless Mentally Ill," *American Journal of Psychiatry* 154 (1997): 1302–4. **reduces hospitalization days:** D. J. Luchins, P. Hanrahan, K. J. Conrad, et al., "An Agency-Based Representative Payee Program and Improved Community Tenure of Persons with Mental Illness," *Psychiatric Services* 49 (1998): 1218–22. **substance abuse:** R. Rosenheck, J. Lam, and F. Randolph, "Impact of Representative Payees on Substance Use among Homeless Persons with Serious Mental Illness and Substance Abuse," *Psychiatric Services* 48 (1997): 800–806. **days spent homeless:** M. R. Stoner, "Money Management Services for the Homeless Mentally Ill," *Hospital and Community Psychiatry* 40 (1989): 751–53. **the court ruled:** Brown v. Bowen, 845 F2d 1211, 3rd Circuit, 1988. **27 percent of patients:** P. Gorman, New Hampshire Department of Health and Human Services, personal communication, September 11, 1998. **In the only study:** C. O'Keefe, D. P. Potenza, K. T. Mueser, "Treatment Outcomes for Severely Mentally Ill Patients on Conditional Discharge to Community-Based Treatment," *Journal of Nervous and Mental Disease* 185 (1997): 409–11. **best-known example:** J. D. Bloom, M. H. Williams, J. L. Rogers, et al., "Evaluation and Treatment of Insanity Acquittees in the Community," *Bulletin of the American Academy of Psychiatry and Law* 14 (1986): 231–44. **Additional studies:** J. D. Bloom, M. H. Williams, and D. A. Bigelow, "Monitored Conditional Release of Persons Found Not Guilty by Reason of Insanity," *American Journal of Psychiatry* 148 (1991): 444–48. **Some form of outpatient commitment:** E. F. Torrey and R. J. Kaplan, "A National Survey of the Use of Outpatient Commitment," *Psychiatric Services* 46 (1995): 778–84. **In Washington, D.C.:** G. Zanni and L. deVeau, "Inpatient Stays before and after Outpatient Commitment," *Hospital and Community Psychiatry* 37 (1986): 941–42. **in Ohio:** M. R. Munetz, T. Grande, J. Kleist, et al., "The Effectiveness of Outpatient Civil Commitment," *Psychiatric Services* 47 (1996): 1251–53. **and in Iowa:** B. M. Rohland, "The Role of Outpatient Commitment in the Management of Persons with Schizophrenia," Iowa Consortium for Mental Health, Services, Training, and Research, May 1998. **In one study in North Carolina:** G. A. Fernandez and S. Nygard, "Impact of Involuntary Outpatient Commitment on the Revolving-Door Syndrome in North Carolina," *Hospital and Community Psychiatry* 41 (1990): 1001–4. **In another study:** M. S. Swartz, J. W. Swanson, H. R. Wagner, et al., "Can Involuntary Outpatient Commitment Reduce Hospital Recidivism?: Findings from a Randomized Trial with Severely Mentally Ill Individuals," *American Journal of Psychiatry* 156 (1999): 1968–75. **only 30 percent:** V. A. Hiday and T. L. Scheid-Cook, "The North Carolina Experience with Outpatient Commitment: A Critical Appraisal," *International Journal of Law and Psychiatry* 10 (1987): 215–32. **In Ohio, outpatient commitment:** Munetz, Grande, Kleist, et al., "The Effectiveness of Outpatient Civil Commitment." **"71 percent":** R. A. Van Putten, J. M. Santiago, and M. R. Berren, "Involuntary Outpatient Commitment in Arizona: A Retrospective Study," *Hospital and Community Psychiatry* 39 (1988): 953–58. **"it appears"**: Rohland, "The Role of Outpatient Commitment." **"the results were striking"**: J. W. Swanson, M. S. Swartz, R. Borum, et al., "Involuntary Outpatient Commitment and Reduction of Violent Behaviour in Persons with Severe Mental Illness," *British Journal of Psychiatry* 176 (2000): 224–31. **66 percent reduction:** J. C. Phelan, M. Sinkewicz, D.M. Castille, et al. "Effectiveness and Outcomes of Assisted Outpatient Treatment in New York State," Psychiatric Services 61 (2010): 137-43. **Kendra's Law:** *Kendra's Law: An Interim Report on the Status of Assisted Outpatient Treatment* (New York State Office of Mental Health, 2003). **"of the 35 patients"**: H. R. Lamb and L. E. Weinberger, "Conservatorship for Gravely Disabled Psychiatric Patients: A Four-Year Follow-up Study," *American Journal of Psychiatry* 149 (1992): 909–13. **six-month study:** J. Geller, A. L. Grudzinskas Jr., M. McDermett, et al., "The Efficacy of Involuntary Outpatient Treatment in Massachusetts," *Administration and Policy in Mental Health* 25 (1998): 271–85. **"In one of the more"**: J. L. Geller, "On Being 'Committed' to Treatment in the Community," *Innovations and Research* 2 (1993): 23–27. **"if the lithium level"**: J. L. Geller, "Rights, Wrongs, and the Dilemma of Coerced Community Treatment," *American Journal of Psychiatry* 143 (1986): 1259–64. **Recent studies:** H. J. Steadman, A. Redlich, L. Callahan, et al., "Effect of Mental Health Courts on Arrests and Jail Days," *Archives of General Psychiatry* 68 (2011): 167–72; V. A. Hiday and B. Ray, "Arrests Two Years after Exiting a Well-Established Mental Health Court," *Psychiatric Services* 61 (2010): 463–68. **one observer:** H. R. Lamb and L. E. Weinberger, "Mental Health Courts as a Way to Provide Treatment to Violent Persons with Severe Mental Illness," *Journal of the American Medical Association* 300 (2008): 722–24. **Baltimore PACT study:** A. F. Lehman, personal communication, October 12, 1998. **riboflavin:** S. Kapur, R. Ganguli, R. Ulrich, et al., "Use of Random-Sequence Riboflavin as a Marker of Medication Compliance in Chronic Schizo-phrenics," *Schizophrenia Research* 6 (1992): 49–53. **isoniazid:** G. A. Ellard, P. J. Jenner, and P. A. Downs, "An Evaluation of the Potential Use of Isoniazid, Acetylisoniazid and Isonicotinic Acid for Monitoring the Self-Administration of Drugs," *British Journal of Clinical Pharmacology* 10 (1980): 369–81. **27 outpatients:** A. Lucksted and R. D. Coursey, "Consumer Perceptions of Pressure and Force in Psychiatric Treatments," *Psychiatric Services* 46 (1995): 146–52. **30 patients:** W. M. Greenberg, L. Moore-Duncan, and R. Herron, "Patients' Attitudes toward Having Been Forcibly Medicated," *Bulletin of the American Academy of Psychiatry and the Law* 24 (1996): 513–24. **"freedom to be"**: R. Reich, "Care of the Chronically Mentally Ill: A National Disgrace," *American Journal of Psychiatry* 130 (1997): 912. **"reported that their"**: Cited in A. B. Hatfield, *Family Education in Mental Illness* (New York: Guilford Press, 1990), p. 124. **A 1990 NAMI:** D. M. Steinwachs, J. D. Kaspar, and E. A. Skinner, "Family Perspectives on Meeting the Needs for Care of Severely Mentally Ill Relatives: A National Survey" (Arlington, Va.: National Alliance for the Mentally Ill, 1992). **"arrest and conviction"**: J. Rabkin, "Criminal Behavior of Discharged Mental Patients: A Critical Appraisal of the Research," *Psychological Bulletin* 86 (1979): 1–27. **fifteen of twenty**: D. A. Martell and P. E. Dietz, "Mentally Disordered Offenders Who Push or Attempt to Push Victims onto Subway Tracks in New York City," *Archives of General Psychiatry* 49 (1992): 472–75. **"that 27 percent"**: J. Monahan, "Mental Disorder and Violent Behavior," *American Psychologist* 47 (1992), 511–21. **study by Link et al.**: B. G. Link, H. Andrews, and F. T. Cullen, "The Violent and Illegal Behavior of Mental Patients Reconsidered," *American Sociological Review* 57 (1992) 275–92. **(ECA) study**: J. W. Swanson, C. E. Holzer, V. K. Ganju, et al., "Violence and Psychiatric Disorder in the Community: Evidence from the Epidemiologic Catchment Area Surveys," *Hospital and Community Psychiatry* 41 (1990): 761–70. **"The data"**: J. Monahan, "Mental Disorder and Violent Behavior," *American Psychologist* 47 (1992): 511–21. **"In the last"**: P. M. Marzuk, "Violence, Crime, and Mental Illness," *Archives of General Psychiatry* 53 (1996): 481–86. **A 2015 summary**: J. W. Swanson, E. E. McGinty, S. Fazel, et al., "Mental Illness and Reduction of Gun Violence and Suicide: Bringing Epidemiologic Research to Policy," *Annals of Epidemiology* 25 (2015): 366–76. **20 percent**: All references in this section, unless otherwise noted, are taken from E. F. Torrey, *Out of the Shadows: Confronting America's Mental Illness Crisis* (New York: John Wiley, 1997), chapter 3, pp. 25–42. **5 percent**: B. A. Palmer, V. S. Pankratz, and J. M. Bostwick, "The Lifetime Risk of Suicide in Schizophrenia," *Archives of General Psychiatry* 62 (2005): 247–53. **within the first ten years**: C. P. Miles, "Conditions Predisposing to Suicide: A Review," *Journal of Nervous and Mental Disease* 164 (1977): 231–46. **Finnish study**: H. Heilä, "Suicide in Schizophrenia—A Review," *Psychiatria Fennica* 30 (1999): 59–79. **Belgian study**: M. De Hert, K. McKenzie, and J. Peuskens, "Risk Factors for Suicide in Young People Suffering from Schizophrenia: A Long-Term Follow-up Study," *Schizophrenia Research* 47 (2001): 127–34.

Chapter 11

"The wretchedness": H. M. Hurd, *The Institutional Care of the Insane in the United States and Canada*, vol. 2 (New York: Arno Press, 1973), p. 95, quoting S. B. Woodward; originally published in 1917. **"gets emotional support"**: "Compassion and Love for One Son; Fear and Anger for the Other," *Ontario Friends of Schizophrenics Newsletter,* Summer 1987; reprinted from the *Alliance for the Mentally Ill of Southern Arizona Newsletter.* **An excellent description**: L. Wilson, *This Stranger, My Son* (New York: Putnam, 1968). **"You know, Dad"**: J. Wechsler, N. Wechsler, and H. Karpf, *In a Darkness* (New York: Norton, 1972), p. 27. **"I read a book"**: Wilson, *This Stranger, My Son*, pp. 123–24. **"Badly treated families"**: W. S. Appleton, "Mistreatment of Patients' Families by Psychiatrists," *American Journal of Psychiatry* 131 (1974): 655–57. **"Once you have"**: A. C., personal communication, Maryland. **Cogentin tablet:** C. Adamec, *How to Live with a Mentally Ill Person* (New York: John Wiley, 1996), p. 52. **"One of our"**: H. B. M. Murphy, "Community Management of Rural Mental Patients," Final Report of USPHS Grant (Rockville, Md.: National Institute of Mental Health, 1964). **"I am haunted"**: E. Leete, "The Treatment of Schizophrenia: A Patient's Perspective," *Hospital and Community Psychiatry* 38 (1987): 486–91. **"There came the morning"**: J. Baum, "Mental Illness: Acceptance Is the Key," originally published in the *Alabama Advocate* and reprinted in the *Utah AMI Newsletter*, Oct./Dec. 1993, p. 4. **"I cry"**: R. Carter, *Helping Someone with Mental Illness* (New York: Times Books, 1998), pp. 6–7. **"Well, I guess"**: G. L., personal communication, Maryland. **Several observers have noted:** W. W. Michaux, et al., *The First Year Out: Mental Patients After Hospitalization* (Baltimore: Johns Hopkins University Press, 1969). **"Several relatives mentioned"**: C. Creer and J. K. Wing, *Schizophrenia at Home* (London: Institute of Psychiatry, 1974), p. 33. **"You've got to reach"**: Laffey, p. 40. **"Recognizing that a person"**: H. R. Lamb and Associates, *Community Survival for Long-Term Patients* (San Francisco: Jossey-Bass, 1976), p. 7. **"A neutral"**: Wing, *Schizophrenia*, p. 29. **"Superficially she *was*"**: O. Sacks, *The Man Who Mistook His Wife for a Hat* (New York: Summit Books, 1985), pp. 70–74. **"My advice"**: E. Francell, "Medication: The Foundation of Recovery," *Innovations and Research* 3 (1994): 31–40. **"family-to-family"**: L. Dixon, B. Stewart, J. Burland, et al., "Pilot Study of the Effectiveness of the Family-to-Family Education Program," *Psychiatric Services* 52 (2001): 965–67. **"a controlled environment"**: E. Leete, "How I Perceive and Manage My Illness," *Hospital and Community Psychiatry* 15 (1989): 197–200. **"recognizing when"**: E. Leete, "The Treatment of Schizophrenia: A Patient's Perspective," *Hospital and Community Psychiatry* 38 (1987): 486–91. **study of exercise:** G. Faulkner and A. Sparkes, "Exercise as Therapy for Schizophrenia: An Ethnographic Study," *Journal of Sport and Exercise Psychology* 21 (1999): 52–69. **"a seat where"**: E. Leete, "How I Perceive and Manage My Illness." **"to help restore"**: J. Walsh, "Schizophrenics Anonymous: The Franklin County, Ohio, Experience," *Psychosocial Rehabilitation Journal* 18 (1994): 61–74. **"peer counselors"**: C. W. McGill and C. J. Patterson, "Former Patients as Peer Counselors on Locked Psychiatric Inpatient Units," *Hospital and Community Psychiatry* 41 (1990): 1017–20. **case management aides:** P. S. Sherman and R. Porter, "Mental Health Consumers as Case Management Aides," *Hospital and Community Psychiatry* 42 (1991): 494–98. **twenty-eight such studies:** A.-M. Baronet, "Factors Associated with Caregiver Burden in Mental Illness: A Critical Review of the Research Literature," *Clinical Psychology Review* 19 (1999): 819–41. **"Sometimes I feel"**: "Thoughts from a NAMI Mother," *NAMI Oklahoma News* 15

(1999), p. 1. **A 2018 online:** D. Lerner, H. Chang, W. H. Rogers, "Psychological Distress Among Caregivers of Individuals with a Diagnosis of Schizophrenia or Schizoaffective Disorder," *Psychiatric Services* 69 (2018): 169–78. **in Australia:** J. Farhall, B. Webster, B. Hocking, et al., "Training to Enhance Partnerships between Mental Health Professionals and Family Caregivers: A Comparative Study," *Psychiatric Services* 49 (1998): 1488–90. **"Look at the person":** Anonymous, personal communication, Davis, California. **"My son seemed":** A. H., personal communication, Washington, D.C. **"Patients tended to":** Wing, *Schizophrenia*, p. 27. **"I would have been":** H. R. Rollin, ed., *Coping with Schizophrenia* (London: Burnett, 1980), p. 158. **"A more realistic":** Creer and Wing, p. 71. **"One patient returned home":** Ibid., p. 22. **"One young man":** Ibid., p. 11. **"One lady said":** Ibid., p. 8. **"Leave me alone":** B. B., personal communication, New York. **"When our son was":** L.Y., personal communication, San Jose, California. **"The most remarkable lesson":** L.M., personal communication, Florida. **"While admiring":** P. Earle, "Popular Fallacies in Regard to Insanity and the Insane," *Journal of Social Science* 26 (1890): 113. **"I found structure":** A.H., personal communication, Washington, D.C. **"My wife will cook":** Creer and Wing, p. 30. **"The second practical":** Anonymous, personal communication, California. **"It's so annoying":** Creer and Wing, p. 10. **"convinced that":** R. Lanquetot, "First Person Account: On Being Daughter and Mother," *Schizophrenia Bulletin* 14 (1988): 337–41. **"and sit us":** M. Fichtner, "Children of Madness," *Miami Herald*, September 15, 1991, pp. J-1–4. **Meg Livergood:** M. Blais, "Trish," *Miami Herald Sunday Magazine*, May 24, 1987, pp. 7–16. **"suddenly both":** W. Kelley, "Unmet Needs," *Journal of the California Alliance for the Mentally Ill* 3 (1992): 28–30. **"envious watching":** J. Mozham, "Daddy and Me: Growing Up with a Schizophrenic," *Reflections of AMI of Michigan*, May/June 1991, pp. 18–19. **"That day":** A. S. Brodoff, "First Person Account: Schizophrenia through a Sister's Eyes—The Burden of Invisible Baggage," *Schizophrenia Bulletin* 14 (1988): 113–16. **"I feel such":** M. Wasow, *The Skipping Stone* (Palo Alto, Calif.: Science and Behavior Books, 1995), p. 72. **"My husband's":** D. T. Marsh, *Serious Mental Illness and the Family* (New York: John Wiley, 1998), p. 239. **"It's funny":** P. Aronowitz, "A Brother's Dreams," *New York Times Magazine*, January 24, 1988, p. 355. **"superkids":** C. Kauffman, H. Grunebaum, B. Cohler, et al., "Superkids: Competent Children of Psychotic Mothers," *American Journal of Psychiatry* 136 (1979): 1398–1402. **"Growing up":** Lanquetot. **Moorman:** M. Moorman, *My Sister's Keeper* (New York: Norton, 1992). **"She once knew":** Mozham. **"was aware that":** Fichtner. **Julie Johnson:** J. Johnson, *Hidden Victims—Hidden Healers* (New York: Doubleday, 1988). **in one of the largest studies:** C. D. Swofford, J. W. Kasckow, G. Scheller-Gilkey, et al., "Substance Use: A Powerful Predictor of Relapse in Schizophrenia," *Schizophrenia Research* 20 (1996): 145–51. **145 patients:** M. I. Herz and C. Melville, "Relapse in Schizophrenia," *American Journal of Psychiatry* 137 (1980): 801–5. **"it is extremely":** M. Herz,

"Prodromal Symptoms and Prevention of Relapse in Schizophrenia," *Journal of Clinical Psychiatry* 46 (1985): 22–25. **In England:** M. Birchwood, J. Smith, F. MacMillan, et al., "Predicting Relapse in Schizophrenia: The Development and Implementation of an Early Signs Monitoring System Using Patients and Families as Observers," *Psychological Medicine* 19 (1989): 649–56. **"Warning Signals Scale":** P. Jørgensen, "Schizophrenic Delusions: The Detection of Warning Signals," *Schizophrenia Research* 32 (1998): 17–22. **"In the first stage":** M. Lovejoy, "Recovery from Schizophrenia: A Personal Odyssey," *Hospital and Community Psychiatry* 35 (1984): 809–12. **videotapes:** S. A. Davidoff, B. P. Forester, S. N. Ghaemi, et al., "Effect of Video Self-Observation on Development of Insight in Psychotic Disorders," *Journal of Nervous and Mental Disease* 186 (1998): 697–700.

Chapter 12

"There is": R. Mead, *Medical Precepts and Cautions* (London: J. Brindley, 1751). **identical twins:** D. L. DiLalla and I. I. Gottesman, "Normal Personality Characteristics in Identical Twins Discordant for Schizophrenia," *Journal of Abnormal Psychology* 104 (1995): 490–99. **"The daughter":** B. Bick, "Love and Resentment," *New York Times Magazine*, March 25, 1990, p. 26. **"Part of the":** J. K. Wing, *Schizophrenia and Its Management in the Community* (pamphlet published by National Schizophrenic Fellowship, 1977), pp. 28–29. **"Almost all crimes":** S. Brill, "A Dishonest Defense," *Psychology Today*, November 1981, pp. 16–19. **"the line between":** C. Holden, "Insanity Defense Reexamined," *Science* 222 (1983): 994–95. **small loss of IQ:** A. J. Russell, J. C. Munro, P. B. Jones, et al., "Schizophrenia and the Myth of Intellectual Decline," *American Journal of Psychiatry* 154 (1997): 635–39. **in Finland:** I. Isohanni, M. R. Jarvelin, P. Jones, et al., "Can Excellent School Performance Be a Precursor of Schizophrenia? A 28-Year Follow-Up in the Northern Finland 1966 Birth Cohort," *Acta Psychiatrica Scandinavica* 100 (1999): 17–26. **in childhood:** J. S. Bedwell, B. Keller, A. K. Smith, et al., "Why Does Postpsychotic IQ Decline in Childhood-Onset Schizophrenia?" *American Journal of Psychiatry* 156 (1999): 1996–97. **a 1989 study:** M. J. Edlund, C. Conrad, and P. Morris, "Accidents among Schizophrenic Outpatients," *Comprehensive Psychiatry* 30 (1989): 522–26. **Two earlier studies:** L. E. Hollister, "Automobile Driving by Psychiatric Patients," letter, *American Journal of Psychiatry* 149 (1992): 274; see also D. O'Neill, "Driving and Psychiatric Illness," letter, *American Journal of Psychiatry* 150 (1993): 351. **"an increase":** G. Kirov, R. Kemp, K. Kirov, et al., "Religious Faith after Psychotic Illness." *Psychopathology* 31 (1998): 234–45. **the clergy:** D. B. Larson, A. A. Hohmann, L. G. Kessler, et al., "The Couch and the Cloth: The Need for Linkage," *Hospital and Community Psychiatry* 39 (1988): 1064–69. **religious cult:** See M. Galanter, "Psychological Induction into the

Large Group: Findings from a Modern Religious Sect," *American Journal of Psychiatry* 137 (1980): 1574–79; see also M. Galanter, et al., "The 'Moonies': A Psychological Study of Conversion and Membership in a Contemporary Religious Sect," *American Journal of Psychiatry* 136 (1979): 165–70; for a particularly cogent analysis, see also S. V. Levine, "Role of Psychiatry in the Phenomenon of Cults," *Canadian Journal of Psychiatry* 24 (1979): 593–603. **there may be some advantages:** See S. V. Levine, "Role of Psychiatry." **"that you respond":** F. J. Frese, "Twelve Aspects of Coping for Persons with Schizophrenia," *Innovations and Research* 2 (1993): 39–46. **28 and 29 percent:** E. Kringlen, "Adult Offspring of Two Psychotic Parents, with Special Reference to Schizophrenia," in L. C. Wynne, R. L. Cromwell, and S. Matthysse, *The Nature of Schizophrenia* (New York: John Wiley, 1978), pp. 9–24; K. Modrzewska, "The Offspring of Schizophrenic Parents in a Swedish Isolate," *Clinical Genetics* 17 (1980): 191–201. **28 percent:** E. F. Torrey, "Are We Overestimating the Genetic Contribution to Schizophrenia?" *Schizophrenia Bulletin* 18 (1992): 159–70.

Chapter 13

"But the brilliance": F. S. Fitzgerald, *Tender Is the Night* (New York: Charles Scribner's Sons, 1934), pp. 191–92. **"the quintessential film":** J. Mahler, "Fully Committed," *Talk*, March 2000, pp. 134–35. **a "must see":** Although he occasionally misses the mark, as in his review of *Shine*, Roger Ebert usually writes about mental illness with sensitivity and understanding; see www.suntimes.com/ebert/index.html or *Roger Ebert's Video Companion* (Kansas City: Andrews and McMeel, updated annually since 1986). **"[Although] most viewers":** M. Martin and M. Porter, *Video Movie Guide 2000* (New York: Ballantine Books, 1999). **"Two centuries ago":** T. Teachout, "The Music and the Mayhem," *New York Daily News*, March 20, 1997 (www.nydailynews.com). Thanks to Darlene Bakk for her article "David Helfgott—Poster Boy for the Mental Illness Myth," which was published in the *AMI Cooke County North Suburban Newsline* in early 1998. **"bone-chillingly bleak":** S. Holden, "Into Sinister Webs of a Jumbled Mind," *New York Times*, February 28, 2003, E-1. **"one of the oldest":** E. L. Altschuler, "One of the Oldest Cases of Schizophrenia in Gogol's *Diary of a Madman*," *British Medical Journal* 323 (2001): 1475–77. **"Berenice":** Quotes are taken from E. A. Poe, "Berenice," in *The Works of the Late Edgar Allan Poe*, vol. 1, N. P. Willis, J. R. Lowell, and R. W. Griswold, eds. (New York: J. S. Redfield, 1850), pp. 437–45. **"Yes!—a madman's!":** C. Dickens, "A Madman's Manuscript," in *The Works of Charles Dickens: The Pickwick Papers* (New York: Books, Inc., 1868), p. 134. **"In the deep shade":** C. Brontë, *Jane Eyre* (New York: Penguin Books, 1982), p. 295. **"in which all":** H. Small, *Love's Madness: Medicine, the Novel, and Female Insanity, 1800–1865* (New York: Oxford University Press, 1996), p. 165, quoting Brontë's letter of January 4, 1848.

" 'Well,' returned Mr. Dick": C. Dickens, *The Oxford Illustrated Dickens: The Personal History of David Copperfield* (London: Oxford University Press, 1966), p. 202. **Bartleby:** H. Melville, *Herman Melville: Four Short Novels* (New York: Bantam Books, 1959), pp. 3–41. **"At home":** Excerpted in A. A. Stone and S. S. Stone, eds., *The Abnormal Personality through Literature* (Englewood Cliffs, N.J.: Prentice-Hall, 1966), p. 5. **"But they beckoned":** V. Woolf, *Mrs. Dalloway* (New York: Knopf, 1993), p. 23. **"Other people":** V. Woolf, *The Waves* (New York: Harcourt Brace, 1988), pp. 43–45, 107. **"a sense as of":** C. Aiken, "Silent Snow, Secret Snow," in *The World Within: Fiction Illuminating Neuroses of Our Time*, Mary Louise Aswell, ed. (New York: McGraw-Hill, 1947), p. 241. **"Lie down":** Ibid, p. 258. **"The walls of the room":** Z. Fitzgerald, *Save Me the Waltz* (New York: Signet, 1968), p. 186. **"my great worry":** Letter from F. S. Fitzgerald to Dr. J. Slocum, April 8, 1934 (www.poprocks.com/zelda/scott letters/fitz4.html). **"It was necessary":** F. S. Fitzgerald, *Tender Is the Night* (New York: Scribners, 1934), pp. 191–92. **"I Am Lazarus":** A. Kavan, in *The World Within: Fiction Illuminating Neuroses of Our Time*, Mary Louise Aswell, ed. (New York: McGraw-Hill, 1947), pp. 270–81. **"The Headless Hawk":** T. Capote, in *The World Within: Fiction Illuminating Neuroses of Our Time*, Mary Louise Aswell, ed. (New York: McGraw-Hill, 1947), pp. 270–81. **dopamine-2 receptors:** O. de Manzano, S. Cervenka, A. Karabanov, et al., "Thinking Outside a Less Intact Box: Thalamic Dopamine D2 Receptor Densities Are Negatively Related to Psychometric Creativity in Healthy Individuals," *PLoS One* 5 (2010): e10670. **one study has suggested:** J. L. Karlson, "Genetic Association of Giftedness and Creativity with Schizophrenia," *Hereditas* 66 (1970): 177. **A biography:** R. Ellmann, *James Joyce: New and Revised Edition* (New York: Oxford University Press, 1982), p. 685. **A psychiatrist:** N.J.C. Andreasen, "James Joyce: A Portrait of the Artist as a Schizoid," *Journal of the American Medical Association* 224 (1973): 67–71. **"Joyce had":** Ellmann, p. 650. **"this sickness":** *Antonin Artaud: Selected Writings* (New York: Farrar, Straus and Giroux, 1976), p. 423. **"If I am":** A. A. Davidson, "The Wretched Life and Death of an American Van Gogh," *Smithsonian Magazine*, December 1987, pp. 80–91. **"his brain":** This and other quotes about Gurney are from M. Hurd, *The Ordeal of Ivor Gurney* (Oxford: Oxford University Press, 1978), pp. 43, 122, and 158. **"To God":** From P. J. Kavanagh, ed., *Collected Poems of Ivor Gurney* (Oxford: Oxford University Press, 1982), p. 156; reprinted by permission of the editor. **"his career":** These quotes are from S. Nasar, *A Beautiful Mind* (New York: Simon & Schuster, 1998), pp. 243 and 244. **"I love life":** R. Nijinsky, ed., *The Diary of Vaslav Nijinsky* (Berkeley: University of California Press, 1968), pp. 185–86. **"Oh, if I":** B. Schiff, "Triumph and Tragedy in the Land of 'Blue Tones and Gay Colors,'" *Smithsonian Magazine*, October 1984, p. 89. **college freshmen:** O. Wahl, "Public vs. Professional Conceptions of Schizophrenia," *Journal of Community Psychiatry* 15 (1987): 285–91. **A 1986 poll:** C. Holden, "Giving Mental Illness Its Research Due," *Science* 232 (1986): 1084–86. **a 1996 survey:**

J. C. Phelan, B. G. Link, A. Stueve, et al., "Public Conceptions of Mental Illness in 1950 and 1996: What Is Mental Illness and Is It to Be Feared?," *Journal of Health and Social Behavior* 41 (2000): 188–207. **"Why is stigma"**: *Report on Mental Health of the United States Surgeon General* (Washington, D.C.: U.S. Department of Health and Human Services, 1999). A **2006 follow-up**: B. A. Pescolsolido, J. K. Martin, J. S. Long, et al., "A Disease Like Any Other? A Decade of Change in Public Reactions to Schizophrenia, Depression, and Alcohol Dependence," *American Journal of Psychiatry* 167 (2010): 1321–30. **A 2016 study**: E. E. McGinty, A. K. Hendricks, S. Chosky, et al., "Trends in the News Media Coverage of Mental Illness in the United States: 1995–2014," *Health Affairs* 35 (2016): 1121–29. **"negative attitudes"**: J. A. Thorton and O. F. Wahl, "Impact of a Newspaper Article on Attitudes toward Mental Illness," *Journal of Community Psychology* 24 (1996): 17–25. **"marked increase"**: M. C. Angermeyer and H. Matschinger, "The Effect of Violent Attacks by Schizophrenic Persons on the Attitude of the Public Towards the Mentally Ill," *Social Science and Medicine* 43 (1996): 1721–28. **"A mass shooting"**: M. S. McGinty, D. W. Webster, C. L. Barry, "Effects of News Media Message About Mass Shootings on Attitudes Toward Persons With Serious Mental Illness and Public Support for Gun Control Policies," American Journal of Psychiatry 170 (2013): 494–501. **"the proportion"**: E. E. Ginty et al., op cit. **"within hours"**: E. Jarvik, "Mental Health Clients Fear Growing Stigma," *Deseret News*, April 24, 1999, p. A-1.

Chapter 14

"Schizophrenia is": W. Hall, G. Andrews, and G. Goldstein, "The Costs of Schizophrenia," *Australian and New Zealand Journal of Psychiatry* 19 (1985): 3–5. **"one of the most sinister"**: L. Wilson, *This Stranger, My Son* (New York: Putnam, 1968), p. 174. **Studies of homeless:** E. F. Torrey, *Out of the Shadows: Confronting America's Mental Illness Crisis* (New York: John Wiley, 1997); **15 percent:** D. J. James and L. E. Glaze, *Mental Health Problems of Prison and Jail Inmates* (Washington, D.C.: U.S. Department of Justice, 2006). **1991 survey:** D. M. Steinwachs, J. D. Kasper, E. A. Skinner, et al., *Family Perspectives on Meeting the Needs for Care of Severely Mentally Ill Relatives* (Arlington, Va.: NAMI, 1992). **one thousand homicides:** J. M. Dawson and P. A. Langan, *Murder in Families* (Washington, D.C.: U.S. Department of Justice, 1994). **In Los Angeles:** A. F. Lehman and L. S. Linn, "Crimes against Discharged Mental Patients in Board-and-Care Homes," *American Journal of Psychiatry* 141 (1984): 271–74. **In New York:** S. Friedman and G. Harrison, "Sexual Histories, Attitudes, and Behavior of Schizophrenic and Normal Women," *Archives of Sexual Behavior* 13 (1984): 555–67. **In Des Moines:** T. Alex, "Summer in the City: Violent Crime in D.M.," *Des Moines Register*, August 3, 1989, p. 1. **the police removed:** "21 Ex-Mental Patients Taken from 4 Private Homes," *New York Times*, August 5, 1979, p. A-33. **in 1990:** S. Raab, "Mental Homes Are Wretched, A Panel Says," *New York Times,* August 6, 1990. **in Mississippi:** "9 Ex-Patients Kept in Primitive Shed," *New York Times,* October 21, 1982, p. A-21. **In Illinois:** R. Davidson, "A Mental Health Crisis in Illinois," *Chicago Tribune,* December 9, 1991. **In New York:** C. F. Muller and C.L.M. Caton, "Economic Costs of Schizophrenia: A Postdischarge Study," *Medical Care* 21 (1983): 92–104. **A study of readmissions:** J. L. Geller, "A Report on the 'Worst' State Hospital Recidivists in the U.S.," *Hospital and Community Psychiatry* 43 (1992): 904–8. **24,787 such calls:** E. Bumiller, "In Wake of Attack, Giuliani Cracks Down on Homeless," *New York Times,* November 20, 1999, p. 1. **only 3 percent:** M. Olfson, H. A. Pincus, and T. H. Dial, "Professional Practice Patterns of U.S. Psychiatrists," *American Journal of Psychiatry* 151 (1994): 89–95. **only 60 percent:** D. A. Regier, W. E. Narrow, D. S. Rae, et al., "The De Facto U.S. Mental and Addictive Disorders Service System," *Archives of General Psychiatry* 50 (1993): 85–94. **survey in Baltimore:** M. Von Korff, G. Nestadt, A. Romanoski, et al., "Prevalence of Untreated *DSM-III* Schizophrenia," *Journal of Nervous and Mental Disease* 173 (1985): 577–81. **in Wisconsin:** D. A. Treffert, "The Obviously Ill Patient in Need of Treatment," *Hospital and Community Psychiatry* 36 (1985): 259–64. **1.5 percent:** "Health Care Reform for Americans with Severe Mental Illnesses: Report of the National Advisory Mental Health Council," *American Journal of Psychiatry* 150 (1993): 1447–65. **study in Baltimore:** J. C. Anthony, M. Folstein, A. J. Romanoski, et al., "Comparison of the Lay Diagnostic Interview Schedule and a Standardized Psychiatric Diagnosis," *Archives of General Psychiatry* 42 (1985): 667–75. **revised its estimate:** W. E. Narrow, D. S. Rae, L. N. Robins, "Revised Prevalence Estimates of Mental Disorders in the United States," *Archives of General Psychiatry* 59 (2002): 115–23. **Five separate studies:** See M. Kramer, B. M. Rosen, and E. M. Willis, "Definitions and Distribution of Mental Disorders in a Racist Society," in C. V. Willie, B. M. Kramer, and B. S. Brown, eds., *Racism and Mental Health* (Pittsburgh: University of Pittsburgh Press, 1973); and M. Kramer, "Population Changes and Schizophrenia, 1970–1985," in L. Wynne, et al., eds., *The Nature of Schizophrenia* (New York: Wiley, 1978). **careful study in Rochester:** *Report of the President's Commission on Mental Health* (Washington, D.C.: U.S. Government Printing Office, 1978). **in Texas and in Louisiana:** Kramer, Rosen, Willis. **Hispanic residents:** M. A. Burnam, R. L. Hough, J. I. Escobar, et al., "Six-Month Prevalence of Specific Psychiatric Disorders among Mexican Americans and Non-Hispanic Whites in Los Angeles," *Archives of General Psychiatry* 44 (1987): 687–94. **study of Mexican-American residents:** E. G. Jaco, *The Social Epidemiology of Mental Disorders: A Psychiatric Survey of Texas* (New York: Russell Sage Foundation, 1960). **Hutterites:** J. W. Eaton and R. J. Weil, *Culture and Mental Disorders: A Comparative Study of the Hutterites and Other Populations* (Glencoe: Free Press, 1955). **schizophrenia elsewhere in the world:** Unless otherwise indicated, all studies mentioned in this section are reviewed in E. F. Torrey, *Schizophrenia and Civilization* (New York: Jason Aronson, 1980); and E. F. Torrey, "Prevalence Studies in Schizophrenia," *British Journal of Psychiatry* 150 (1987): 598–608. **McGrath and his colleagues:** S. Saha, D. Chant, J. Welham, and J. McGrath, "A Systematic Review of the Prevalence of Schizophrenia," *PLoS Medicine* 2 (2005): e141-e433. *fivefold difference:* J. J. McGrath, "Myths and Plain Truths about Schizophrenia Epidemiology—the NAPE Lecture 2004," *Acta Psychiatrica Scandinavica* 111 (2005): 4–11. **Micronesia:** F. X. Hezel and A. M. Wylie, "Schizophrenia and Chronic Mental Illness in Micronesia: An Epidemiological Survey," *ISLA: A Journal of Micronesian Studies* 1 (1992): 329–54. **"insanity is a disease":** A. Halliday, *Remarks on the Present State of the Lunatic Asylums in Ireland* (London: John Murray, 1808). **Caribbean immigrants:** S. Wessely, D. Castle, G. Der, et al., "Schizophrenia and Afro-Caribbeans," *British Journal of Psychiatry* 159 (1991): 795–801. **twofold risk:** E. Cantor-Graae and J.-P. Selten, "Schizophrenia and Migration: A Meta-Analysis and Review," *American Journal of Psychiatry* 162 (2005): 12–24. **Since 1985 similar:** R. E. Kendell, D. E. Malcolm, and W. Adams, "The Problem of Detecting Changes in the Incidence of Schizophrenia," *British Journal of Psychiatry* 162 (1993): 212–18. **In Baltimore:** R. Lemkau, C. Tietze, and M. Cooper, "Mental-Hygiene Problems in an Urban District," *Mental Hygiene* 25 (1941): 624–46; and 26 (1942): 100–19. **in New Haven:** A. B. Hollingshead and F. C. Redlich, *Social Class and Mental Illness* (New York: John Wiley, 1958). **high incidence of *new* cases:** A. Y. Tien and W. W. Eaton, "Psychopathologic Precursors and Sociodemographic Risk Factors for the Schizophrenia Syndrome," *Archives of General Psychiatry* 49 (1992): 37–46. **"schizophrenia has existed":** D. V. Jeste, R. del Carmen, J. B. Lohr, et al., "Did Schizophrenia Exist before the Eighteenth Century?" *Comprehensive Psychiatry* 26 (1985): 493–503; see also N. M. Bark, "On the History of Schizophrenia," *New York State Journal of Medicine* 88 (1988): 374–83. **The other side:** E. F. Torrey, *Schizophrenia and Civilization* (New York: Jason Aronson, 1980). **Poor Mad Tom:** N. M. Bark, "Did Shakespeare Know Schizophrenia? The Case of Poor Mad Tom in King Lear," *British Journal of Psychiatry* 146 (1985): 436–38. **George Trosse:** Jeste, et al., and E. Hare, "Schizophrenia before 1800? The Case of the Revd George Trosse," *Psychological Medicine* 18 (1988): 279–85. **insanity was increasing:** Torrey, *Schizophrenia and Civilization*, and E. Hare, "Was Insanity on the Increase?" *British Journal of Psychiatry* 142 (1983): 439–55. **accompanying graph:** Data are from A. L. Stroup and R. W. Manderscheid, "The Development of the State Mental Hospital System in the United States: 1840–1980," *Journal of the Washington Academy of Sciences* 78 (1988): 59–68. **"insanity is an increasing disease":** E. Jarvis, "On the Supposed Increase in Insanity," *American Journal of Insanity* 8 (1852): 333. **"the successive reports":** Quoted in W. J. Corbet, "On the Increase of Insanity," *American Journal of Insanity* 50 (1893): 224–38. **"the insane have increased":** F. B. Sanborn, "Is American Insanity Increasing? A Study," *Journal of Mental Science* 40 (1894):

214–19. **Deinstitutionalization:** Most of the material in this section is from Torrey, *Nowhere to Go* (New York: Harper and Row, 1988). **"no convictions were had":** Hearings on the National Neuropsychiatric Institute, Subcommittee on Health and Education, United States Senate, March 6–8, 1946, pp. 167 and 169. **"in some of the wards":** A. Deutsch, *The Shame of the States* (New York: Harcourt Brace, 1948), p. 28. **Kennedy's younger sister:** See Torrey, *Nowhere to Go*, pp. 102–6. **"it has been demonstrated":** President Kennedy's 1963 special message to Congress, reprinted in H. A. Foley and S. S. Sharfstein, *Madness and Government* (Washington, D.C.: American Psychiatric Press, 1983). **federal CMHC program:** E. F. Torrey, S. M. Wolfe, and L. M. Flynn, "Fiscal Misappropriations in Programs for the Mentally Ill: A Report on Illegality and Failure of the Federal Construction Grant Program for Community Mental Health Centers" (Washington, D.C.: Public Citizen Health Research Group and National Alliance for the Mentally Ill, 1990). **number of lawyers:** L. Caplan, "The Lawyers Race to the Bottom," *Washington Post*, August 6, 1993, A-24. **A 1980 survey:** C. A. Taube, B. J. Bums, and L. Kessler, "Patients of Psychiatrists and Psychologists in Office-Based Practice: 1980," *American Psychologist* 39 (1984): 1435–47. **In 2000:** The Oregon example is taken from "No Housing, No Recovery," an editorial in the *Oregonian*, March 20, 2000, p. E-12. **$636,000:** A. E. Moran, R. I. Freedman, and S. S. Sharfstein, "The Journey of Sylvia Frumkin: A Case Study for Policymakers," *Hospital and Community Psychiatry* 35 (1984): 887–93. **One study:** D. P. Rice and L. S. Miller, "The Economic Burden of Schizophrenia," *Journal of Clinical Psychiatry* 60 (Suppl. 1) (1999): 4–6. **other study:** R. J. Wyatt, I. de Saint Ghislain, M. C. Leary, et al., "An Economic Evaluation of Schizophrenia—1991," *Social Psychiatry and Psychiatric Epidemiology* 30: 196–205, 1995. **data from 2002:** E. Q. Wu, H. G. Birnbaum, L. Shi, et al., "The Economic Burden of Schizophrenia in the United States in 2002," *Journal of Clinical Psychiatry* 66 (2005): 1122–29. **In Australia:** G. Andrews, W. Hall, G. Goldstein, et al., "The Economic Costs of Schizophrenia," *Archives of General Psychiatry* 42 (1985): 537–43. **$180 billion:** R. J. Wyatt, "Science and Psychiatry," in J. T. Kaplan and B. J. Sadock, eds., *Comprehensive Textbook of Psychiatry*, 4th ed. (Baltimore: Williams and Wilkins, 1984), chapter 53, p. 2027. **"In whatever":** E. Jarvis, *Insanity and Idiocy in Massachusetts: Report of the Commission on Lunacy, 1855* (Cambridge: Harvard University Press, 1971), p. 104.

Chapter 15

"And, once more": R. C. Waterston, "The Insane in Massachusetts," *Christian Examiner* 33 (1843): 338–52. **"They say, 'Nothing'":** F. Tiffany, *Life of Dorothea Lynde Dix* (Ann Arbor: Plutarch Press, 1971), p. 134. **2003 report:** E. F. Torrey, M. T. Zdanowicz, S. M. Wolfe, et al., *A Federal Failure in Psychiat-*

ric Research: Continuing NIMH Negligence in Funding Sufficient Research on Serious Mental Illnesses (Arlington, Va.: Treatment Advocacy Center, November 2003). **SAMHSA:** E. F. Torrey, "Bureaucratic Insanity: The Federal Agency That Wastes Money while Undermining Public Health," *National Review*, June 20, 2011. **"We can reduce":** H. R. Lamb, "Combating Stigma by Providing Treatment," *Psychiatric Services* 50 (1999): 729. **a study in 2009:** H. Takahashi, T. Ideno, S. Okubo, et al., "Impact of Changing the Japanese Term for 'Schizophrenia' for Reasons of Stereotypical Beliefs of Schizophrenia in Japanese Youth," *Schizophrenia Research* 112 (2009): 149–52. **2015 and 2016:** A. Aoki, Y. Aoki, R. Goulden, et al., "Change in Newspaper Coverage of Schizophrenia in Japan Over 20-year Period," *Schizophrenia Research* 175 (2016): 193–97; S. Koike, S. Yamaguchi, Y. Ojie, et al., "Effect of Name Change of Schizophrenia on Mass Media Between 1985 and 2013 in Japan: A Text Data Mining Analysis," *Schizophrenia Bulletin* 42 (2015): 552–9. **"a minority within minorities":** *Report of the President's Commission on Mental Health*, vol. 2 (Washington, D.C.: U.S. Government Printing Office, 1978), p. 362. **"Schizophrenia is":** R. W. Heinrichs, *In Search of Madness: Schizophrenia and Neuroscience* (New York: Oxford University Press, 2001), p. 276.

INDEX

oral administration, 174–75, *175*, 188

polypharmacy, 183–84, 190–93

during pregnancy, 181, 248, 250, *251*

prostate cancer and, 111

record keeping, 186

second-generation, 174–75, *175*

selection process, 174–81

side effects. *See* side effects

smoking and efficacy, 240

supportive psychotherapy with, 198–201

survival strategies, 297

treatment plan for first-break psychosis, 181–84, *183*

antisocial personality disorders, 82

anxiety, 61, 63, 191, 197, 198, 200, 202

apathy, 42, 88, 94, 351

Appeals Council Review Board, 208

Appleton, William S., 287

apps, 428

Aralen (chloroquine), *75*

arched palate, 123

arguments, 300

Arieti, Silvano, 34–35

aripiprazole (Abilify), 173, *175*, *176*, 177, 180, *183*, 188, 190

Arizona, 163, 226, 232, 268

Arkansas, 163, 267

Armat, Virginia C., 407

Aronofsky, Darren, 345

Aronowitz, Paul, 310

arrest, 231, 270, 273, 277–79

arrhythmias, 180

Artaud, Antonin, 357

asenapine (Saphris), *175*, *176*, 177, 180, 240

Asian-Americans, 184

Asperger's disorder, 80

aspirin, 192

assaultive and violent behavior, 273–77

alcohol and drug abuse and, 245

arrest and jail, 277–79

family and, 245, 275–77, 305, 366

need for asylum, 227–28

predictors of, 275

prevention of, 275–77, *276*

studies on prevalence of, 273–75, 365–66

victimization, 252–54

assertive case management, 265–66, 271

Assertive Community Treatment (ACT), 229–30, 265–66

Assisted Outpatient Treatment (AOT), 230–32, 268, 392

assisted treatment, 264–73

astrocytes, 116

asylum care, 100

need for, 227–28

Ativan (lorazepam), 191–92

attention problems, 7–8, 119–20

Attenuated Psychosis Syndrome, 64

attitude of family, 285–94. *See also* SAFE attitude

auditory hallucinations, 30–34

in childhood schizophrenia, 90–91

diagnostic workup, 153

first rank symptom, *56*

from prescription drugs, 74, *75*

responsibility for behavior and, 324–26

schizophrenia spectrum, 62–64

from street drugs, 72

survival strategies, 295

Australia, 139, 187, 202, 229, 250, 298, 368, 375, 388

autism, 80–81, 90, 96

autonomy, 305–7

public crime. *See* crime
public shelters, 209, 211, 228, 253,
    365, 371

Quakers, 380
quality of life measures, 235, *236*
quarter-way houses, 210
quetiapine (Seroquel), *175, 176,*
    177, 178, 180, 181, 182, *183*

Rabkin, J., 273
radio-control of another person, 27
raloxifene, 192
ramelteon (Rozerem), *75*
rape, 82, 211, 253
Reader's Digest, 380
reading, 403–20
    the best (recommended),
        403–15
    the worst (not recommended),
        415–20
Reagan, Ronald, 48, 385
realistic expectations, 292–94
receptive aphasia, 14
Recovered, Not Cured (McLean),
    262, 409
recovery
    case studies of successful
        schizophrenia, 107–10
    in developing countries, 104–5
    possible courses
        ten years later, 96–100, *97*
        thirty years later, *97*, 101–4
    recommended reading, 113–14
    recovery model, 105–6, 205–6
Recovery After an Initial
    Schizophrenia Episode
    (RAISE), 201–3
Recovery Inc., 296
recreational therapy, 158–59
Redlich, Frederick, 375
referral lists, 149
reflexes, 121

"refrigerator mother," 81
rehabilitation, 205–24
    clubhouse programs, 212,
        218–19, 234
    employment, 214–17
    exercise, 221
    friendship and social skills
        training, 217–19
    housing. *See* housing
    medical and dental care, 220–21
    money and food, 206–10
    need for asylum, 227–28
    peer support groups, 221–23
    quality of life measures, 235, *236*
    realistic expectations, 292–94
    recommended reading, 223–24
    recovery model, 105–6, 205–6
rehospitalization rates, 92, 172,
    199, 234, 259, 265
relapse. *See also* noncompliance
    antipsychotics duration, 185–86
    minimization of, 312–15
    Warning Signals Scale, 313, *314*
release-of-information forms, 257
religion (religious issues), 329–31
    changes in affect, 38
    contraception use and, 248–49
    culturally sanctioned psychotic
        behavior, 83
    educating the public, 397–98
    evaluation of hallucinations, 330
    excessive preoccupation with, 11
    "peak experiences," 10–11, 11,
        38, 330
religious cults, 330–31
religious ecstasy, 38
religious hallucinations, 34–35
remission, 43
    possible courses
        ten years later, 96–100, *97*
        thirty years later, *97*, 101–4
    suicide following, 280–81
Renaudin, E., 377–78

ABOUT THE AUTHOR

E. FULLER TORREY, M.D., is a research psychiatrist specializing in schizophrenia and bipolar disorder. He is the research director of the Stanley Medical Research Institute, the founder of the Treatment Advocacy Center, and a professor of psychiatry at the Uniformed Services University of the Health Sciences. He is also the author and editor of twenty books, including *The Roots of Treason: Ezra Pound and the Secret of St. Elizabeths*, which was nominated by the National Book Critics Circle as one of the five best biographies of 1983. He has lectured extensively and has appeared on *Oprah*, *60 Minutes*, and *20/20*. Dr. Torrey lives in the Washington, D.C., area.